中医五 病机学

Pathomechanisms of the

Zhōng Yī Wǔ Zàng Bì

腎病之病機

Pathomechanisms of the KIDNEY

Shèn Bìng Zhī Bìng Jī

Yán Shí-Lín, Lǐ Zhèng-Huá

Edited by Nigel Wiseman and Anthony Venuti

Translated by Sabine Wilms

Paradigm Publications
Taos, New Mexico

Pathomechanisms of the Five Viscera
Volume Five
Pathomechanisms of the Kidney

Yán Shí Lín 严石林 Lǐ Zhèng-Huá 李正华
Translated by Sabine Wilms
Edited by Nigel Wiseman and Anthony Venuti

202 Bendix Drive, Taos, New Mexico 87571 USA
www.paradigm-pubs.com
Distributed by Redwing Book Company
www.redwingbooks.com
COMP Designation: Original Chinese work in English translation

Library of Congress Cataloging-in-Publication Data

Yan, Shi Lin, 1943-
[Zhong Yi Wu Zang Bing Ji Xue: Xin Bing Zhi Bing Ji. English]
Pathomechanisms of the five viscera: pathomechanisms of the heart / Yan Shi Lin, Li Zheng-Hua ; with
the assistance of Yan Yan ... [et al.] ; translated by Wang Ying and Sabine Wilms ; edited by Eric Brand and Zhang Yu Huan.
p. ; cm.
Includes bibliographical references and index.
ISBN 0-912111-79-8
1. Heart--Pathophysiology. 2. Medicine, Chinese. I. Li, Zheng-Hua,
1942- . II. Brand, Eric, 1978- . III. Wiseman, Nigel. IV. Title.
[DNLM: 1. Heart--physiopathology. 2. Medicine, Chinese Traditional.
WG 200 Y21z 2005a]
RC682.9.Y36125 2005
616.1'2--dc22 2005023189

Library of Congress Number: 2005023189

International Standard Book Number (ISBN-13): 978-0912111-86-5

Printed in the United States of America

Table of Contents

Introduction

Pathomechanisms of the Kidney

The kidney is the root of earlier heaven, and the residence of water and fire. It is positioned in the lumbar region, with one kidney each on the right and left. Being a key viscus for maintaining the vital activities in the human body, it has three major physiological functions, namely storing essence, governing water, and absorbing qì.

Regading the first of these, the kidney stores earlier heaven essence (reproductive essence) and later heaven essence (bowel and visceral essence), and it houses original yīn and original yáng. The life gate, which is the source of life and the root of bowel and visceral yīn and yáng, is attached to it. The kidney stores essential qì and manages the reproductive functions of growth and development. Its original yīn provides the material foundation for human development and reproduction, and its original yáng promotes and activates the vital functions of the bowels and viscera. Thus, it brings into play important physiological functions for every stage in human life, from birth to growth, maturity, aging, and death.

Secondly, of the five phases the kidney belongs to water. As such, it is able to transform qì by steaming, control fluid metabolism, promote the circulation of the fluids, and maintain a balanced fluid metabolism inside the body. This leads to its functions of regulating stool and urine as well as the waterways throughout the body.

Thirdly, the kidney governs the absorption of qì. Original qì is formed from original yáng in the kidney and is rooted and bound in the cinnabar field. The kidney reaches upward to lung-metal, governs sinking and downbearing, and contains and absorbs the clear qì inhaled by the lung. It regulates the rhythm of respiration, controls the outflow of original qì, and safeguards the depth of breathing.

In the body, the kidney corresponds to the bones, engenders marrow, is linked to the brain, has its external bloom in the hair of the head, and opens at the ears and the two yīn. Its emotion is fear and its humor is spittle. At the same time, the foot lesser yīn kidney channel and the foot greater yáng bladder channel are connected and stand in an exterior-interior relationship with each other.

Pathomechanisms related to abnormal physiological functioning of the kidney can be divided into the two major categories of vacuity and repletion. Since storing essential qì is the kidney's main role, pathomechanisms of vacuity detriment are most common, manifesting in insufficiency of kidney essence, qì, yīn, or yáng. Progressing further into yīn-yáng disharmony, the pathomechanical changes of reciprocal detriment of yīn and yáng can occur.

Actual mention of the pathomechanism of kidney repletion in the literature appeared rather late. After the initial recognition of the phenomenon of kidney repletion patterns, during the early Spring and Autumn period, Chinese medicine went through a long developmental stage from the Sòng period onward, during which authors either stated that the kidney never suffered from repletion patterns at all, or mostly from vacuity and only rarely from repletion. Thus, the pathomechanism of kidney repletion only gradually gained wide-spread acceptance. Nevertheless, invading evil qì of the six excesses, accumulated pathologic byproducts, or cold, heat, dampness, phlegm, water, stagnant qì, static blood, or lumps and stones can all obstruct the channels and network vessels of the kidney and the free flow of qì and blood in this viscus, and form the pathomechanism of kidney repletion.

肾病病机

肾为先天之本，水火之宅，位于腰部，左右各一，是维持人体生命活动的重要脏腑。肾有藏精、主水、纳气三大生理功能。肾中藏有先天之精（生殖之精）、后天之精（脏腑之精），内舍元阴元阳，命门附于其中，为生命之本源，脏腑阴阳之根本。肾藏精气，有主持人的生长、发育与生殖的作用，其元阴能提供人体生长发育及生殖的物质基础，其元阳又能促进、激发脏腑的生命活动，在人的生、长、壮、老、已整个生命活动过程中发挥重要的生理作用。肾在五行属水，能蒸腾气化，主司水液代谢，促进水液循环，维持体内水液代谢平衡，从而起到调节二便，通调全身水道的作用。肾又主纳气，肾中元阳化生元气，根结于丹田，上达于肺金，主沉主降，能摄纳肺吸入的清气，调节呼吸的节律，控制元气的流失，保持呼吸的深度。肾在体为骨，生髓通脑，外荣于发，开窍于耳及前后二阴，在志为恐，在液为唾。同时，足少阴肾经与足太阳膀胱经相互联络，互为表里。肾脏的生理功能失调，其病机变化可分为虚、实两大类。肾以藏精气为主，故虚损的病机最为多见，表现在肾的精、气、阴、阳诸虚不足，进而阴阳失调，发展为阴阳互损的病机变化。肾实的病机正式提出较晚，在经历了春秋早期肾有实证，宋代以后肾无实证，或多虚少实的漫长发展阶段后，肾实的病机逐渐获得大家的公认。六淫邪气的侵犯，病理产物的停留，寒、热、湿、痰、水、气滞、血瘀、结石，均能阻滞肾的经络和本脏的气血流通，形成肾实的病机变化。

1. Pathomechanisms of Kidney Vacuity

Pathomechanisms of kidney vacuity include aspects like loss of storage, loss of warming, loss of enrichment, loss of replenishment, loss of absorption, and reciprocal detriment of yīn and yáng.

(1) Loss of storage: The kidney is the root of earlier heaven and the viscus of storage. It stores true yīn and hosts original yáng. The essential qì that is stored in the kidney is the motivating force that maintains the normal physiological functions in the body. It must be stored securely, may not leak out, and should be abundant at all times. When the kidney viscus is injured and loses its ability to store, it manifests primarily in a loss of kidney yīn, essence, yáng, and qì. This means that the vital activities in the body are weakened at the root and that yīn and yáng become disharmonious, which causes the hundred diseases to break out and the various symptoms to arise everywhere.

(2) Loss of warming: The kidney stores original yáng. When yáng qì is plentiful, the vital activities are exuberant and the physiological functions of the organism are normal. When kidney yáng is depleted, however, it fails to propel and activate, causing reduced functioning in the whole body. When kidney yáng debilitation prevents it from restraining yīn, the generation of heat is insufficient; warming and nourishing are impaired, and vacuity cold arises internally. This can lead to an abnormal exuberance of yīn cold in the organism. When kidney yáng insufficiency causes a debilitation of life gate fire and a loss of stimulation, this leads to a decline in sexual and reproductive functions. When kidney yáng debilitation leads to fire failing to engender earth, the spleen loses its ability to move and transform. Kidney yáng insufficiency causes a loss of warmth in the blood vessels and cold evil congeals in the channels. This can prevent blood from flowing freely, resulting in stasis obstruction in the blood vessels. When kidney yáng debilitation prevents the transformation of qì by steaming, thereby affecting fluid metabolism, this can lead to indiscriminate flooding and upward intimidation by water qì. Kidney yáng debilitation and resulting exuberance of yīn due to yáng vacuity can further lead to pathomechanical changes like repelling yáng to the outside and upward counterflow surging of qì.

(3) Loss of enrichment: The kidney is the place where earlier heaven original yīn is stored. When original yīn is plentiful, the material foundation necessary for the body's survival is generously available and the source of transformation is uninterrupted. Kidney yīn depletion, however, causes a shortage of yīn liquid and loss of enrichment, so that there are no substances for nourishing the entire body or for enriching the formal body. This results in limp aching lower back and knees and emaciation. When kidney yīn depletion deprives the bone and marrow, the brain, and the intestinal tract of proper nourishment and moistening, this can lead to pathologies in the skeleton, head and face, offices and orifices, and the stool and urine. Kidney yīn depletion can prevent yīn from restraining yáng, causing loss of restraint of the life gate fire and frenetic stirring of the ministerial fire. In men, this results in harassment of the essence chamber and vacuity-type hyperactivity of sexual function; in women, it results in harassment of the thoroughfare and controlling vessels and resultant menstrual disorders and vaginal discharge. In either gender, this can progress further into disordered reproductive functions. When kidney yīn depletion prevents yīn from restraining yáng and makes yáng qì abnormally hyperactive, pathomechanical changes apper, such as effulgent yīn vacuity fire, vacuity heat harassing internally, and upward flaming of vacuity fire appear.

(4) Loss of replenishment: The kidney stores essence and governs bones, engenders marrow, and links up with the brain. The kidney also stores yīn essence in men and essence-blood in women, governing growth, development, and reproduction. An insufficiency of kidney essence and loss of replenishing can prevent essence from engendering marrow, fortifying the skeleton, nourishing the sinews and bones, and filling the brain marrow. In addition, it can cause retarded growth and development in infants and premature debilitation in adults. Lastly, depletion of yīn essence and insufficiency of essence-blood can manifest in disturbed childbearing functions.

(5) Loss of absorption: Original qì within the kidney is able to promote the normal performance of vital activities. In addition, it can also secure and contain the coming and going of qì in the body, coordinate with the lung in accomplishing the basic respiratory functions, and control and contain stool and urine, as well as reproductive essence. When kidney qì is depleted and unable to propel, this manifests as decreased functioning of the entire body. Lack of strength in containment manifests as the kidney failing to absorb qì, which causes the symptoms of panting counterflow and shortness of breath. A breakdown of containment manifests as symptoms like enuresis, insecurity of the essence gate, and stirring fetus.

(6) Reciprocal detriment of yīn and yáng: Both original yīn and original yáng are entrusted to the kidney. Thus it functions as the residence of water and fire. Kidney yīn and kidney yáng exist, grow, and decline in interdependence, balancing one to the other. Together, they maintain the normal physiological functions of the body. In physiology, yīn and yáng constitute each other's cause and effect; in pathology, they damage each other. Thus, an insufficiency of one aspect commonly affects the other aspect, ultimately resulting in a dual vacuity of yīn and yáng. When kidney yīn is vacuous, yáng qì is deprived of engenderment by yīn essence and also becomes deficient. This manifests in a dual vacuity of yīn and yáng that is predominantly characterized by yīn vacuity. When kidney yáng is vacuous, yīn essence has difficulty engendering yáng qì and has nothing to increase. This creates a dual vacuity of yīn and yáng that is predominantly characterized by yáng vacuity. Dual vacuity of yīn and yáng then leads to vanquishing of yīn and yang and to detriment in all five viscera.

肾虚的病机

肾虚的病机包括失于封藏，失于温煦，失于滋养，失于充填，失于摄纳，阴阳互损等方面的变化。

（1）失于封藏：肾为先天之本，封藏之脏，藏真阴而寓元阳。肾藏之精气是维持人体正常生理功能的原动力，只能固藏而不宜泄露，力求常常满盛。肾脏受损，失于封藏，主要表现于肾中阴、精、阳、气之流失，造成人体生命活动之根本虚衰，阴阳失调，引起百病丛生，诸证四起。

（2）失于温煦：肾藏元阳，阳气充沛，则生命活动旺盛，机体生理功能正常。肾阳亏损，失于推动、激发，则全身机能活动减退；肾阳虚衰，阳不制阴，产热不足，失却温养，虚寒内生，可致机体阴寒偏盛；肾阳不足，命门火衰，失于振奋，引起性功能衰退，生殖功能下降；肾阳虚衰，火不生土，则脾失健运；肾阳不足，血脉失温，寒邪凝滞经脉，可致血行不畅，血脉瘀阻；肾阳虚衰，失于蒸腾气化，影响水液代谢，可致水气泛滥、水气上凌；肾阳虚衰，阳虚阴盛，还可进一步引起格阳于外、冲气上逆等病机改变。

（3）失于滋养：肾为先天元阴固藏之处，元阴充沛，则人体赖以生存的物质基础丰厚，化源不断。肾阴亏损，阴津匮乏，失于滋养，无物以养全身，无质以滋形体，则腰膝酸软，形体消瘦；肾阴亏虚，骨髓失滋，脑海失养，肠道失濡，则可引起骨骼、头面、官窍、二便的病变；肾阴亏虚，阴不制阳，命门之火失制，相火妄动，男子则扰乱精室，引起性功能虚性亢进，女子则扰乱冲任，引起经带失调，进而导致生殖功能异常；肾阴亏虚，阴不制阳，阳气偏亢，则出现阴虚火旺，虚热内扰、虚火上炎等病机改变。

（4）失于充填：肾藏精，主骨生髓通于脑。肾藏男子阴精、女子精血，主生长发育、生殖。故肾精不足，失于充填，既可导致精不生髓，骨骼不健，筋骨失养，脑髓失充；又可引起小儿生长发育迟缓，成人早衰；还可因阴精亏虚，精血不足，出现生育功能障碍。

（5）失于摄纳：肾中元气既可推动生命活动的正常进行，又可固摄人体的出入之气，与肺脏协调完成基本的呼吸功能，还能统摄二便及生殖之精。故肾气亏损，推动无能，则表现为全身功能减退；固摄乏力，则表现为肾不纳气，出现喘逆、短气等症；统摄失司，则可出现小便遗失、精关不固、胎动不安等病机改变。

（6）阴阳互损：元阴元阳同寄肾中，使肾成为水火之宅。肾阴肾阳相互依存，相互消长，相对平衡，共同维持人体的正常生理功能。阴阳在生理上互根互用，病理上则相互损伤。一方不足常累及另一方，最终导致阴阳两虚的病机变化。肾阴虚，则阳气无阴精之化生而随之匮乏，表现为以阴虚为主的阴阳两虚病机变化；肾阳虚，则阴精难得阳气之化生而无以增长，形成以阳虚为主的阴阳两虚病机变化。阴阳俱虚，则引起阴阳衰败，五脏俱损的病机改变。

Summary of Kidney Vacuity

1. Loss of storage

   Kidney viscus is injured and loses its ability to store: loss of kidney yīn, essence, yáng, and qì.

   Vital activities in the body are weakened at the root: yīn and yáng become disharmonious; the hundred diseases manifest and various symptoms arise everywhere.

2. Loss of warming

   Kidney yáng debilitation: vacuity cold arises internally.

   Debilitation of life gate fire: decline in sexual/reproductive functions.

   Fire failing to engender earth: spleen loses ability to move and transform.

   Loss of warmth in the blood vessels: blood prevented from flowing freely, resulting in stasis obstruction in the blood vessels .

   Prevents the transformation of qì by steaming: indiscriminate flooding and upward intimidation by water qì.

3. Loss of enrichment

   Kidney yīn depletion results in limp aching lower back and knees and emaciation, It deprives the brain, the bone and marrow, and the intestinal tract of proper nourishment and moistening.

   Loss of restraint of the life gate fire and frenetic stirring of the ministerial fire: In men, vacuity-type hyperactivity in sexual functions; in women, menstrual disorders and vaginal discharge.

   Prevents yīn from restraining yáng: effulgent yīn vacuity fire, vacuity heat harassing internally, and upward flaming of vacuity fire.

4. Loss of replenishment

   Prevents essence from engendering marrow: Retarded growth and development in infants and premature debilitation in adults.

   Insufficiency of essence-blood: disturbed childbearing functions.

5. Loss of absorption

   Unable to propel: decreased functioning of the entire body.

   Lack of strength in containing: panting counterflow and shortness of breath, enuresis, insecurity of the essence gate, and stirring fetus.

6. Reciprocal detriment of yīn and yáng

   Dual vacuity of yīn and yáng: predominantly characterized by yáng vacuity.

   Vanquishing of yīn and yang: detriment in all five viscera.

肾虚的病机

失于封藏

肾脏受损，失于封藏—— 中阴、精、阳、气之流失

造成人体生命活动之根本虚衰——阴阳失调，引起百病丛生，诸证四起

失于温煦

肾阳虚衰——阳不制阴，产热不足，失却温养，虚寒内生，可致机体阴寒偏盛

命门火衰——失于振奋，引起性功能衰退

火不生土—— 则脾失健运

寒邪凝滞经脉——可致血行不畅，血脉瘀阻

失于蒸腾气化——影响水液代谢，可致水气泛滥，水气上凌

失于滋养

肾阴亏损—— 阴津匮乏，失于滋养，无物以养全身，无质以滋形体，则腰膝酸软，形体消瘦,骨髓失滋，脑海失养，肠道失濡

命门之火失制，相火妄动——男子则扰乱精室，引起性功能虚性亢进，女子则扰乱冲任，引起经带失调

阴不制阳—— 阳气偏亢，则出现阴虚火旺，虚热内扰

失于充填

精不生髓——骨骼不健，筋骨失养，脑髓失充

精血不足——出现生育功能障碍

失于摄纳

推动无能——则表现为全身功能减退

固摄乏力—— 出现喘逆，短气,小便遗失，精关不固，胎动不安

阴阳互损

阴阳两虚—— 阳虚为主

阴阳衰败—— 五脏俱损

2. Pathomechanisms of Kidney Repletion

Pathomechanisms of kidney repletion include aspects like wind evil pouring in, dampness obstructing the channels and network vessels, cold congealing channel qì, heat congesting the qì dynamic, phlegm turbidity collecting in the channels, qì stagnation and blood stasis, and obstruction by lumps and stones.

For a long time, the belief that the kidney did not exhibit repletion patterns exerted great influence and people thought at the least that kidney disease was mostly a case of vacuity and only rarely of repletion. However, the fact that the kidney's functions of governing hibernation and storing essential qì can easily be damaged merely reflects the natural tendency of the kidney to be susceptible to this type of vacuity detriment pathomechanism. In fact, evil qì and pathologic byproducts can invade the kidney channel at any time, resulting in a variety of pathomechanical changes of kidney repletion.

(1) External invasion of the six excesses: The evil qì of wind, cold, dampness, heat, dryness, and fire can enter through the fleshy exterior and the skin and body hair. Wind qì likes to move and can pour into the kidney channel. Dampness is by nature sticky and stagnating and can impede the kidney channel. Cold by nature causes contraction and tautness and can congeal in the kidney channel. Heat is by nature inflating and can congest the kidney channel. As such, these evils can either act on their own or they can combine with each other to invade the kidney viscus, channels and network vessels, and lower back, obstructing channel qì and the movement of qì and blood. The resulting impediment by wind-cold, wind-damp, cold-damp, and damp-heat results in pathologic change or kidney repletion that is in fact extremely common in clinic.

(2) Phlegm turbidity collecting in the channels: Phlegm turbidity and water qì are pathologic byproducts that arise internally. They can scurry around the whole body, collect in the lower back, obstruct the channels and network vessels, and form new pathologic factors, resulting in the pathomechanism of kidney repletion.

(3) Qì stagnation and blood stasis: Depression from anxiety and thought or affect-mind dissatisfaction can inhibit the qì dynamic. Knocks and falls and damage from physical activity can cause an obstructed blood flow. In enduring illness, evil qì can invade or pathological substances can pour in and enter the network vessels. All these can form the pathomechanism of qì stagnation and blood stasis in the kidney.

(4) Obstruction by lumps and stones: When damp-heat brews and boils, it can form grit and stones, which sink and accumulate in the kidney. This can form the pathomechanism of kidney repletion, impeding the movement of channel qì and of the fluids.

肾实的病机

肾实的病机包括风邪流注、湿阻经络、寒凝经气、热壅气机、痰浊停经、气滞血瘀、结石阻滞等变化。

长期以来，肾无实证之说影响很大，至少也认为肾病多虚少实。肾主蛰，藏精气，容易损伤，仅反映肾病易于发生虚损一类病机的自然倾向。其实，邪气和病理产物随时均可侵犯肾经，引起多种肾实的病机变化。

（1）六淫侵犯：风、寒、湿、热等六淫邪气从肌表、皮毛而入，风气善行，流注肾经；湿性粘滞，阻碍肾经；寒性收引，凝滞肾经；热性膨胀，壅塞肾经，既可单独，亦可相互结合，侵犯肾脏、经络、腰府，阻碍经气、气血运行，形成风寒、风湿、寒湿、湿热之痹，是临床十分常见的肾实病机变化。

（2）痰浊停经：痰浊、水气作为内生的病理产物，可以流窜全身，停留腰府，阻滞经络，成为新的致病因素，引起肾实的病机变化。

（3）气滞血瘀：忧思抑郁，情志不遂，气机不畅；跌仆击打，运动损伤，血行瘀阻；邪气侵犯，病理产物流注，久病入络，均会形成肾脏气滞血瘀的病机变化。

（4）结石内停：湿热之邪蕴蒸、煎熬，形成砂石，沉积于肾，阻碍经气和水液运行，可形成肾实的病机。

Summary of Kidney Repletion
1. External invasion of the six excesses *Evil qì entering externally.* Wind, cold, dampness, heat, dryness, and fire: any of these six can enter through the fleshy exterior and the skin and body hair.

The six excesses act alone or in combination, invading the kidney viscus, channels and network vessels, and lower back, obstructing channel qì and the movement of qì and blood.

2. Phlegm turbidity collecting in the channels

Pathologic byproducts that arise internally scurry around the whole body, collect in the lower back, and obstruct the channels and network vessels.

Phlegm turbidity forms new pathologic factors.

3. Qì stagnation and blood stasis

Inhibition of the qì dynamic leads to depression from anxiety and thought or affect-mind dissatisfaction. Evil qì can invade or pathological substances can pour in, and in enduring illness, enter the network vessels.

Obstructed blood flow: knocks and falls and damage from physical activity.

4. Obstruction by lumps and stones

Damp-heat brews and boils, forming grit and stones, which sink and accumulate in the kidney.

肾实的病机

六淫侵犯

邪气 —— 风，寒，湿，热，燥，火

可单独可相互结合 —— 从肌表、皮毛而入, 风气善行, 流注肾经

痰浊停经

内生的病理 —— 可以流窜全身, 停留腰府, 阻滞经络

成为新的致病因素

气滞血瘀

气机不畅 —— 忧思抑郁, 情志不遂，邪气侵犯, 病理产物流注, 久病入络

血行瘀阻 —— 跌仆击打, 运动损伤

结石内停

湿热之邪蕴蒸，煎熬 ——形成砂石, 沉积于肾

Overview of Pathomechanisms of the Kidney

Kidney disease can have several causes. Firstly, it can arise from an invasion of external evil of the six excesses, of which wind, cold, dampness, and heat are most likely to invade the kidney. Secondly, it can be caused by pathologic byproducts that collect and impede the movement of channel qì. Lastly, a variety of disease factors like insufficiency of earlier heaven, impaired nourishment of later heaven, excessive sexual taxation, frequent childbirth and pregnancy, excessive fear, essence depletion in old age, enduring or severe illness, lack of or inappropriate treatment, and disease in the other viscera affecting the kidney can all give rise to kidney disease.

Pathomechanisms of kidney disease can affect many different aspects such as growth and development, the reproductive system, respiratory system, digestive system, kinetic system, and neuroendocrine immune system, as well as fluid metabolism and energy metabolism.

Guided by the main principles of vacuity and repletion, the pathomechanisms of kidney disease can reflect conditions of exuberance and debilitation of evil and right in the process of arising and developing diseases. Beginning with the authors of the ancient medical classic *Huáng Dì Nèi Jīng* ("The Yellow Emperor's Inner Canon"), numerous texts separately discussed the pathomechanical changes of kidney vacuity and kidney repletion.

The chapter, "Forms of Disease from Evil Qì in the Viscera and Bowels" in the *Líng Shū* ("The Magic Pivot") states: "If people exert themselves lifting heavy weights, engage in excessive sexual intercourse, or sweat while bathing, this causes kidney damage." This quotation is an early mention of the notion of "kidney damage" and contains an elementary recognition of the pathomechanism of kidney vacuity.

The treatise, "On Seas" in the *Líng Shū* states: "Insufficiency in the sea of marrow results in spinning brain and ringing ears." What this source calls "insufficiency in the sea of marrow" is a condition that is caused by kidney vacuity and depletion of essential qì, so that it is unable to nourish the head. Thus this quotation already distinguishes the pathomechanism of kidney vacuity.

The chapter, "Dreams Caused by Excesses and Evils" in the *Líng Shū* ("The Magic Pivot") states: "Kidney qì exuberance results in dreams of the lower back and spine separating instead of connecting." This quotation points out that kidney qì exuberance is one of the key factors in forming pathomechanisms of kidney repletion.

The chapter, "The Spirit" in the *Líng Shū* ("The Magic Pivot") states: "Vacuity of kidney qì leads to reversal; repletion leads to distention." This text thus set a precedent for dividing pathomechanisms of the kidney into the two categories of vacuity and repletion.

The chapter, "Discussing the Pulses and Patterns of Vacuity and Repletion, Cold and Heat, Life and Death, and Favorable and Unfavorable Shifts in the Kidney" in the Hàn period text, *Zhōng Zàng Jīng* ("Central Treasury Canon") attributed to Huà Tuó, states the following:

> "[Kidney] vacuity results in dreams of boats and drowning people; and when it flourishes, dreams of being submerged in water, and of that which a person fears. Exuberant repletion results in dreams of the lower back and spine separating instead of connecting. Reverting evil lodging in the kidney results in dreams of being next to deep water and being thrown in."

This source differentiated the pathomechanisms of kidney repletion and vacuity into yīn and yáng, vacuity and repletion, and cold and heat.

In the chapter, "Normal Pulses in Front and Back of Shén-Mén and Qì-Kǒu" [ancient pulse positions] from Wáng Shū-Hé's Jìn period text, *Mài Jīng* ("The Pulse Canon"), it states:

> "Kidney repletion: The pulse behind Spirit Gate (*shén mén,* HT-7) on the left hand will indicate yīn repletion. This is the foot lesser yīn channel. Such a patient will suffer from bladder distention and block and from pain stretching from the smaller abdomen to the lumbar spine... The patient will suffer from a dry tongue, swollen pharynx, heart vexation, dry throat, intermittent chest and rib-side pain, panting and cough with sweating, smaller-abdominal fullness and distention, rigidity in the back and lower back, heaviness of the body and heat in the bones, reddish yellow urine, tendency to anger and forgetfulness, heat and pain on the underside of the feet, blackness of the four limbs, and deafness.
>
> "Kidney vacuity: The cubit pulse behind Spirit Gate (*shén mén,* HT-7) on the left hand will indicate yīn vacuity. This is the foot lesser yīn channel. Such a patient will suffer from oppression in the heart, lower-body heaviness, and swelling in the feet that does not tolerate pressure."

This source thus launched an extremely detailed investigation into the pathomechanisms of kidney disease with vacuity and repletion as the guiding principles.

Subsequently, numerous authors of famous classics like the *Qiān Jīn Yào Fāng* ("A Thousand Gold Pieces Prescriptions"), *Yán Shì Jì Shēng Fāng* ("Yan's Remedies for Curing All People"), *Shèng Jì Zǒng Lù* ("Sages' Salvation Records"), *Jǐng Yuè Quán Shū* ("Jǐng-Yuè's Complete Compendium"), and *Yī Zōng Bì Dú* ("Indispensable Medical Reading") analyzed vacuity and repletion in kidney disease from different angles.

The kidney is mostly affected by vacuity, which is embodied in depletion of the kidney's yáng qì or yīn essence. The resulting insufficiency of kidney qì, kidney yáng, kidney essence, or kidney yīn leads to a loss of the physiological functions in the viscera and bowels. Kidney repletion, on the other hand, means that evil qì is exuberant. In cases without right qì vacuity, evil and right struggle and produce pathological changes, whether these are caused by externally contracted evil or by congestion from internal pathologic byproducts. For this reason, it is meaningful to discuss pathomechanisms of kidney disease on the basis of the guiding principles of vacuity and repletion.

肾病的病因

可由六淫外邪内侵而致，特别是风、寒、湿、热之邪最易犯肾。 也可因病理产物停留，阻碍经气引起。 先天不足，后天失养，房劳过度，多产多孕，恐惧过度，年老精亏，久病重病，失治误治，它脏患病累及肾脏等多种因素均可引起肾病的发生。

肾病的病机涉及到生长发育，泌尿、生殖系统，呼吸系统，消化系统，运动系统，神经内分泌免疫系统，水液代谢，能量代谢失调等诸多方面。

肾病病机以虚实为纲，体现了邪正双方在疾病发生发展过程中的盛衰状态。从古老的医学经典著作《黄帝内经》开始，多处分别论述了肾虚肾实的病机变化。如《灵枢•邪气脏腑病形》曰："有所用力举重，若入房过度，汗出浴水，则伤肾。"较早地提出了"伤肾"的概念，对肾虚的病机有了基本的认识。《灵枢•海论》曰："髓海不足，则脑转耳鸣。"其中髓海不足，是因肾虚精气亏损，不能上养于头所致，已包含肾虚的病机。《灵枢•淫邪发梦》曰："肾气盛，则梦腰脊两解不属。"指出肾气盛是形成肾实病机的其本要素之一。《灵枢•本神》曰："肾气虚则厥，实则胀。"开创了把肾的病机分为虚实两端的先例。汉代华佗《中藏经•论肾脏虚实寒热生死逆顺脉证之法》曰："虚，则梦舟溺人，得其时，梦伏水中，若有所畏。盛实，则梦腰脊离解不相属。厥邪客于肾，则梦临深投水中。"从阴阳虚实寒热分析了肾实、肾虚的病机变化。晋代王叔和《脉经•平人迎神门气口前后脉》亦说："肾实：左手神门以后脉阴实者，足少阴经也。病苦膀胱胀闭，少腹与腰脊相引痛。左手尺中神门以后脉阴实者，足少阴经也。病苦舌燥，咽肿，心烦，嗌干，胸胁时痛，喘咳汗出，小腹胀满，腰背强急，体重骨热，小便赤黄，好怒好忘，足下热疼，四肢黑，耳聋。肾虚：左手尺中神门以后脉阴虚者，足少阴经也。病苦心中闷，下重，足肿不可以按地。"极为详细地以虚实为纲开展对肾病病机的研究。其后，《千金要方》、《济生方》、《圣济总录》、《景岳全书》、《医宗必读》等多部经典名著也都从不同的角度对肾病的虚实变化进行了剖析。肾病多虚，体现在肾之阳气阴精亏损，肾气、肾阳、肾精、肾阴的不足，导致了脏腑生理功能的减退；肾实，则为邪气方盛，正气不虚的状态下，邪正相争而出现的病理改变，或由感受外邪，或因内部病理产物的堵塞而引起。因此，以虚实为纲论述肾病病机的规律有着重要的意义。

Literature Review of Pathomechanisms of the Kidney

📖 *Sù Wèn* ("Plain Questions"), "Methods of Treating Visceral Qì in Accordance with the Seasons"

> "Kidney disease manifests in enlarged abdomen and swelling of the shins, panting and cough, generalized heaviness, night sweating, and abhorrence of wind. Vacuity manifests in pain in the chest and in the greater and smaller abdomen, reversal cold, and depression."

The first half of this source describes the pathomechanism of kidney repletion, the second half the pathomechanism of kidney vacuity.

📖 *Nàn Jīng* ("The Classic of Difficult Issues"), "Forty-Ninth Difficult Issue"

> "Prolonged sitting on damp ground or exerting great strength while in water damage the kidney."

This quotation indicates the pathomechanical changes of kidney vacuity due to taxation detriment.

📖 *Qiān Jīn Yào Fāng* ("A Thousand Gold Pieces Prescriptions"), "Treatise on the Pulse in Kidney Disease"

> "Vacuity of kidney qì leads to reverse flow; repletion leads to distention and fullness, and to blackness of the four limbs. Vacuity causes a person

to dream of boats and drowning people, and when it flourishes, of being submerged in water, and of that which the person fears. Kidney qì exuberance results in dreams of the lower back and spine separating instead of connecting. Reverse qì settling in the kidney results in dreams of being next to abysses and of sinking into and being held under water."

This quotation describes the types of clinical manifestations caused by the pathomechanisms of kidney repletion and vacuity.

🕮 *Tài Píng Shèng Huì Fāng* ("The Great Peace Sagacious Benevolence Formulary"), "Treatise on the Kidney"

"Kidney qì exuberance makes the mind superabundant. Such a patient will suffer from abdominal distention and itching, heaviness of the body and swelling of the shins, panting and cough with sweating, aversion to wind, a black face and eyes, and yellow urine. These signs are caused by kidney qì repletion. Thus it is appropriate to drain it. When kidney qì is insufficient, the patient will suffer from coldness in the back and lower back, pain inside the chest, tinnitus or deafness, reversal cold in the feet, and pain in the smaller abdomen. These signs are caused by vacuity of kidney qì. Thus it is appropriate to supplement it."

This quotation discusses the pathomechanical changes in kidney vacuity and repletion from the angle of kidney qì exuberance and debilitation.

🕮 *Yán Shì Jì Shēng Fāng* ("Yan's Remedies for Curing All People"), "Section on the Five Viscera: On the Treatment of Vacuity and Repletion in the Kidney and Bladder"

"First, in kidney vacuity, vacuity engenders cold. This results in cutting pain in the back and lower back, inability to bend forward and backward, aching and weakness of the feet and lower legs, increased aversion to wind and cold, reversal cold of the extremities, shortage of qì, vexing pain in the joints, binding pain in the umbilical region, a soot-black facial complexion, vacuity ringing in both ears, desiccated flesh and bones, frequent uncontrolled urination, and a fine rapid floating pulse. These are the symptoms of kidney vacuity.

Secondly, in kidney repletion, repletion engenders heat. This results in dry tongue with swollen throat, heart vexation with dry throat, intermittent chest and rib-side pain, panting and cough with sweating, smaller-abdominal fullness and distention, hypertonicity of the back and lower back, heaviness of the body and heat in the bones, reddish yellow urine, heat and pain on the underside of the feet, and a tight floating pulse. These are the symptoms of kidney repletion. A pulse that is sunken, soggy, and slippery is not a pathological pulse."

This quotation offers a detailed description of the clinical manifestations and special tongue characteristics for the pathomechanisms of kidney vacuity and repletion. Hence it reflects the high level of knowledge about the pathomechanisms of kidney vacuity and repletion that was reached already at this time.

🕮 *Shèng Jì Zǒng Lù* ("Sages' Salvation Records"), "Section on the Kidney: Systematic Treatise on the Kidney"

> "When a patient presents with smaller-abdominal fullness and distention, and urination that is marked by reddish yellow urine, dripping at the end, frequency, and pain, these are the signs of kidney repletion. If a patient presents with block and repulsion [urinary stoppage and continuous vomiting], rigid back and lower back, decreased intake of food and drink, and fatigued qì and lack of bodily strength, these are the signs of kidney vacuity."

This quotation describes and differentiates the special clinical characteristics of kidney repletion and vacuity.

🕮 *Dān Xī Shǒu Jìng* ("Dān-Xī's Hand Mirror"), "Vacuity and Repletion of the Five Viscera: The Kidney"

> "Vacuity manifests in cutting pain in the back and lower back, inability to bend forward and backward, aching feet and lower legs, cold hands and feet, shortage of qì, joint pain, binding pain in the abdomen, black face, tinnitus, frequent urination, and a fine rapid floating pulse. Repletion manifests in dry tongue and swollen dry throat, heart vexation, intermittent pain in the chest and diaphragm, panting and cough, smaller-abdominal fullness, stiffness and pain in the lower back, heaviness of the body, heat under the joints, yellow urine, swelling of the abdomen and lower back, night sweating, and distention and diarrhea."

This quotation comprehensively sums up the clinical manifestations caused by the pathomechanisms of kidney vacuity and repletion.

🕮 *Jǐng Yuè Quán Shū* ("Jǐng-Yuè's Complete Compendium"), "Record of Transmitting Loyalty: Vacuity and Repletion"

> "Kidney repletion is mostly related to a block in the lower burner, and possibly manifests with pain, distention, or with heat effusion that occurs when defecating and urinating. Kidney vacuity manifests with two yīn stoppage, possibly with incontinence in urine and stool, increased seminal emission, or inability to bend forward and backward in the lumbar spine, and with aching and wilting reversal in the bones."

This quotation describes the key features for pattern differentiation in kidney vacuity and repletion.

文献评述

《素问•藏气法时论》曰："肾病者，腹大胫肿，喘咳身重，寝汗出，憎风。虚则胸中痛，大腹、小腹痛，清厥意不乐。"文中前半段论述肾实，后半段论述肾虚的病机。

《难经•四十九难》曰："久坐湿地，强力入水则伤肾。"指出劳损而致肾虚的病机变化。

《千金要方•肾脏病脉论》曰："肾气虚则厥逆，实则胀满，四肢正黑。虚则使人梦见舟船溺人，得其时，梦伏水中，若有畏怖。肾气盛，则梦腰脊两解不相属。厥气客于肾，则梦临渊，没居水中。"描述了肾实肾虚病机引起的多种临床表现。

《太平圣惠方•肾脏论》曰："肾气盛为志有馀，则病腹胀发痒，体重胫肿，喘咳汗出，恶风，面目黑，小便黄，是为肾气之实也，则宜泻之。肾气不足则腰背冷，胸内痛，耳鸣或聋，足冷厥，小腹痛，是为肾气之虚也，则宜补之。"从肾气盛衰的角度讨论肾病虚实的病机变化。

《济生方•五脏门•肾膀胱虚实论治》曰："方其虚也，虚则生寒，寒则腰背切痛，不能俯仰，足胫酸弱，多恶风寒，手足厥冷，呼吸少气，骨节烦疼，脐腹结痛，面色黧黑，两耳虚鸣，肌骨干枯，小便滑数，诊其脉浮细而数者，是肾虚之候也；及其实也，实则生热，热则舌燥咽肿，心烦咽干，胸胁时痛，喘嗽汗出，小腹胀满，腰背拘急，体重骨热，小便赤黄，足下热痛，诊其脉浮紧者，是肾实之候也。脉沉濡而滑者，不病之脉也。"详细论述了肾病虚实病机的临床表现及舌象特征，对肾病虚实病机的认识已经达到了相当的水准。

《圣济总录•肾脏门•肾脏统论》曰："其证少腹胀满，小便黄赤，末有余沥，数而痛者，此肾实也。若关格塞，腰背强直，饮食减少，气力疲乏者，此肾虚也。"论述辨别肾实肾虚病机的临床特征。

《丹溪手镜•五脏虚实•肾》曰："虚：腰背切痛，不得俯仰，足腿酸，手足冷，呼吸少气，骨节痛，腹结痛，面黑，耳鸣，小便数，脉浮细而数。实：舌燥咽干肿，心烦，胸膈时痛，喘嗽，小腹满，腰强痛，体重，骨节下热，小便黄，腹腰肿，盗汗，胀泄。"全面总结肾病虚实病机所致的临床表现。

《景岳全书•传忠录•虚实》曰："肾实者，多下焦闭，或痛或胀，或热见于二便。肾虚者，或为二阴不通，或为两便失禁，或多遗泄，或腰脊不可以俯仰，而骨酸痿厥。"论述了肾病虚实病机的辨证要点。

Part One

Pathomechanisms of Kidney Repletion

肾实的病机

Introduction

Kidney Repletion

The kidney is the root of earlier heaven. It likes fullness and is averse to depletion. When the constitutional origin is abundant and the body suddenly suffers an invasion by external evil or an obstruction from internal pathologic byproducts, if right qì is not yet debilitated, right qì and evil qì will struggle. This manifests in the pathomechanical changes of kidney repletion.

The *Huáng Dì Nèi Jīng* ("Yellow Emperor's Inner Canon") already contains abundant information regarding the pathomechanism of kidney repletion. The chapter, "The Spirit" in the *Líng Shū* ("The Magic Pivot") states: "Vacuity of kidney qì leads to reversal; repletion leads to distention." Thus, this quotation describes the pathomechanism by which kidney repletion can lead to kidney distention, even if it does not yet explicitly mention the term "kidney repletion."

The "Jade Swivel Treatise on True Visceral Pulses" in the *Sù Wèn* ("Plain Questions") also states: "Exuberance in the pulse, heat in the skin, distention in the abdomen, stoppage in the anterior and posterior yīn, and depression with visual distortion: these are called the five repletions." Zhāng Zhì-Cōng's commentary on this section stated: "The kidney opens at the two yīn, and stoppage in the anterior and posterior means kidney qì repletion." This quotation also contains the notion of "kidney qì repletion."

The chapter, "Methods of Treating Visceral Qì in Accordance with the Seasons" in the *Sù Wèn* ("Plain Questions") explains: "Kidney disease manifests in an enlarged abdomen and swelling of the shins, panting and cough, generalized heaviness, night sweating, and abhorrence of wind."

The chapter, "Five Evils" in the *Líng Shū* ("The Magic Pivot") states:

> "When evil is located in the kidney, the patient suffers from bone pain and yīn impediment. Yīn impediment is not resolved when pressure is applied and is accompanied by abdominal distention, lumbar pain, difficult defecation, pain in the shoulder, back, and neck, and intermittent dizziness."

This text offers a description of the pathomechanism by which external evils like cold or dampness invade the kidney and cause kidney repletion.

Further, "Treatise on the Essential Subtleties of the Pulse" in the *Sù Wèn* ("Plain Questions") also discussed the pulse manifestations in the pathomechanism of kidney repletion: "When the kidney pulse is virulent, hard, and long, and the patient's complexion is reddish yellow, the patient will suffer from splitting pain in the lower back." Virulent, hard, and long describe a pulse with a substantial, forceful, and long quality. This is mostly seen in heat repletion patterns. Gāo Shì-Zōng commented: "When the kidney pulse is virulent, hard and long, there is evil repletion in the kidney."

The chapter, "Forms of Disease from Evil Qì in the Viscera and Bowels" in the *Líng Shū* ("The Magic Pivot") points out: "Extreme urgency in the kidney pulse indicates the disease of bone withdrawal; slight urgency indicates deep reversal, running piglet, loss of use of the legs, and inability to urinate or defecate." Zhāng Jiè-Bīn commented thus on this passage:

> "When the kidney pulse is extremely urgent, wind-cold is lodged in the kidney. The kidney governs the bones; therefore this causes bone withdrawal disease. When the pulse is slightly urgent, deep reversal and loss of use of the legs are caused by the presence of cold evil in the channels; running piglet is caused by cold evil in the viscus; and inability to urinate or defecate is caused by cold evil in yīn."

These quotations provide descriptions of the numerous pathomechanical changes in kidney repletion that are caused by wind evil or cold evil settling in the kidney.

Subsequent generations of physicians conducted more and more extensive and in-depth research on the pathomechanism of kidney repletion. In the *Jīn Guì Yào Lüe* ("Essential Prescriptions of the Golden Coffer"), Zhāng Zhòng-Jǐng of the Hàn dynasty recorded in detail pathomechanical changes of kidney repletion such as kidney fixity, kidney water, and running piglet. Furthermore, he established their treatment with formulas like *gān jiāng líng zhú tāng* (Licorice, Ginger, Poria and White Atractylodes Decoction) and *líng guì gān zǎo tāng* (Poria, Cinnamon Twig, Jujube, and Licorice Decoction).

In the Jìn period, Wáng Shū-Hé articulated the pathomechanism of "kidney repletion" by name in the chapter, "Normal Pulses in Front and Back of Shén-Mén and Qì-Kǒu" in the *Mài Jīng* ("The Pulse Canon"). He described the pathomechanical changes of kidney and bladder repletion in this way:

"Kidney repletion: The cubit pulse behind Spirit Gate (*shén mén,* HT-7) on the left hand will indicate yīn repletion. This is the foot lesser yīn channel. Such a patient will suffer from bladder distention and block and from pain stretching from the smaller abdomen to the back and lower back… The patient will suffer from a dry tongue, swollen pharynx, heart vexation, dry throat, intermittent chest and rib-side pain, panting and cough, sweating, smaller-abdominal fullness and distention, rigidity in the back and lower back, heaviness of the body and heat in the bones, reddish yellow urine, tendency to anger and forgetfulness, heat and pain on the underside of the feet, blackness of the four limbs, and deafness."

In the following Suí dynasty, author Cháo Yuán-Fāng pointed out the following in the chapter, "Various Symptoms of Diseases of the Five Viscera and Six Bowels; Symptoms of Kidney Disease" in the *Zhū Bìng Yuán Hòu Lùn* ("Origin and Indicators of Disease"):

"The kidney is the viscus that governs the interior. Exuberant kidney qì makes the mind superabundant. This results in abdominal distention and swill diarrhea, swelling of the body and panting and cough, sweating and abhorrence of wind, black face and eyes, and yellow urine. These are the signs of kidney qì repletion."

This quotation also analyzed the pathomechanical changes of kidney repletion.

In the Táng period, Sūn Sī-Miǎo, the peerless king of medicine, examined in further detail the pathomechanism of kidney repletion heat mentioned in the *Mài Jīng* ("The Pulse Canon"). In his "Treatise on the Pulse in Kidney Disease; Kidney Repletion Heat" in the *Qiān Jīn Yào Fāng* ("A Thousand Gold Pieces Prescriptions"), he stated:

["When the cubit pulse behind Spirit Gate (*shén mén,* HT-7) on the left hand indicates yīn repletion, this [refers to] the foot lesser yīn kidney channel. Such a patient will suffer from dry tongue with swollen pharynx, heart vexation with dry throat, intermittent chest and rib-side pain, panting and cough, sweating, smaller-abdominal fullness and distention, rigidity in the back and lower back, heaviness of the body, bone heat, reddish yellow urine, tendency to anger and forgetfulness, heat and pain on the underside of the feet, blackness of the four limbs, and deafness. This is called kidney repletion heat…

"When the cubit pulse behind Spirit Gate (*shén mén,* HT-7) on the right hand indicates yīn repletion, this [indicates] the foot lesser yīn channel. The patient will suffer from impediment, generalized heat effusion and heart pain, pain stretching from the spine to the rib-side, and counterflow and vexing heat in the feet. This is called kidney repletion heat."

Subsequently, clinically adept Sòng dynasty physicians recognized the existence of kidney repletion patterns and originated several formulas for treating kidney repletion, such as *xiè shèn xuán shēn sǎn* (Kidney Draining Scrophularia Powder) and *xiè shèn gān dì huáng sǎn* (Kidney and Liver Draining Rehmannia Powder) from the *Tài Píng Shèng Huì Fāng* ("Great Peace Sagacious Benevolence Formulary") and *xiè shèn dà huáng tāng* (Drain the Kidney Rhubarb Decoction) and *zé xiè tāng* (Alisma Decoction) from the *Shèng Jì Zǒng Lù* ("Sages' Salvation Records").

Despite this recognition, Sòng period authors began to question the existence of the pathomechanism of kidney repletion like never before. To the Sòng physician Qián Yǐ is attributed the expression, "The kidney is without repletion." In the chapter, "What the Five Viscera Govern" in his work, *Xiǎo Ér Yào Zhèng Zhí Jué* ("Key to Diagnosis and Treatment of Children's Diseases"), he stated: "The kidney governs vacuity and is without repletion." Later physicians were influenced by this statement and therefore focused mostly on kidney vacuity while neglecting kidney repletion. They accepted statements like "the kidney is without repletion and may not be drained," "draining the bladder equals draining the kidney," and "for kidney repletion, drain the liver."

Yet while Qián Yǐ had stated that "the kidney is without repletion," it is worth noting that Qián Yǐ himself never denied the existence of pathomechanical changes in the kidney related to repletion. In the chapter, "Swelling Conditions" in the *Xiǎo Ér Yào Zhèng Zhí Jué* ("Key to Diagnosis and Treatment of Children's Diseases"), he remarked: "When the kidney is greatly exuberant, the spleen and stomach are vacuous and unable to restrain the kidney, so that water instead restrains earth." From this comment, the notion that the kidney is without repletion can be construed as a one-sided comprehension of Qián Yǐ's theories by his followers.

Arriving in the Yuán period, the famous physician Zhū Dān-Xī broke through the confinement of the stricture that the kidney is without repletion. He broadened the study of the pathomechanism of kidney repletion by positing that damp-heat in the kidney channel can lead to pathomechanical changes like urinary turbidity, seminal emission, or genital pain.

In the "Record on Transmitting Loyalty; Vacuity, and Repletion" in the *Jǐng Yuè Quán Shū* ("Jǐng-Yuè's Complete Compendium"), the Míng period physician Zhāng Jiè-Bīn stated unequivocally that evil qì congestion in the lower burner had the special characteristic of manifesting in the pathomechanism of kidney repletion: "Kidney repletion is mostly related to a block in the lower burner and manifests possibly with pain or distention, or with heat effusion that occurs when defecating and urinating."

Subsequently, during the Qīng dynasty, Zhāng Xī-Chún originated a treatment method using *qīng shèn tāng* (Clear the Kidney Decoction) to clear and drain repletion heat in the kidney. He stated: "Seminal emission, white turbidity, urinary frequency, and a forceful pulse when applying heavy pressure to the two cubit positions mean that the kidney channel is certain to have repletion heat." This statement comes from the text *Yī Xué Zhōng Zhōng Cān Xī Lù* ("Records of Chinese Medicine with Reference to Western Medicine"), "Medical Formulas; *Qīng Shèn Tāng* (Clear the Kidney Decoction)."

As we can see from the above discussion, conditions of sole exuberance of evil qì without vacuity of right qì can fully manifest with the pathomechanical changes of kidney repletion and are for the most part caused by contraction of external evils, by seven-affect internal damage, or by an amassment of pathologic byproducts.

Contraction of external evil is predominantly characterized by the evils of wind, cold, dampness, and heat, which impair the fluid metabolism or storage functions of the kidney. Seven-affect internal damage is predominantly caused by great anger damaging the liver or by emotional changes like great fright or sudden fear, which trigger kidney qì depression bind. Lastly, amassment of pathologic byproducts is predominantly seen when dampness evil, static blood, phlegm turbidity, or stones settle in the kidney channel or viscus, causing the pathomechanical changes of qì stagnation and blood stasis. Thus, wind, cold, dampness, heat, anger, fear, phlegm, and stasis are the basic factors that create the pathomechanisms of kidney repletion.

Because of differences in the pathogenic factors that cause kidney repletion, we can further divide this pathomechanism into the following ten categories: Kidney channel wind-cold, kidney channel wind-heat, kidney channel wind-damp, kidney channel cold-damp, kidney channel damp-heat, kidney channel repletion fire, kidney channel static blood, kidney channel phlegm turbidity, kidney channel stones, and kidney channel qì stagnation.

肾饱食

肾为先天之本，喜满盈而恶亏损。素体先元充沛，突遇外邪之侵袭，或体内病理产物之阻滞，正气未衰，正气与邪气相争，则表现出肾实的病机变化。早在《黄帝内经》中对肾实的病机就有了较丰富的认识。如《灵枢•本神》曰: "肾气虚则厥，实则胀。"已论述了肾实可致肾胀的病机，只未明确提出"肾实"的病机称谓。《素问•玉机真脏论》又曰: "脉盛，皮热，腹胀，前后不通，闷瞀，此谓五实。"张志聪在此条下批注道: "肾开窍于二阴，前后不通，肾气实也"。再次提出了"肾气实"的概念。《素问•脏气法时论》则说: "肾病者，腹大胫肿，咳喘身重，寝汗出，憎风。"《灵枢•五邪》又曰: "邪在肾，则病骨痛，阴痹。阴痹者，按之而不得，腹胀，腰痛，大便难，肩背颈痛，时眩。" 对寒湿等外邪犯肾导致肾实的病机进行了论述。此外，《素问•脉要精微论》还论及肾实病机的脉象: "肾脉搏坚而长，其色黄而赤者，当病折腰。"搏坚而长是脉象坚实有力且长的表现，多见于实热证，故高士宗注: "肾脉搏坚而长，则邪实于肾"。《灵枢•邪气脏腑病形》则指出: "肾脉急甚为骨癫疾; 微急为沉厥，奔豚，足不收，不得前后。" 张介宾注此条曰: "肾脉急甚者，风寒在肾，肾主骨，故为骨癫疾。若微急而为沉厥足不收者，寒邪在经也。为奔豚者，寒邪在脏也。为不得前后者，寒邪在阴也。"对风邪、寒邪客肾引起的多种肾实病机的改变进行了描述。

此后，历代医家对"肾实"的病机变化相继进行了更为广泛深入的探讨和研究。汉代张仲景在《金匮要略》中详尽记载了肾著、肾水、奔豚等多种肾实的病机变化，并设有甘姜苓术汤、苓桂甘枣汤等治疗方药。晋代王叔和《脉经•平人迎神门气口前后脉》明确提出了"肾实"的病机名称，论述了肾及膀胱实的病机变化："肾实：左手尺中神门以后脉阴实者，足少阴经也。病苦膀胱胀闭，少腹与腰脊相引痛。...病苦舌燥，咽肿，心烦，嗌干，胸胁时痛，喘咳，汗出，小腹胀满，腰背强急，体重骨热，小便赤黄，好怒好忘，足下热疼，四肢黑，耳聋。"此后，隋代巢元方在《诸病源候论•五脏六腑病诸候•肾病候》指出："肾为脏，主里，肾气盛为志有余，则为腹胀飧泄、体肿喘咳、汗出憎风、面目黑、小便黄，是为肾气之实也。"也剖析了肾实的病机变化。唐代药王孙思邈则对《脉经》中肾实热的病机进行了更详细地分析，如《千金要方•肾脏病脉论•肾实热》云："左手尺中神门以后脉阴实者，足少阴肾也。病苦舌燥咽肿，心烦嗌干，胸胁时痛，喘咳，汗出，小腹胀满，腰背强急，体重，骨热，小便黄赤，好怒好忘，足下热痛，四肢黑，耳聋，名曰肾实热。 …右手尺中神门以后脉阴实者，足少阴经也。病苦痹，身热心痛，脊胁相引痛，足逆热烦，名曰肾实热也。”继之，宋代医家对肾实证的认识从临床实践出发，又创立了许多治疗肾实的方剂，如《太平圣惠方》之泻肾玄参散、泻肾肝地黄散；《圣济总录》之泻肾大黄汤、泽泻汤等。

但是，肾实病机变化的进一步认识在此时却受到了前所未有的阻碍。宋代著名医家钱乙提出了“肾无实”的说法，如《小儿药证直诀•五脏所主》曰：“肾主虚，无实也。”后世医家受其影响，多强调肾虚而忽视肾实，接受“肾无实不可泻”、“泻膀胱即泻肾”、“肾实泻肝”等理论。实际上，钱乙虽有“肾无实”一说，但在《小儿药证直诀•肿病》中又有：“肾大盛，脾胃虚而不能制肾，水反克土 …”的论述，可见钱乙本人并不否认肾有属实的病机变化，“肾无实”只是后人对钱乙之说的片面理解。

到了元代，著名医家朱丹溪突破“肾无实”学说的禁锢，又进一步扩大了肾实病机的研究，认为肾经湿热可导致尿浊、遗精、阴痛等病机变化。明代医家张介宾在《景岳全书•传忠录•虚实》中明确提出邪气壅闭下焦可出现肾实的病机特征：“肾实者，多下焦壅闭，或痛、或胀、或热，见于二便。”继而，清代张锡纯又创立清肾汤，以清泻肾中实热，治疗：“遗精白浊，小便频数 …，两尺重按有力 …，肾经确有实热也。”（《医学衷中参西录•医方•清肾汤》）。因此，在邪气方盛正气未虚的情况下，完全可以出现肾实的病机改变，多由感受外邪、七情内伤及病理产物堆积而引起。感受外邪，多以风、寒、湿、热等邪为主，导致肾脏水液代谢及封藏功能失调；七情内伤，多因大怒伤肝，或大惊卒恐等情绪变化引发肾气郁结；病理产物堆积则多见湿邪、瘀血、痰浊、砂石等停留肾经、肾府导致气滞血瘀的病机变化。因此，风、寒、湿、热、怒、恐、痰、瘀是造成肾实病机的基本因素。肾实的病机由于致病因素的不同，进一步分为肾经风寒、肾经风热、肾经风湿、肾经寒湿、肾经湿热、肾经实火、肾经瘀血、肾经痰浊、肾经砂石、肾经气滞等十种病机类型。

Chapter One

Kidney Channel Wind-Cold

Wind evil is the leader of the hundred diseases, and wind-cold is most likely to invade the exterior and the lung. However, when the lumbar region is sweating and then exposed to wind, or when wind-cold directly strikes the kidney channel, wind-cold accumulates in the kidney, and the qì-transforming and warming functions of the kidney break down. This can result in the pathomechanical changes of kidney channel wind-cold.

The chapter, "Longevity and Premature Death, Hardness and Softness" in the *Líng Shū* ("The Magic Pivot) states:

> "Wind-cold damaging the physical body occurs like this: Fear and anger damage qì and qì damages the viscera. Thus the viscera fall sick. Cold damages the physical body and so the physical body responds. Wind damages the sinews, and so the sinews respond."

This quotation describes the effect of wind-cold damaging the five viscera in the body, as well as the physical body and sinews. Of course it therefore also refers to the pathomechanical changes of kidney channel wind-cold.

Because the kidney channel can be affected by wind and cold in different strengths, we can further divide this pathomechanism into three types: Wind-cold assailing the kidney, fulminant strike of cold evil, and kidney channel cold mounting.

肾经风寒

风为百邪之首，风寒之邪最易袭表及肺，但如遇腰间汗出当风，或风寒之邪直中肾经，风寒蕴积于肾，肾之气化温煦失职，则可表现为肾经风寒的病机变化。《灵枢•寿夭刚柔篇》曰："风寒伤形，忧恐忿怒伤气，气伤脏，乃病脏，寒伤形，乃应形，风伤筋脉，筋脉乃应。"论述了风寒对人体五脏及形体筋脉的伤害，当然包括肾经风寒的病机变化在内。而因肾经受风受寒的偏重有所不同，可进一步分为风寒袭肾、寒邪暴中、肾经寒疝等三种病机变化。

1.1 Wind-Cold Assailing the Kidney

The kidney is the root of earlier heaven. It is the viscus that stores original yáng so that the entire body receives warmth from yáng qì and does not show signs of cold. However, if the body in a moment of carelessness suffers damage from the evil qì of the six excesses and wind-cold, or if a habitual vacuity of kidney yáng allows wind-cold to exploit this vacuity, enter, and congeal in the kidney channel, either of these can form the pathomechanism of wind-cold assailing the kidney.

In the initial stage of wind-cold assailing the kidney, defensive yáng is obstructed. Furthermore, since cold governs contracture and tautness, the flesh is pressed together securely and densely. This manifests in symptoms like absence of sweating, extreme aversion to cold, and heat effusion.

The lesser yīn kidney channel reaches straight up to the vertex. When cold congeals in the channels and obstructs channel qì, this results in headache and body pain.

Cold is a yīn evil and it represses yáng qì and impairs warming. This results in fatigued spirit and desire to sleep, and lack of warmth in the limbs.

Wind-cold invading the kidney results in a pale tongue with thin white tongue fur, and sunken pulse.

As stated in the "Treatise on Needling Malaria" in the *Sù Wèn* ("Plain Questions"), "Kidney malaria makes a person manifest with shivering as after soaking, pain in the lumbar spine and difficulty turning sides, difficult defecation, dizzy vision, and cold extremities." This quotation presented basic knowledge regarding the pathomechanical changes of wind-cold assailing the kidney.

The chapter, "Identifying Pulse Symptoms and Treatments of Lesser Yīn Disease" in the *Shāng Hán Lùn* ("On Cold Damage") also explained: "When lesser yīn disease in the beginning stage of contraction manifests with paradoxical heat effusion and a sunken pulse, *má huáng xì xīn fù zǐ tāng* (Ephedra, Asarum, and Aconite Decoction) governs it." Lesser yīn homes to the kidney, and since the disease is located in the interior, the pulse is sunken. Lesser yīn disease should not manifest with heat effusion, but when wind-cold assails the exterior, defense yáng is obstructed; hence we see heat effusion. In this quotation, Zhāng Zhòng-Jǐng thus pointed directly at the pathomechanism of wind-cold damaging the kidney.

The treatment method for wind-cold assailing the kidney consists of warming the kidney and dispersing cold. The recommended formula is *má huáng fù zǐ xì xīn tāng* (Ephedra, Aconite, and Asarum Decoction) from the *Shāng Hán Lùn* ("On Cold Damage").

Má Huáng Fù Zǐ Xì Xīn Tāng 麻黄附子细辛汤 Ephedra, Aconite, and Asarum Decoction
má huáng (麻黄 Ephedrae Herba, ephedra)
fù zǐ (附子 Aconiti Radix Lateralis Praeparata, aconite)
xì xīn (细辛 Asari Herba, asarum)

风寒袭肾

肾为先天之本，为元阳存贮之脏，全身得阳气之温煦，不见寒象。但如疏忽之间，受六淫风寒邪气所伤，或肾阳素虚，风寒乘虚而入，凝滞肾经，均可形成风寒袭肾的病机变化。风寒邪气袭肾之初，卫阳受遏，加之寒主收引，肌凑固密，则表现为无汗，恶寒较重，发热等症；少阴肾经脉直达头顶，寒凝经脉，阻滞经气，则头身疼痛；寒为阴邪，抑遏阳气，失于温煦，则神疲欲卧，四肢不温。风寒犯肾，则舌质淡、苔薄白，脉沉。如《素问•刺疟论》曰："肾疟者，令人洒洒然，腰脊痛宛转，大便难，目眴眴然（眴，音 *xuàn* 眩。目眴眴然，指目眩），手足寒。"初步认识到风寒袭肾的病机变化。《伤寒论•辨少阴病脉证并治》也说："少阴病，始得之，反发热，脉沉者，麻黄细辛附子汤主之。"少阴属肾，病位在里，故其脉沉。少阴病不应发热，风寒袭表，卫阳被遏，才见发热。仲景正式提出风寒伤肾的病机。治法为温肾散寒。方药选用《伤寒论》麻黄附子细辛汤（麻黄、附子、细辛）。

Literature Review of Wind-Cold Assailing the Kidney

📖 *Shèng Jì Zǒng Lù* ("Sages' Salvation Records"), "Section on the Kidney"

> "When the kidney is vacuous, yáng qì becomes insufficient and is struck by cold qì. As a result, disharmony of the origin viscus arises."

This quotation describes the pathomechanism by which the evil qì of wind-cold exploits vacuity and enters, resulting in repletion in the kidney channel and exterior.

📖 *Lèi Zhèng Zhì Cái* ("Systematized Patterns with Clear-Cut Treatments"), "Discussing the Treatment of Pain in the Lumbar Spine, Legs, and Feet"

> "When the six qì exploit vacuity and invade greater yáng…cold damage [manifests in] icy coldness in the lower back, a pulse that is invariably tight, and relief when exposed to heat. Use *jiāng fù tāng* (Ginger and Aconite Decoction) with the addition of *ròu guì* (Cinnamomi Cortex) and *dù zhòng* (Eucommiae Cortex) in a topical application by rubbing it onto the lower back as a paste."

Cold damage means that an external contraction of cold evil has occurred. Lumbar pain means that wind-cold has invaded the kidney. Thus this quotation describes how wind-cold invading the kidney results in lumbar pain.

📖 *Yī Xué Xīn Wù* ("Medical Insights"), "Lumbar Pain"

> "Icy coldness in the lower back, liking for heat and for hot friction rubbing with the hands, and a slow sunken or tight pulse are signs of cold. Use *dú huó tāng* (Pubescent Angelica Decoction) to govern it."

When wind-cold assails, it fetters yáng qì. This is the reason for icy coldness in the lower back and a slow sunken pulse.

文献评述

《圣济总录•肾脏门》曰："肾脏虚弱，阳气不足，为寒气所中，元脏不和而成"。阐述了风寒邪气乘虚而入，引起肾经表实的病机。

《类证治裁•腰脊腿足痛论治》曰："其六气乘虚，侵犯太阳，…伤寒腰冷如冰，脉必紧，得热则减，姜附汤加肉桂、杜仲，外用摩腰膏。" 伤寒为外感寒邪，腰痛为风寒犯肾，论述风寒犯肾引起腰痛的病机变化。

《医学心悟•腰痛》曰："腰冷如冰，喜得热手熨，脉沉迟，或紧者，寒也，并用独活汤主之。"风寒侵袭，束缚阳气，故腰部冰冷，脉象沉迟。

Summary of Wind-Cold Assailing the Kidney
1. Obstruction of Defensive Yáng Absence of sweating, rather serious aversion to cold, heat effusion. 2. Cold Congealing in the Channels Headache and body pain. 3. Cold Evil Damaging Yáng Fatigued spirit and desire to sleep, lack of warmth in the limbs. 4. Wind-Cold Invading the Kidney Pale tongue with thin white fur, sunken pulse.

风寒袭肾
卫阳受遏—无汗，恶寒较重，发热 寒凝经脉—头身疼痛 寒邪伤阳—神疲欲卧，四肢不温 风寒犯肾—舌质淡、苔薄白，脉沉

1.2 Fulminant Strike of Cold Evil

The kidney stores original yáng and is the soil in which the entire body's yáng qì grows. Thus it is able to warm the viscera in the entire body. If it suddenly encounters fulminant cold, and cold evil directly strikes the kidney channel, original yáng inside the body is obstructed and warming breaks down. This manifests in the pathomechanical changes of fulminant strike of cold evil.

The lower back is the house of the kidney, and the whole area below the lower back and umbilicus is governed by the kidney. Cold evil striking fulminantly and assailing the lower back results in heavy pain and cold pain in the lower back and legs.

When fulminant cold attacks the abdomen, since cold governs congealing and contracture, this results in cold pain in the umbilicus and abdomen, intermittent hypertonicity with fulminant pain, and hypertonicity in the four limbs.

When yīn cold exuberates internally and obstructs yáng qì, preventing it from reaching the four limbs, this results in a cold body, shivering, and cold pain in the extremities.

Cold evil directly striking and damaging the kidney manifests in a pale tongue and fine sunken pulse.

The "Great Treatise on the Essentials of Supreme Truth" in the *Sù Wèn* ("Plain Questions") had stated: "All contracture and tautness by cold is related to the kidney." This text thus firmly recognized a relationship between the kidney and pathomechanisms of cold evil.

The chapter, "Cold Strike Patterns in the Five Viscera" in the *Sān Yīn Jí Yī Bìng Zhèng Fāng Lùn* ("A Unified Treatise on Diseases, Patterns, and Remedies According to the Three Causes") also explained: "Kidney cold strike … manifests in a black complexion, weak qì, shortage of qì in breathing, deafness, lumbar pain, coldness below the knee, hypertonicity and pain, and clouding loss of consciousness." This quotation describes the pathomechanism and clinical manifestations of cold evil fulminantly striking the kidney.

This condition is treated by warming the kidney and expelling cold. The recommended formula is *bā jǐ wán* (Morinda Pill) from the *Shèng Jì Zǒng Lù* ("Sages' Salvation Records").

Bā Jǐ Wán 巴戟丸
Morinda Pill

fù zǐ (附子 Aconiti Radix Lateralis Praeparata, aconite) [blast-fried]
ròu guì (肉桂 Cinnamomi Cortex, cinnamon bark)
gān jiāng (干姜 Zingiberis Rhizoma, dried ginger)
bā jǐ tiān (巴戟天 Morindae Officinalis Radix, morinda)
ròu cōng róng (肉苁蓉 Cistanches Herba, cistanche)
hú lú bā (胡芦巴 Trigonellae Semen, fenugreek)
tù sī zǐ (菟丝子 Cuscutae Semen, cuscuta)
shú dì huáng (熟地黄 Rehmanniae Radix Praeparata, cooked rehmannia)
wǔ wèi zǐ (五味子 Schisandrae Fructus, schisandra)
huáng qí (黄芪 Astragali Radix, astragalus)
bái zhú (白朮 Atractylodis Macrocephalae Rhizoma, white atractylodes)

寒邪暴中

肾藏元阳，为全身阳气生发之地，可温煦全身脏器。如突遇暴寒，寒邪直中肾经，体内元阳被遏，温煦失职，则出现寒邪暴中的病机变化。腰为肾之府，腰脐以下皆由肾所主，寒邪暴中，攻袭于腰，则腰脚重痛冷痛；暴寒攻腹，寒主凝滞、收引，则脐腹冷痛，时而拘急暴痛，四体拘挛；阴寒内盛，阳气被遏，不达四肢，则身冷战栗，手足冷痛。寒邪直中伤肾，则舌质淡，脉沉细。如《素问•至真要大论》提到："诸寒收引，皆属于肾。"对肾与寒邪的病机关系有一定认识。《三因极一病证方论•五脏中寒症》又说："肾中寒， ... 色黑，气弱，呼吸少气，耳聋，腰痛，膝下清，拘挛而痛，昏不知人。"论述了寒邪暴中于肾的病机及临床表现。治法为温肾驱寒。方药选用《圣济总录》巴戟丸（炮附子、肉桂、干姜、巴戟天、肉苁蓉、葫芦巴、菟丝子、熟干地黄、五味子、黄芪、白术）。

Literature Review of Fulminant Strike of Cold Evil

📖 *Jǐng Yuè Quán Shū* ("Jǐng-Yuè's Complete Compendium"), "Schema of Miscellaneous Patterns: Aversion to Cold and Heat Effusion"

> "Whenever the yīn toxin of cold evil directly strikes the three yīn, this refers to yīn patterns in which evils of the cold damage category directly strike the yīn channels. In these cases, a sudden contraction of cold leads to a cold body and shivering, possibly hypertonicity in the four limbs, heart and intestinal pain, clenched jaw and loss of voice, stupor and reverse flow, vomiting and diarrhea with fatigue and sleeping, and a fine faint or tight sunken spiritless pulse. All these are its symptoms.
>
> Be sure to avoid reckless use of wind medicinals, which will only further disperse the patient's qì. Instead, I recommend to quickly warm the center so that wind evil disperses on its own. In mild cases, use *lǐ zhōng tāng* (Center-Rectifying Decoction) or *wēn wèi yǐn* (Stomach-Warming Beverage); in severe cases, use *sì nì tāng* (Counterflow Cold Decoction), *dà wēn zhōng yǐn* (Major Warm the Center Decoction), or *fù zǐ lǐ yīn jiān* (Aconite Yīn-Rectifying Brew) to govern this condition. ...Cold strike in lesser yīn results in umbilical and abdominal pain and is best treated with *guī qì yǐn* (Angelica Qi Beverage)."

This quotation clearly elucidates a series of pathomechanical changes and the treatment method for cold evil fulminantly striking the kidney channel.

📖 *Zá Bìng Yuán Liú Xī Zhú* ("Incisive Light on the Source of Miscellaneous Disease"), "The Origin and Development of Cold Disease"

> "Whenever people get caught in rain or snow, wade in icy or deep water, walk through open spaces in the morning, sit in dew late at night, fail to cover up sufficiently for a period of time, or force themselves to gulp down cold food and drink, they can thereby contract cold evil. If this enters the interior from the outside and is not immediately outthrust, it can pass through many places and fall deep down, possibly becoming deep-lying in the channels and network vessels or viscera and bowels. …
>
> If cold evil is deep-lying in lesser yīn, it will manifest in diarrhea, reverse flow with no pulse, dry retching and vexation, abdominal pain, heaviness and pain in the four limbs, inhibited urination, and possibly vexation and agitation verging on death, or fifth-watch diarrhea."

This quotation also distinctly analyzes how cold evil striking and damaging the kidney channel can lead to changes like abdominal pain, limb pain, or reverse flow.

文献评述

《景岳全书•杂证谟•寒热》曰："凡阴毒寒邪直中三阴者，此即伤寒类所谓直中阴经之阴证也。其于仓卒受寒，以致身冷战栗，或四体拘挛，或心肠疼痛，或口噤失音，昏迷厥逆，或吐泻倦卧，脉来微细，或沉紧无神者，皆其证也。切不可妄用风药，再散其气，但速宜温中，则寒邪自散。轻则理中汤、温胃饮，甚则四逆汤、大温中饮，或附子理阴煎之类主之。 …寒中少阴，则脐腹疼痛，宜归气饮。"明确指出了寒邪暴中肾经所引起的一系列病机变化和治法。

《杂病源流犀烛•寒病源流》曰："凡人或冒雨雪，或涉冰渊，或晨行旷野，或夜深露坐，或衣被一时不及，或饮食耐冷强吞，而一股寒冷之邪，自外入里，又一时不即透发，以致辗转深陷，或伏于经络，或伏于脏腑。及其发也， …或寒冷之邪伏于少阴，下利，厥逆无脉，干呕而烦，腹痛，四肢沉重痛，小便不利，或烦躁欲死，或五更泄泻。"也清楚分析了寒邪中伤肾经所导致的腹痛、肢痛、厥逆等病机变化。

Summary of Fulminant Strike of Cold Evil
1. Cold Assailing the Lower Back Heavy pain and cold pain in the lower back and legs.
2. Fulminant Cold Attacking the Abdomen Umbilical and abdominal cold pain, intermittent hypertonicity with fulminant pain, hypertonicity in the four limbs.
3. Obstruction of Yáng Qì Cold body and shivering, cold pain in the extremities.
4. Cold Evil Damaging the Kidney Pale tongue, fine sunken pulse.

寒邪暴中
寒袭于腰—腰脚重痛冷痛
暴寒攻腹—脐腹冷痛，时而拘急暴痛，四体拘挛
阳气被遏—身冷战栗，手足冷痛
寒邪伤肾—舌质淡，脉沉细

1.3 Kidney Channel Cold Mounting

The kidney opens at the two yīn, and its channel enters the smaller abdomen from the inner side of the leg and skirts around the genitals. If cold evil invades from the outside and directly invades the kidney channel, yīn cold binds inside. This can form the pathomechanism of kidney channel cold mounting.

When cold strikes the kidney channel, the qì dynamic in the channels of the lower back, umbilicus, abdomen, and genitals is obstructed and fails to course freely so that channel qì stops. This results in lumbar pain, hypertonicity and pain in the smaller abdomen, and possibly pain around the umbilicus spreading towards the testicles. When cold obstructs the inner body, yáng qì fails to reach the four limbs. This results in reversal cold of the extremities.

The kidney controls stool and urine. When cold evil congeals in the kidney channel and causes a breakdown of qì transformation, this results in dry bound stool and inhibited urination.

Congealing cold in the kidney channel manifests in a pale fat tongue and a sunken tight, stringlike tight, or rough sunken pulse.

The "Treatise on Needling Joints" in the *Sù Wèn* ("Plain Questions") states: "When the disease is in the smaller abdomen, the patient experiences abdominal pain and inability to urinate or defecate. This disease is called mounting and it is contracted through cold." This quotation clearly points out how an invasion of cold evil can lead to mounting qì.

The "Point-by-Point Treatise on Mounting" in the *Sān Yīn Jí Yī Bìng Zhèng Fāng Lùn* ("A Unified Treatise on Diseases, Patterns, and Remedies According to the Three Causes") also explains: "Generally speaking, when blood is congealed due to cold, it forms conglomeration qì; when blood gathers due to coldness, it forms mounting." This quotation also indicates that mounting arises as a result of contracting cold.

Beginning with Zhāng Zhòng-Jǐng, most physicians attributed mounting to the liver. For example, the chapter, "Mounting Pain" in the *Dān Xī Xīn Fǎ* ("Dān Xī's Heart-Approach") states:

> "Mounting pain arises generally as a result of cold depression. Even if it is caused by phlegm-rheum, food accumulations, and dead blood, these are hosted especially in the liver channel and have absolutely no relationship with the kidney channel."

However, this statement is subject to debate. By contrast, the chapter, "Mounting Qì" in the *Jǐng Yuè Quán Shū* ("Jǐng-Yuè's Complete Compendium"), "Schema of Miscellaneous Patterns" points out:

> "Mounting qì is not related to only one channel… Even if the sinews are governed by reverting yīn, they are nevertheless scattered throughout all the channels, constituting the sinews of all the channels. If disease can affect all the channels, it is certainly possible that the channels are disabled by the sinews. The channels in the smaller abdomen and genitals involve reverting yīn, lesser yīn, greater yīn, yáng brightness, lesser yáng, and greater yáng, as well as the thoroughfare, controlling, and governing vessels."

This quotation indicates that the pathomechanism of cold mounting can be caused by contraction of cold in the kidney channel.

The chapter, "Origin and Development of the Seven Mountings" in the *Zá Bìng Yuán Liú Xī Zhú* ("Incisive Light on the Source of Miscellaneous Disease") also explains:

> "The theory that the condition of mounting disease in the channels is ascribed to the liver and controlling vessels is admittedly valid. Yet this is not the end of it. Such a person is also bound to suffer from vacuity

> cold in the kidney, as dampness has been allowed to exploit the vacuity, settle there, and consequently form mounting. When Dān-Xī states that this condition has absolutely no relationship with the kidney channel, he is mistaken."

This passage asserts that mounting is necissarily related to the kidney channel.

Furthermore, the "Section on Mounting Qì" in the *Piàn Yǜ Xīn Shū* ("Jade Tablet of Heart Insights") expounds:

> "All pain in the smaller abdomen with swelling and hardness in the external kidney [the male genitals], is called mounting. When children sit on damp ground for a longer period of time, this allows cold evil to invade the kidney. This results in stabbing pain in the smaller abdomen and swelling and hardness in the external kidney."

This quotation directly refers to the pathomechanism of kidney channel cold mounting.

This condition is treated by warming the kidney and dispersing cold. The recommended formulas are *wū tóu guì zhī tāng* (Aconite Main Tuber and Cinnamon Twig Decoction) from the *Jīn Guì Yào Lüe* ("Essential Prescriptions of the Golden Coffer") for mild cases or *dà wū tóu jiān* (Major Aconite Decoction) from the same text for severe cases.

Wū Tóu Guì Zhī Tāng 乌头桂枝汤 Aconite Main Tuber and Cinnamon Twig Decoction
chuān wū (川乌 Aconiti Radix, aconite main root)
guì zhī (桂枝 Cinnamomi Ramulus, cinnamon twig)
bái sháo (白芍 Paeoniae Radix Alba, white peony)
shēng jiāng (生姜 Zingiberis Rhizoma Recens, fresh ginger)
dà zǎo (大枣 Jujubae Fructus, jujube)
gān cǎo (甘草 Glycyrrhizae Radix, licorice)

Dà Wū Tóu Jiān 大乌头煎 Major Aconite Decoction
wū tóu (乌头 Aconiti Radix Wutou, aconite)

肾经寒疝

肾开窍于二阴，其经脉从下肢内侧入少腹，绕阴器。如寒邪外侵，直犯肾经，阴寒内结，则可形成肾经寒疝的病机变化。寒中肾经，腰、脐腹、前阴经脉气机阻滞，疏泄不利，经气不通，则腰痛，少腹拘急疼痛，或绕脐疼痛并牵引睾丸而痛；寒阻于内，阳气不达四肢，则手足厥冷；肾司二便，寒邪凝结肾经，气化失司，则大便干结，小便不利。肾经寒凝，则舌淡胖，脉沉紧或弦紧，或沉涩。如《素问•长刺节论》云："病在少腹，腹痛不得大小便，病名曰疝，得之寒。"明确指出了寒邪侵犯，可引起疝气的病机改变。《三因极一病证方论•疝叙论》又说："大抵血因寒泣则为瘕气，因寒聚而为疝。"指出疝病多因受寒而起。虽然仲景以来，医家多归属于肝，如《丹溪心法•疝痛》曰："疝痛，…大概因寒郁而作，即是痰饮食积并死血，专主肝经，与肾经绝无相干。"但事实并非如此，如《景岳全书•杂证谟•疝气》指出："疝气所属，本非一经。…且筋虽主于厥阴，然散见诸经，即为诸经之筋矣，若病在诸经，固可因筋而废经乎？…然而小腹前阴之经，则厥阴、少阴、太阴、阳明、少阳、太阳，以至冲、任、督脉皆有所涉。"对肾经受寒，可引起寒疝的病机变化进行了分析论证。《杂病源流犀烛•七疝源流》也说："且经以疝症属肝任，理固然已。而犹有未尽者，必其人肾虚寒，湿邪乘虚客之，遂成疝病。丹溪谓与肾经绝无相干者，误也。"指出疝病与肾经有必然联系。更有《片玉心书•疝气门》说："凡小腹疼痛，外肾肿硬者，此名疝。盖由小儿久坐湿地，以致寒邪内侵于肾而得，所以小腹刺痛，外肾肿硬。"明确提出肾经寒疝的病机。治法为温肾散寒。方药轻则选用《金匮要略》乌头桂枝汤(制川乌蜜煮、桂枝、芍药、生姜、大枣、甘草)。重则选用《金匮要略》大乌头煎（乌头，蜜煮煎）。

Literature Review of Kidney Channel Cold Mounting

📖 *Biàn Zhèng Lù* ("Records on Pattern Differentiation"), "Section on Mounting Qì"

"In cases where a person's testicles hurt with a feeling as if soaked in cold water, the cold causes unbearable pain. This means that damp qì has entered the kidney channel. But when dampness assails the kidney, the disease should be in the lower back. How is it that the lower back does not hurt and that the pain is located in the testicles? Don't you know that the testicles are linked to the kidney and that when kidney qì fails to reach the testicles, this external force is unable to invigorate them? Now if the kidney suffers from cold as a result of contracting dampness, this cold in the kidney directly causes cold in the testicles and, as a result of qì binding inside the kidney and lower back, prevents the testicles from repelling. The pain in the testicles is caused by the formation of mounting qì.

"Although this is caused by coldness of kidney qì, it can also be caused by dampness in the testicles. The patient must have sat in a cold damp area after seminal discharge on the same day, causing a double contraction of outside and inside, and the testicles alone were affected by this. This condition is treated by warming the cold inside the kidney and by dispersing the dampness inside the testicles. In this way, you get rid of the disease in one sweep… This condition is a disease of the lesser yīn kidney channel, namely extreme cold inside the kidney that is stopping the flow of kidney qì. When dampness inside the kidney is severe, kidney qì becomes even more stagnant. Eliminate the cold-damp, and kidney qì will spontaneously flow into the testicles. Furthermore, *ròu guì* (Cinnamomi Cortex) and *jú hé* (Citri Reticulatae Semen) are particularly good for entering the testicles and thus will naturally achieve success."

This quotation describes in detail how cold evil invading the lesser yīn channel results in mounting qì pain.

🕮 *Biàn Zhèng Qí Wén* ("Exceptional Pattern Differentiation"), "Mounting Qì"

"When the testicles hurt from contraction of cold-damp, this condition erupts and the pain is unbearable. People assume that it is caused by damp qì entering the testicles, but who knows that it is in fact dampness entering the kidney channel? ... Treat it by warming the kidney and dispersing cold."

This quotation directly points to the pathomechanism of cold evil assailing the kidney.

🕮 *Qī Sōng Yán Jí* ("Records of *Qī Sōng-Yán*"), "Identification and Treatment of Common Diseases: Mounting Qì"

"Kidney mounting is generally found in patients with sexual taxation and excessive desires, which cause a prior vacuity of interior qì. In such patients, cold-damp is able to invade, and after a prolonged period of lying depressed, it can cause mounting. The pain feels as if linked from the lower back and kidney to the penis, and the pulse is rough and sunken, or slight, fine, soggy and soft."

This quotation describes the pathomechanism and manifestations of cold lying depressed in the kidney channel, causing cold mounting.

文献评述

《辨证录•疝气门》曰："人有感浸寒湿，睾丸作痛者，冷即发痛不可忍，此湿气之入于肾经也。夫湿侵于肾，宜病在腰，何以腰不痛而痛在睾丸乎?不知睾属肾，肾气不至睾丸，则外势不能振兴。盖因肾得湿则寒，寒在肾即寒在睾丸，而气结于腰肾之中，宜睾丸之不应矣。其睾丸作痛者，因疝气之成，虽成于肾气之寒，亦成于睾丸之湿也。当日泄精之后，人坐于寒湿之区，内外两感，睾丸独受之矣。治法温其肾中之寒，消其睾丸之湿，病去如扫矣。 ...此症乃少阴肾经之病，肾中寒极，而肾气不通；肾中湿重，而肾气更滞。去其寒湿，而肾气自行于睾丸之内。况肉桂、橘核尤善入睾丸，自然收到功成也。"对寒邪侵犯少阴经脉引起疝气疼痛的病机变化进行了深入的剖析。

《辨证奇闻•疝气》曰："感寒湿睾丸作痛，遇冷即发，痛难忍。人谓湿气入睾丸，谁知湿入肾经乎？ ...法宜温肾散寒。"明确指出寒邪袭肾的病机。

《七松岩集•常见病辨治•疝气》曰："肾疝者，大略房劳多欲之人，里气先虚，寒湿得而入侵，久郁为疝。其痛如连腰、肾、阴茎，其脉沉涩，或微细而濡软。"论述寒郁肾经引起寒疝的病机和表现。

Summary of Kidney Channel Cold Mounting

1. Cold Obstructing the Qì Dynamic
   Lumbar pain, hypertonicity and pain in the smaller abdomen, possibly pain around the umbilicus, and pulling and pain in the testicles.
2. Yáng Qì Failing to Move
   Reversal cold in the extremities.
3. Breakdown of Qì Transformation
   Dry bound stool, inhibited urination.
4. Congealing Cold in the Kidney Channel
   Pale fat tongue, sunken tight, stringlike tight, or rough sunken pulse.

肾经寒疝

寒阻气机—腰痛，少腹拘急疼痛，或绕脐疼痛，并牵引睾丸而痛

阳气不运—手足厥冷

气化失司—大便干结，小便不利

肾经寒凝—舌淡胖，脉沉紧或弦紧，或沉涩

Chapter Two

Kidney Channel Wind-Heat

Wind is the precursor of the hundred diseases. Every year, when spring turns into summer or when there is exuberant heat in the summer season, people like to ingest cold things and expose their bodies. In such a situation, if wind complicated by heat evil goes straight into the kidney channel, this manifests in the pathomechanical changes of kidney channel wind-heat.

The lower back is the house of the kidney. When wind-heat invades the kidney, channel qì in the house of the kidney is inhibited. The result is heat and scorching pain in the lower back.

Wind-heat can follow the channels and harass the upper body, steaming in the face and binding in the throat. This results in a red face and eyes, thirst, and redness, swelling, heat, and pain in the throat.

When wind evil lies depressed in the fleshy exterior, this can lead to headache and body pain, stiffness and pain in the neck and nape, and generalized fever and sweating.

When wind-heat damages the kidney and causes a breakdown of qì transformation, urine becomes concentrated, resulting in short voidings of scant reddish urine.

Kidney channel wind-heat manifests in a red tongue with thin yellow fur and a replete rapid pulse.

The chapter, "Lumbar Pain" in the *Yī Zōng Bì Dú* ("Indispensable Medical Reading") explains:

> "What the *Nèi Jīng* ("The Inner Canon") calls greater yáng lumbar pain refers to an external contraction of the six qì… Whenever there is cold-damp, wind-heat, contusion and wrenching, static blood, stagnant qì, or phlegm accumulation, all of these are signs."

This quotation points out that externally contracted wind-heat can lead to lumbar pain.

"Treatise on Needling Heat" in the *Sù Wèn* ("Plain Questions") states: "In the condition of kidney heat, the jowl will first redden." This is a reference to the reddening of the face and eyes that occurs when wind-heat evil invades the kidney.

Kidney channel wind-heat is treated by clearing, light diffusion and transformation, and by dispelling wind and dispersing heat. The recommended formula is *má huáng xìng rén yì yǐ gān cǎo tāng* (Ephedra, Apricot Kernel, Coix, and Licorice Decoction) from the *Jīn Guì Yào Lüe* ("Essential Prescriptions of the Golden Coffer") with the addition of *yín huā téng* (Lonicerae Caulis), *qín jiāo* (Gentianae Macrophyllae Radix), *fáng jǐ* (Stephaniae Tetrandrae Radix), and *wēi líng xiān* (Clematidis Radix).

Má Huáng Xìng Rén Yì Yǐ Gān Cǎo Tāng 麻黄杏仁薏苡甘草汤
Ephedra, Apricot Kernel, Coix, and Licorice Decoction

má huáng (麻黄 Ephedrae Herba, ephedra)
xìng rén (杏仁 Armeniacae Semen, apricot kernel)
yì yǐ rén (薏苡仁 Coicis Semen, coix)
gān cǎo (甘草 Glycyrrhizae Radix, licorice)

Plus:

rěn dōng téng (忍冬藤 Lonicerae Caulis, lonicera stem)
qín jiāo (秦艽 Gentianae Macrophyllae Radix, large gentian)
fáng jǐ (防己 Stephaniae Tetrandrae Radix, fangji)
wēi líng xiān (威灵仙 Clematidis Radix, clematis)

An alternative choice is *bài dú sǎn* (Toxin-Vanquishing Powder) from the *Xiǎo Ér Yào Zhèng Zhí Jué* ("Key to Diagnosis and Treatment of Children's Diseases") with the addition of *xù duàn* (Dipsaci Radix), *tiān má* (Gastrodiae Rhizoma), *mù guā* (Chaenomelis Fructus), and *bò hé* (Menthae Herba).

Bài Dú Sǎn 败毒散 Toxin-Vanquishing Powder
qiāng huó (羌活 Notopterygii Rhizoma et Radix, notopterygium) *dú huó* (独活 Angelicae Pubescentis Radix, pubescent angelica) *qián hú* (前胡 Peucedani Radix, peucedanum) *zhǐ qiào (ké)* (枳壳 Aurantii Fructus, bitter orange) *jié gěng* (桔梗 Platycodonis Radix, platycodon) *fú líng* (茯苓 Poria, poria) *chuān xiōng* (川芎 Chuanxiong Rhizoma, chuanxiong) *gān cǎo* (甘草 Glycyrrhizae Radix, licorice) Plus: *xù duàn* (续断 Dipsaci Radix, dipsacus) *tiān má* (天麻 Gastrodiae Rhizoma, gastrodia) *mù guā* (木瓜 Chaenomelis Fructus, chaenomeles) *bò hé* (薄荷 Menthae Herba, mint)

肾经风热

风为百病之先，每逢春夏之交，或夏季盛热之时，人喜贪凉取冷，裸露身体，风挟热邪直奔肾经，则出现肾经风热的病机变化。腰为肾之府，风热犯肾，腰府经气不利，则为腰热灼痛；风热循经上扰，熏蒸于面，郁结于咽喉，则面目红赤，口渴，咽喉红肿热痛；风邪郁结肌表，可引起头身疼痛，颈项强痛，身热汗出；风热伤肾，气化失司，小便浓缩，则尿少短赤。肾经风热，则舌红苔薄黄，脉实数。如《医宗必读•腰痛》说："<内经>言太阳腰痛者，外感六气也。 …有寒湿，有风热，有挫闪，有瘀血，有滞气，有痰积，皆标也。"指出外感风热可引起腰痛。《素问•刺热篇》曰："肾热病者颐先赤。"对风热之邪犯肾引起的面红目赤的病机改变进行了描述。治则为轻清宣化，祛风散热。方药选用《金匮要略》麻黄杏仁薏苡甘草汤（麻黄、杏仁、薏苡仁、甘草）加银花藤，秦艽，防己，威灵仙。或用《小儿药证直诀》败毒散（羌活、独活、前胡、枳壳、桔梗、茯苓、川芎、甘草）加续断、天麻、木瓜、薄荷。

Literature Review of Kidney Channel Wind-Heat

📖 *Jǐng Yuè Quán* Shū ("Jǐng-Yuè's Complete Compendium"), "Schema of Miscellaneous Patterns: Lumbar Pain"

> "All exterior patterns of lumbar pain are caused by wind-cold-damp stagnation damaging the greater yáng and lesser yīn channels. If wind-cold is present in the channels, it invariably manifests with aversion to cold and heat effusion, a tight rapid pulse that arrives with great haste, and pain that is characterized by hypertonicity with concurrent soreness that usually stretches to the spine and back... Yáng patterns with increased heat should be treated with formulas like *yī chái hú yǐn* (Bupleurum Beverage) or *zhèng chái hú yǐn* (Bupleurum Righting Beverage)."

Lumbar pain belongs to the kidney, although it can be concurrent with an exterior pattern. Exterior patterns refer to wind-cold, but can also refer to wind-heat. Thus, Jǐng-Yuè not only mentions the pathomechanism of kidney channel wind-heat causing lumbar pain, e.g., "yáng patterns and increased heat," but also advocates treatment with *yī chái hú yǐn* (Bupleurum Drink) (*chái hú* (Bupleuri Radix), *huáng qín* (Scutellariae Radix), *bái sháo* (Paeoniae Radix Alba), *shēng dì huáng* (Rehmanniae Radix), *chén pí* (Citri Reticulatae Pericarpium), and *gān cǎo* (Glycyrrhizae Radix)) to cool, disperse, and clear heat.

📖 *Jǐng Yuè Quán Shū* ("Jǐng-Yuè's Complete Compendium"), "Schema of Miscellaneous Patterns: Lumbar Pain"

> "In patterns of lumbar pain... when the patient experiences pain upon encountering any heat and has a liking for cold and aversion to heat, this means heat."

When wind-heat invades the kidney, the house of the kidney receives the evil, thus there is pain and scorching heat, liking for cold, and aversion to heat.

📖 *Lín Chuáng Zhōng Yī Nèi Kē Xué* ("Clinical Chinese Internal Medicine"), "Lumbar Pain"

> "Wind-heat lumbar pain: In wind-heat assailing greater yáng, heat is a yáng evil. Thus there is generalized heat effusion with sweating, dry mouth and thirst, sore swollen throat, and lumbar pain and heat. The tongue is red with a thin yellow fur and the pulse sunken and rapid. These are the signs of wind-heat on the exterior."

This quotation clearly describes the pathomechanism and symptoms of wind-heat evil invading the kidney, resulting in lumbar pain of the kidney channel wind-heat type.

文献评述

《景岳全书•杂证谟•腰痛》曰："腰痛之表证，凡风寒湿滞之邪伤于太阳少阴之经者，皆是也。若风寒在经，其证必有寒热，其脉必见紧数，其来必骤急，其痛必拘急，兼酸而多连脊背。 ...阳证而多热者，宜一柴胡饮或正柴胡饮之类。"腰痛属肾，可兼表证，表证既有风寒，亦有风热，故景岳不仅提出腰痛"阳证而多热"的肾经风热病机，而且主张用凉散清热的一柴胡饮（柴胡、黄芩、白芍、生地、陈皮、甘草）治疗。

《景岳全书•杂证谟•腰痛》曰："腰痛证， ...遇诸热而痛，及喜寒而恶热者，热也"。风热犯肾，腰府受邪，故疼痛灼热，喜寒而恶热。

《临床中医内科学•腰痛》曰："风热腰痛：风热侵袭，犯及太阳，热为阳邪，故身热有汗，口干口渴，咽喉肿痛，腰痛而热。舌质红苔薄黄，脉浮数，是风热在表之征。"明确论述了风热之邪犯肾，引起肾经风热性腰痛的病机和证候。

Summary of Kidney Channel Wind-Heat

1. Wind Heat Invading the Kidney

    Heat and scorching pain in the lower back.

2. Wind Heat Harassing the Upper Body

    Red face and eyes; thirst; redness, swelling, heat, and pain in the throat.

3. Wind Heat Invading the Exterior

    Headache and body pain, stiffness and pain in the neck and nape, generalized fever and sweating.

4. Wind-Heat Damaging the Kidney

    Short voidings of scant reddish urine.

5. Kidney Channel Wind-Heat

    Red tongue with thin yellow fur, replete rapid pulse.

肾经风热
风热犯肾—腰热灼痛
风热上扰—面目红赤，口渴，咽喉红肿热痛
风热犯表—头身疼痛，颈项强痛，身热汗出
风热伤肾—尿少短赤
肾经风热—舌红苔薄黄，脉实数

Chapter Three

Kidney Channel Wind-Damp

Wind is the head of the hundred diseases. The "Treatise on Wind" in the chapter, "Miscellaneous Theories" from the *Wēn Bìng Tiáo Biàn* ("Systematized Identification of Warm Diseases") states: "Wind is the commander of the six qì and the leader of all diseases." This quotation points out that wind is the forerunner of externally contracted diseases and that the other types of evil qì rely on wind evil to invade the body.

Dampness is the qì that steams and moistens yīn and yáng between heaven and earth. Caused by an invasion of fog or dew, by overcast and rainy weather settling in the body, or by sweat sticking to clothing, it usually binds with wind when invading the body. This forms the combined evil of wind-damp.

The kidney is the water viscus. Therefore the evil of wind-damp can easily invade the kidney channel, forming the pathomechanism of kidney channel wind-damp.

Because a combination of wind and dampness can manifest either as water qì or as damp evil, kidney channel wind-damp can be differentiated into two types: wind water assailing the kidney and wind-damp damaging the kidney.

肾经风湿

风为百病之首。《温病条辨•杂说•风论》曰："风也者，六气之帅也，诸病之领袖也。"指出风为外邪致病的先导，其它邪气依附风邪侵入人体。湿为天地间阴阳蒸润之气，或因雾露之侵，或因阴雨所客，或因汗出粘衣，多常与风相结，侵犯人体，成为风湿合邪。肾为水脏，故风湿之邪，容易侵犯肾经，形成肾经风湿的病机。由于风与湿合，有与水气和湿邪之别，故肾经风湿可分为风水袭肾和风湿伤肾两大类型。

3.1 Wind Water Assailing the Kidney

The kidney governs water and regulates the fluid metabolism of the body. If the lower back, back, and soles of the feet are exposed to external dew, or a constitutional insufficiency of yáng qì allows wind evil to directly strike the kidney, this can derange qì transformation in the kidney and disorder the fluid metabolism. If external wind binds with internal water and moves transversely inside the body, the fluids are not distributed and instead inundate the skin. This manifests in the pathomechanical changes of wind water assailing the kidney.

When the kidney is assailed by wind water, it is unable to transform qì or move water, and water qì inundates the skin. This manifests in puffy swelling in the face, limbs, and skin that is particularly pronounced above the lower back, and inhibited urination.

When channel qì in the lower back is impeded by wind evil, movement is inhibited. The result is pain in the lumbar spine and inability to stand erect.

Wind is a yáng evil and by nature freely coursing and scattering. Insecurity of the defensive exterior results in sweating and aversion to wind.

The kidney governs water and its color is black. When wind water assails the kidney, the fluid metabolism is disordered and the kidney's color shows on the outside, making the facial complexion black.

Wind water assailing the kidney results in a fat pale tongue with a glossy white fur, and a large tight pulse.

The "Treatise on Points for Water and Heat" in the *Sù Wèn* ("Plain Questions") states:

> "Tenacious action to the point of severe taxation makes the kidney sweat. When wind is encountered during kidney sweating, [wind] is unable to enter the bowels and viscera on the inside or stray into the skin on the outside. Instead, it intrudes into the mysterious mansion, moves into the interior of the skin, and spreads to cause skin swelling. Rooted in the kidney, this condition is called wind water."

This quotation indicates how a direct strike of wind water on the kidney can prevent it from opening and closing, and from transforming qì or moving water. As a result, the fluids are not retained and instead inundate the skin transversely, forming water swelling.

The chapter, "Origin and Development of Wind Disease" in the *Zá Bìng Yuán Liú Xī Zhú* ("Incisive Light on the Source of Miscellaneous Disease") also states:

> "When the kidney contracts wind, it manifests in spontaneous sweating and aversion to wind. Huge puffy swelling of the face is caused by evil invading the kidney and upbearing with water qì. Pain in the spine and inability to stand erect is due to the fact that the kidney is located in this area."

This quotation clearly points out the pathomechanism by which an invasion of wind water into the kidney channel can manifest in puffy swelling in the face and eyes, and lumbar pain.

Wind water assailing the kidney is treated by warming the kidney, expelling wind, and disinhibiting water. The recommended formula is *yuè bì jiā zhú tāng (*Spleen-Effusing Decoction Plus White Atractylodes*)* from the *Jīn Guì Yào Lüe ("Essential Prescriptions of the Golden Coffer")* with the addition of *fù zǐ* (Aconiti Radix Lateralis Praeparata).

Yuè Bì Jiā Zhú Tāng 越婢加术汤 Spleen-Effusing Decoction Plus White Atractylodes
má huáng (麻黄 Ephedrae Herba, ephedra)
bái zhú (白术 Atractylodis Macrocephalae Rhizoma, white atractylodes)
shí gāo (石膏 Gypsum Fibrosum, gypsum)
shēng jiāng (生姜 Zingiberis Rhizoma Recens, fresh ginger)
dà zǎo (大枣 Jujubae Fructus, jujube)
gān cǎo (甘草 Glycyrrhizae Radix, licorice)
Plus:
fù zǐ (附子 Aconiti Radix Lateralis Praeparata, aconite)

风水袭肾

肾主水，调节人体水液代谢。如腰背足底外露，或素体阳气不足，风邪直中于肾，导致肾之气化失司，水液代谢失常，外风与内水相结，横行体内，水津失布，泛滥肌肤，出现风水袭肾的病机变化。风水袭肾，不能化气行水，水气泛滥于肌肤，表现为颜面四肢皮肤浮肿，腰以上尤甚，小便不利；腰府经气受风邪阻碍，运行不畅，则腰脊疼痛，不能直立；风为阳邪，其性疏散，卫表不固，则汗出恶风；肾主水，其色黑，风水袭肾，水液代谢失常，肾色外露，则面色黑。风水袭肾，则舌质淡胖，苔白滑，脉大而紧。如《素问•水热穴论》曰："勇而劳甚则肾汗出，肾汗出逢于风，内不得入脏腑，外不得越于皮肤，客于玄府，行于皮里，传为胕肿，本之于肾，名曰风水。"指出了风水直中肾脏，导致肾失开阖，不能化气行水，水液失去约束，泛滥横溢于肌肤，形成水肿的病机变化。《杂病源流犀烛•风病源流》也云："肾受风，自汗恶风。面庞然浮肿，以邪入肾，挟水气上升，故肿也。脊痛不能正立，以肾在其部也。"明确指出了肾经受风水邪气所犯，可出现面目浮肿腰痛的病机。治则为温肾驱风利水。方药选用《金匮要略》越婢加术汤（麻黄、白术、石膏、生姜、大枣、甘草）加附子。

Literature Review of Wind Water Assailing the Kidney

🕮 *Sù Wèn* ("Plain Questions"), "On Wind"

> "The symptoms of kidney wind are profuse sweating and aversion to wind, huge puffy swelling of the face, pain in the spine and inability to stand erect, a soot-black complexion, inhibited urination, and blackness when examining the surface of the flesh."

This quotation clearly indicates the pathomechanical changes of wind water assailing the kidney that result from a contraction of wind water when the disease evil enters the interior and passes from the fleshy exterior along the channels and network vessels into the kidney.

🕮 *Wài Tái Mì Yào* ("Essential Secrets from Outside the Metropolis"), "Formulas for Wind Deafness"

> "The source of this disease is in the foot lesser yīn channel, the gathering place of ancestral qì. Its qì penetrates to the ears and when the channel is vacuous, wind evil can exploit it. Consequently, wind enters the ear vessel and blocks channel qì, preventing it from perfusing. This causes wind deafness."

This quotation indicates how wind assailing the lesser yīn kidney channel can induce the pathomechanical change of ear deafness.

📖 *Yī Xué Xīn Wù* ("Medical Insights"), "Lumbar Pain"

> "Lumbar pain and hypertonicity, pulling in the legs and feet, and a floating stringlike pulse mean wind."

The lower back is the house of the kidney, and the kidney channel runs upward from the sole of the feet. When wind evil invades the kidney, it inhibits channel qì in the lower back, legs, and feet, causing pain and hypertonicity.

文献评述

《素问•风论》曰："肾风之状，多汗出恶风，面庞然浮肿，脊痛不能正立，其色炲（指煤烟），隐曲不利，诊在肌上，其色黑。"明确指出了感受风水之邪，病邪入里，由肌表循经络，传入肾脏，引起风水袭肾的病机变化。

《外台秘要•风聋方》曰："病源足少阴之经，宗气之所聚，其气通于耳，其经脉虚，风邪乘之，风入于耳之脉，使经气痞塞不宣，故为风聋。"指出了风袭少阴肾经，可引起耳聋的病机变化。

《医学心悟•腰痛》曰："腰痛拘急，牵引腿足，脉浮弦者，风也。"腰为肾之府，肾经循足底而上走，风邪犯肾，则腰腿足经气不利，疼痛拘急。

Summary of Wind Water Assailing the Kidney

1. Water Spilling into the Skin

   Puffy swelling in the face, limbs, and skin that is particularly pronounced above the lower back; inhibited urination.
2. Stoppage of Channel Qì

   Pain in the lumbar spine, inability to stand erect.
3. Insecurity of the Fleshy Exterior

   Spontaenous sweating with aversion to wind.
4. Kidney's Color Showing on the Outside

   Black facial complexion.
5. Wind Water Assailing the Kidney

   Fat pale tongue with glossy white fur, large tight pulse.

风水袭肾
水泛肌肤—颜面四肢皮肤浮肿，腰以上尤甚，小便不利
经气不通—腰脊疼痛，不能直立
卫表不固—汗出恶风
肾色外露—面色黑
风水袭肾—舌质淡胖，苔白滑，脉大而紧

3.2 Wind-Damp Invading the Kidney

The lower back is the house of the kidney. Conditions like damp rainy years, living in damp places, getting soaked by rain or exposed to dew, having an occupation related to water, or sweating when exposed to wind can all allow the evil of wind-damp to invade the lumbar region and settle in the kidney channel. This forms the pathomechanism of wind-damp invading the kidney.

The chapter, "Treatment Methods for Lumbar Pain" in the *Sān Yīn Jí Yī Bìng Zhèng Fāng Lùn* ("A Unified Treatise on Diseases, Patterns, and Remedies According to the Three Causes"), for example, discusses indications for *dú huó jì shēng tāng* (Pubescent Angelica and Mistletoe Decoction):

> "Lumbar pain is always caused by kidney qì vacuity that is contracted from sleeping in cold damp places and being exposed to wind. If it is not treated in a timely manner, it is likely to flow into the foot and knee. This causes hemilateral withering, cold impediment, slackening and weakening, pain and heaviness, possibly lumbar pain and hypertonicity, and heaviness and glomus in the feet. I recommend that the patient urgently take this formula."

This quotation is an incisive description of the pathomechanism by which a damp sleeping place and exposure to wind allow wind and dampness to combine, exploit vacuity to enter the body, and invade the kidney channel, resulting in pain in the lower back and legs.

It is the nature of wind to cause hypertonicity; dampness is by nature heavy and fixed. When wind and dampness combine to invade the kidney, they block the channels and network vessels in the house of the kidney. This results in hypertonicity of the back and lower back, aching heavy pain, inability to turn sides, and inhibited physical movement.

Dampness is a yīn evil. In cold weather on overcast rainy days, wind-damp can contract cold and congeal, which further aggravates congestion in the qì dynamic. This changes in response to the weather, so that lumbar pain is more severe on rainy overcast days.

Wind is a yáng evil, and its nature is to cause opening and discharge. When the interstices of the flesh are loosened, the result is heat effusion with aversion to wind, and spontaneous sweating with generalized heaviness.

An invasion of wind-damp can cause water-damp to spill outward. This results in puffy swelling in the face and limbs.

Wind-damp collecting internally manifests in a thin slimy tongue fur and a fine soggy pulse.

All this is stated directly in the chapter, "Wind-Damp Lumbar Pain" in the *Zhèng Yīn Mài Zhì* ("Pathoconditions: Causes, Pulses, and Treatments"):

> "The symptoms of wind-damp lumbar pain are heat effusion with aversion to wind, spontaneous sweating with generalized heaviness, heavy pain in the back and lower back, and inability to turn sides. These are the symptoms of wind-damp lumbar pain. The causes of wind-damp lumbar pain are as follows. In rainy and damp years wind-damp may have invaded the fleshy exterior. This results in seasonal lumbar pain and [thus] is a disease caused by annual qì. Alternatively, patients may have been drenched by wind and rain, so that they have contracted wind-damp. Lastly, when a person has a profession related to water, water can abide in the skin, and cause the individual to fall ill. In this case, the disease is induced by the unique [work] environment."

Wind-damp invading the kidney is treated by dispelling wind and disinhibiting dampness. The recommended formula is *dú huó jì shēng tāng* (Pubescent Angelica and Mistletoe Decoction) from the *Sān Yīn Jí Yī Bìng Zhèng Fāng Lùn* ("A Unified Treatise on Diseases, Patterns, and Remedies According to the Three Causes").

Dú Huó Jì Shēng Tāng 独活寄生汤
Pubescent Angelica and Mistletoe Decoction

dú huó (独活 Angelicae Pubescentis Radix, pubescent angelica)
sāng jì shēng (桑寄生 Taxilli Herba, mistletoe)
chuān xiōng (川芎 Chuanxiong Rhizoma, chuanxiong)
dāng guī (当归 Angelicae Sinensis Radix, Chinese angelica)

bái sháo (白芍 Paeoniae Radix Alba, white peony)
shú dì huáng (熟地黄 Rehmanniae Radix Praeparata, cooked rehmannia)
dù zhòng (杜仲 Eucommiae Cortex, eucommia)
niú xī (牛膝 Achyranthis Bidentatae Radix, achyranthes)
qín jiāo (秦艽 Gentianae Macrophyllae Radix, large gentian)
fú líng (茯苓 Poria, poria)
rén shēn (人参 Ginseng Radix, ginseng)
guì zhī (桂枝 Cinnamomi Ramulus, cinnamon twig)
xì xīn (细辛 Asari Herba, asarum)
fáng fēng (防风 Saposhnikoviae Radix, saposhnikovia)
gān cǎo (甘草 Glycyrrhizae Radix, licorice)

风湿犯肾

腰为肾之府。若雨湿之年，居处潮湿，冒雨宿露，水中作业，汗出当风，均可因风湿之邪，侵犯腰间，舍于肾经，形成风湿犯肾的病机。如《三因极一病证方论•腰痛治法》在描述独活寄生汤的主治时说："夫腰痛，皆由肾气虚弱，卧冷湿地当风所得，不时速治，喜流入脚膝，为偏枯，冷痹，缓弱，疼重，或腰痛挛，脚重痹，宜急服此。"对卧湿当风，风湿合邪，乘虚而入，侵犯肾经，引起腰腿疼痛的病机作了精辟的论述。风性拘挛，湿性重着，风湿合犯肾经，腰府经络闭塞，则腰背拘急，酸重疼痛，不能转侧，活动不利；湿为阴邪，阴雨天气候寒冷，风湿受寒而凝，气机阻塞加重，则随气候变化，阴雨天腰痛加重；风为阳邪，其性开泄，肌腠疏松，则发热恶风，自汗身重；风湿侵犯，水湿外溢，则颜面及四肢浮肿。风湿内停，则舌苔薄腻，脉濡细。正如《症因脉治•风湿腰痛》曰："风湿腰痛之症，发热恶风，自汗身重，腰背重痛，不能转侧，此风湿腰痛之症也。风湿腰痛之因，或雨湿之年，风湿袭入肌表，则时行腰痛，此因岁气而致病者；或冲风冒雨，风湿感人；或以水为事，水舍皮肤，一人独病，此人自感冒而致病者也。"治宜祛风利湿。方药选《三因极一病证方论》独活寄生汤（独活、寄生、川芎、当归、白芍、熟地、杜仲、牛膝、秦艽、茯苓、人参、桂枝、细辛、防风、甘草。）

Literature Review of Wind-Damp Invading the Kidney

📖 *Zhū Bìng Yuán Hòu Lùn* ("Origin and Indicators of Disease"), "The Various Symptoms of Disease in the Lumbar Spine: Wind-Damp Lumbar Pain"

> "Taxation damages kidney qì and makes the channels and network vessels vacuous. Possibly as a result of a damp sleeping place and exposure to wind, wind-damp exploits the vacuity and overpowers the kidney channel. As it fights with blood and qì, this causes lumbar pain. Therefore it is called wind-damp lumbar pain."

This quotation is an early description of the pathomechanism by which wind-damp assaulting the kidney channel induces lumbar pain.

📖 *Zhù Jiě Shāng Hán Lùn* ("Annotated Cold Damage"), "Identifying Pulse Symptoms and Treatments of Greater Yáng Disease"

> "Wind damages defense; dampness sinks into the joints. When wind and dampness contend with each other, the two evils disorder the channels. This results in vexing pain in the joints, pulling pain, and inability to bend and stretch… If wind prevails, the result is insecurity of defense qì, sweating, shortness of breath, and aversion to wind with reluctance to remove clothing. These are due to wind in the exterior. If dampness prevails, the result is stoppage of water qì, inhibited urination, and possibly slight generalized swelling. These are due to dampness thriving on the outside."

This quotation describes the pathomechanism by which the two evils of wind and dampness in combination cause joint swelling and pain, sweating with aversion to wind, and generalized swelling and reduced urination. Therefore, when the evil of wind-damp invades the house of the kidney, we can also see the symptoms described above.

文献评述

《诸病源候论•腰脊病诸候•风湿腰痛候》曰："劳伤肾气，经络既虚，或因卧湿当风，而风湿乘虚而搏于肾经，与血气相击而腰痛，故云风湿腰痛。"较早地论述了风湿邪气侵犯肾经，引起腰痛的病机。

《注解伤寒论•辨太阳病脉证并治》曰："风则伤卫，湿沉关节，风湿相搏，两邪乱经，故骨节疼烦、掣痛，不得屈伸。 …风胜则卫气不固，汗出，短气，恶风不欲去衣，为风在表；湿胜则水气不行，小便不利或身微肿，为湿外搏也。”论述风湿二邪，合而为患，引起骨节肿痛，汗出恶风，身肿尿少的病机。故风湿之邪，侵犯腰府亦可见到上述症状。

Summary of Wind-Damp Invading the Kidney

1. Wind-Damp Invading the Kidney

   Hypertonicity in the back and lower back, aching heavy pain, inability to turn sides, inhibited physical movement.

2. Dampness Being a Yīn Evil

   Changes in response to the weather, lumbar pain aggravated on rainy overcast days.

3. Wind by Nature Causing Opening and Discharge

   Heat effusion with aversion to wind, spontaneous sweating with generalized heaviness.

4. Wind-Damp Collecting Internally

   Thin slimy tongue fur, fine soggy pulse.

风湿犯肾

风湿犯肾—腰背拘急，酸重疼痛，不能转侧，活动不利

湿为阴邪—随气候变化，阴雨天腰痛加重

风性开泄—发热恶风，自汗身重

风湿内停—舌苔薄腻，脉濡细

Chapter Four

Kidney Channel Cold-Damp

The kidney governs water and manages the fluid metabolism in the entire body. It also governs the bones and has the function of sustaining and coordinating the physical activities of the body. The evils of cold and dampness can combine and together cause trouble, invading the lesser yīn channel. Alternatively, factors like kidney depletion in old age, enduring disease, or sexual taxation can induce kidney yáng vacuity, which allows cold-damp to arise internally. Either of these can lead to the pathomechanism of kidney channel cold-damp.

The chapter, "Origin and Development of Kidney Disease" in the *Zá Bìng Yuán Liú Xī Zhú* ("Incisive Light on the Source of Miscellaneous Disease") states:

> "Water disease is a disaster that arises when the excesses of cold and dampness prevail. It manifests in swelling of the instep, bone pain, yīn impediment, intermittent dizziness and clarity with reversal, abdominal enlargement and swelling of the shins, panting and cough, generalized heaviness, night sweating, pain in the head and nape, hunger with no desire to eat, spontaneous damage from cold qì, and unhappiness. These are the indicators of kidney disease."

This quotation clearly describes the pathomechanical changes resulting from cold-damp invading the kidney.

Cold-damp is a yīn evil and therefore most likely to encumber yáng qì. Loss of yáng qì can directly result in two different types of pathomechanical changes, namely disorders of the organism's fluid metabolism, or deformity of the skeleton and joints and impaired physical activity. Thus, we can further divide the pathomechanism of kidney channel cold-damp into four types: Cold-damp damaging the kidney, cold-damp affixed to the kidney, cold-damp damaging the bones, and cold-damp swelling of the instep.

肾经寒湿

肾主水，司一身水液代谢；肾主骨，对人体的运动起支持和协调的作用。如寒与湿邪交相为患，内侵少阴，或由年老肾亏，久病房劳等多种原因引起肾阳虚衰，寒湿内生，均可导致肾经寒湿的病机变化。《杂病源流犀烛•脏腑门•肾病源流》曰："水病者，寒湿之淫，所胜为灾也，其症有跗肿骨痛阴痹，时眩清厥，腹大胫肿，喘咳身重，寝汗，头项痛，饥不欲食，寒气自伤，意不乐等类，是则肾之病有可指数者。"对寒湿犯肾所引起的病机变化有明确的论述。寒湿为阴邪，多能困阻阳气，阳气一失，则可导致机体的水液代谢失常，或骨骼关节变形及运动障碍等两方面的病机改变。因此，肾经寒湿可进一步分为寒湿伤肾、寒湿着肾、寒湿伤骨、寒湿跗肿等四种病机类型。

4.1 Cold-Damp Damaging the Kidney

The kidney channel starts at the sole of the foot and runs up along the inner thigh to the lower back. If cold-damp evil internally invades the kidney channel and follows the channel route in a sneak attack, it can disorder channel qì, obstruct the qì dynamic, and damage original yáng. This can manifest in the pathomechanical changes of cold-damp damaging the kidney.

When cold-damp internally damages the kidney channel, it can repress yáng qì, so that yáng qì is damaged and unable to warm. This results in coldness in the back region and counterflow cold of the extremities.

When cold-damp congeals and stagnates, it impedes the movement of channel qì. This manifests in heavy fixed pain all over the body and aching joints.

The lower back is the house of the kidney. When cold-damp evil congests the channels and network vessels in the lumbar region, this results in coldness and heavy fixed pain in the lumbar region, with inability to freely turn sides.

Dampness is a yīn evil and by nature sticky and stagnating. When lying down tranquilly, dampness evil is even more likely to collect and stagnate. Thus the pain is aggravated by tranquility. Rainy, overcast, and cold weather aggravates the congealing and stagnating nature of cold-damp. Thus, the pain is worse on rainy overcast days. Since heat is able to disperse cold and overcome dampness, we can see that symptoms are relieved by heat.

Cold-damp damaging the kidney manifests in a slimy white tongue fur and a deep, fine, and slow pulse.

The chapter, "Identifying Pulse Symptoms and Treatments of Lesser Yīn Disease" in the *Shāng Hán Lùn* ("On Cold Damage") states: "When lesser yīn disease manifests with generalized pain, cold extremities, joint pain, and a sunken pulse, *fù zǐ tāng* (Aconite Decoction) governs it." The kidney governs the bones. When this text describes how the disease worsens, giving generalized pain, joint pain, cold extremities, and a sunken pulse, this means that the damage of cold-damp evil has reached the channels and network vessels of the kidney, but not the viscus of the kidney itself. Therefore the commentator Huáng Zhòng-Lǐ explains:

> "This condition is a disease of the lesser yīn kidney channel. The bones belong to the kidney, and kidney cold therefore causes joint pain. *Fù zǐ tāng* (Aconite Decoction) is used to warm the channels, expel cold, and eliminate dampness."

The chapter, "Cold-Damp Lumbar Pain" in the "General Introduction to Lumbar Pain" from the *Zhèng Yīn Mài Zhì* ("Pathoconditions: Causes, Pulses, and Treatments") points out:

> "The symptoms of cold-damp lumbar pain are headache and generalized pain, absence of sweating, hypertonicity, and lumbar pain with inability to turn sides. The causes of cold-damp lumbar pain are as follows. In cold damp years yīn cold may take charge and the people consequently may suffer from generalized heaviness and lumbar pain. [Thus] this is a disease caused by annual qì. Alternatively, patients may have been drenched by cold and rain, and the evils of yīn cold and rain dampness are causing pain. In this case, the disease is caused by an individual catching cold. The pulse of cold-damp lumbar pain manifests in an increased sunken and tight quality. A sunken and tight pulse at the left cubit means cold-damp in greater yáng; a fine tight pulse at the left cubit means cold-damp in lesser yīn."

This quotation analyzes special characteristics of the pathomechanism of cold-damp damaging the kidney, congesting the channels, and causing lumbar pain.

The treatment method for this condition consists of dispelling cold and dispersing dampness, and of supplementing the kidney and quickening the network vessels. Recommended formulas are *fù zǐ tāng*

(Aconite Decoction) from the *Shāng Hán Lùn* ("On Cold Damage"), *wǔ jī sǎn* (Five Accumulations Powder) from the *Tài Píng Huì Mín Hé Jì Jú Fāng* (Tài-Píng Imperial Grace Pharmacy Formulas), or *qū hán sàn shī tāng* (Cold-Dispelling Dampness-Dispersing Decoction) from *Yè Tiān Shì Fāng* ("Ye Tian-Shi's Formulas").

Fù Zǐ Tāng 附子汤 Aconite Decoction
fù zǐ (附子 Aconiti Radix Lateralis Praeparata, aconite)
fú líng (茯苓 Poria, poria)
rén shēn (人参 Ginseng Radix, ginseng)
bái zhú (白术 Atractylodis Macrocephalae Rhizoma, white atractylodes)
bái sháo (白芍 Paeoniae Radix Alba, white peony)

Wǔ Jī Sǎn 五积散 Five Accumulations Powder
bái zhǐ (白芷 Angelicae Dahuricae Radix, Dahurian angelica)
chén pí (陈皮 Citri Reticulatae Pericarpium, tangerine peel)
hòu pò (厚朴 Magnoliae Officinalis Cortex, officinal magnolia bark)
jié gěng (桔梗 Platycodonis Radix, platycodon)
zhǐ qiào (ké) (枳壳 Aurantii Fructus, bitter orange)
chuān xiōng (川芎 Chuanxiong Rhizoma, chuanxiong)
fú líng (茯苓 Poria, poria)
dāng guī (当归 Angelicae Sinensis Radix, Chinese angelica)
cāng zhú (苍术 Atractylodis Rhizoma, atractylodes)
má huáng (麻黄 Ephedrae Herba, ephedra)
sháo yào (芍药 Paeoniae Radix, peony)
gān jiāng (干姜 Zingiberis Rhizoma, dried ginger)
bàn xià (半夏 Pinelliae Rhizoma, pinellia)
ròu guì (肉桂 Cinnamomi Cortex, cinnamon bark)
gān cǎo (甘草 Glycyrrhizae Radix, licorice)

Qū Hán Sàn Shī Tāng 祛寒散湿汤 Cold-Dispelling Dampness-Dispersing Decoction
dú huó (独活 Angelicae Pubescentis Radix, pubescent angelica)
fáng jǐ (防己 Stephaniae Tetrandrae Radix, fangji)
fù zǐ (附子 Aconiti Radix Lateralis Praeparata, aconite) [cooked]
guì zhī (桂枝 Cinnamomi Ramulus, cinnamon twig)
fú líng (茯苓 Poria, poria)
bì xiè (萆薢 Dioscoreae Hypoglaucae seu Semptemlobae Rhizoma, fish poison yam)
zhū líng (猪苓 Polyporus, polyporus)

寒湿伤肾

肾之经脉起于足底，向上沿腿之内侧上行至腰部。如因寒湿之邪内犯肾经，沿经脉循行线路侵袭，扰乱经气，遏阻气机，损伤元阳，可出现寒湿伤肾的病机变化。寒湿内伤肾经，遏郁阳气，阳气受伤，失于温煦，可见背部寒冷，手足逆冷；寒湿凝滞，阻碍经气运行，表现为身体疼痛重着，骨节酸痛；腰为肾之府，寒湿之邪阻塞腰部经络，则腰部冷痛重着，转侧不利；湿为阴邪，其性粘滞，静卧则湿邪更易停滞，则静则疼痛加重；阴雨寒冷，寒湿凝滞加重，则阴雨天疼痛加剧；热能散寒胜湿，则见热则减。寒湿伤肾，则舌苔白腻，脉沉细而迟缓。如《伤寒论•辨少阴病脉证并治》曰："少阴病，身体痛，手足寒，骨节痛，脉沉者，附子汤主之。"肾主骨，条文中身体痛，骨节痛，手足寒，脉沉，病变重点为寒湿之邪伤及肾的经络而非肾之本脏，故注家黄仲理说："此乃少阴肾脏病，骨属肾，肾寒故骨节痛，用附子汤以温经驱寒除湿。"《症因脉治•腰痛总论•寒湿腰痛》指出："寒湿腰痛之症，头痛身痛，无汗拘紧，腰痛不能转侧，此寒湿腰痛之症也。寒湿腰痛之因，或寒湿之年，阴寒司令，民病身重腰痛，此因岁气而成病者，或冲寒冒雨，阴寒雨湿之邪致痛，此人自感冒而成病者。寒湿腰痛之脉，脉多沉紧，左尺沉紧，太阳寒湿，左尺细紧，少阴寒湿。"分析了寒湿伤肾，经脉阻塞而引起腰痛的病机特点。治法为祛寒散湿，补肾活络。方药选用《伤寒论》附子汤（附子、茯苓、人参、白术、芍药）；或选《和剂局方》五积散（白芷、陈皮、厚朴、桔梗、枳壳、川芎、茯苓、当归、苍术、麻黄、芍药、干姜、半夏、肉桂、甘草）；或用《叶天士方》祛寒散湿汤（独活、防已、熟附子、桂枝、茯苓、川萆薢、猪苓）。

Literature Review of Cold-Damp Invading the Kidney

📖 *Dān Xī Xīn Fǎ* ("Dān Xī's Heart-Approach"), "Lumbar Pain"

> "In cold-damp lumbar pain, you will observe relief by heat and aggravation by cold. I recommend *wǔ jī sǎn* (Five Accumulations Powder) with the addition of ½ qián of *wú zhū yú* (Evodiae Fructus) and 1 qián of *dù zhòng* (Eucommiae Cortex)."

This quotation describes how cold-damp damaging the kidney causes stoppage in the channels and network vessels and resulting pain in the lumbar region.

📖 *Zá Bìng Yuán Liú Xī Zhú* ("Incisive Light on the Source of Miscellaneous Disease"), "The Origin and Development of Lumbar and Umbilical Disease"

> "Regarding lumbar pain…it is stated that it arises from greater yáng. It is also stated that great yáng vacuity results in pain in the head, nape, lower back, and back. These two texts refer to the bladder channel, which pinches the back, hits the lower back, and diverges below the nape. Vacuity in this channel allows the evils of the six qì to settle there, which is the cause of pain. Harm by the six qì is mostly limited to cold-damp lodging there."

This text analyzes the pathomechanism by which cold-damp damaging the kidney leads to lumbar and back pain.

📖 *Nèi Jīng Bó Yì* ("Broad Discussion of The Inner Canon"), "Section on Capabilities of Disease: Treatise on Foot Lesser Yīn Kidney Disease"

> "For this reason, kidney disease is not limited to a weakness of water that is allowing earth to restrain it, but furthermore includes a dual disease of water and fire. If excess dampness or excess cold overcome this, the result is swelling of the instep, bone pain, yīn impediment, pain in the head and nape, intermittent dizziness, and hunger with no desire to eat."

This quotation also describes the pathomechanical changes of cold-damp damaging the kidney.

文献评述

《丹溪心法•腰痛》曰："若寒湿腰痛，见热则减，见寒则增，宜五积散加吴茱萸半钱，杜仲一钱。"阐述了寒湿伤肾，经络不通引起腰部疼痛的病机变化。

《杂病源流犀烛•腰脐病源流》曰："腰痛，…又曰：太阳所至为腰痛。又曰：巨阳虚，则头项腰背痛。此二条言膀胱之脉，挟背抵腰，别下项，是经虚则六气之邪客，以致痛也。而六气所害，惟寒湿居多。"对寒湿伤肾引起腰背疼痛的病机进行了分析。

《内经博议•病能部•足少阴肾脏病论》曰："是以肾家之病，不止水衰为土所克，而又有水火两病也。如湿淫、寒淫所胜，则跗肿，骨痛，阴痹，头项痛，时眩，饥不欲食。"也论述了寒湿伤肾的病机变化。

Summary of Cold-Damp Damaging the Kidney

1. Encumbrance of Yáng Qì

   Fear of cold in the lumbar and back regions, counterflow cold of the extremities.

2. Cold-Damp Obstructing the Channels

   Heavy fixed pain all over the body, aching joints.

3. Cold-Damp Obstructing the Lower Back

   Cold and heavy fixed pain in the lumbar region, inability to freely turn sides.

4. Cold-Damp Being a Yīn Evil

   Pain that is aggravated by tranquility and by rainy, overcast, and cold weather and that is relieved by heat.

5. Cold-Damp Damaging the Kidney

   White slimy tongue fur; deep, fine, and slow pulse.

寒湿伤肾

困伤阳气—腰背部畏寒，手足逆冷

寒湿阻经—身体疼痛重着，骨节酸痛

寒湿阻腰—腰部冷痛重着，转侧不利

寒湿阴邪—静则疼痛加重，阴雨寒冷疼痛加剧，得热则减

寒湿伤肾—舌苔白腻，脉沉细而迟缓

4.2 Cold-Damp Affixed to the Kidney

The kidney governs water and is thereby able to regulate the fluid metabolism. The lower back is the house of the kidney and is the pivot for the body's turning, bending, and stretching. Sleeping on damp ground, getting soaked by rain or wading through water, or engaging in sexual intercourse after bathing can allow cold-damp evil to encumber the home of the kidney and furthermore to attach itself only to the region of the kidney's home. This can form the pathomechanism of cold-damp affixed to the kidney, which is also called "kidney fixity."

When cold-damp affixes itself to the kidney, kidney yáng is obstructed. Since dampness is by nature heavy and fixed, this results in coldness in the lower back as if sitting in water and in heaviness as if carrying five thousand coins.

As a result of cold-damp encumbering the kidney, spleen yáng can also become vacuous and the movement of the fluids can become irregular so that they spill into the skin. Consequently, we can observe generalized puffy swelling that is particularly pronounced below the lower back, abdominal enlargement and swelling of the shins, a heavy body, and because the upper burner is without heat, absence of thirst.

If cold-damp in the kidney house has not yet affected qì transformation in the bladder, urination is uninhibited. If qì transformation in the urinary bladder is disordered, urination becomes inhibited. If the kidney fails to warm earth, it damages the spleen, but does no harm to stomach intake. Thus, eating and drinking is as normal.

Cold-damp affixed to the kidney results in a pale tongue with white slimy fur and a slow sunken pulse.

The chapter, "Pulse Symptoms and Treatments of Wind-Cold Accumulations and Gatherings in the Five Viscera" in the *Jīn Guì Yào Lüe* ("Essential Prescriptions of the Golden Coffer") describes this condition as follows:

> "The disease of kidney fixity manifests in a heavy body, coldness in the lower back as if sitting in water, a watery body but absence of thirst, uninhibited urination, and eating and drinking as normal. This disease belongs to the lower burner and is contracted by taxation of the body and sweating, and by prolonged presence of cold-damp inside clothing. It results in cold pain below the lower back and heaviness in the abdomen as if carrying five thousand coins. *Gān jiāng líng zhú tāng* (Licorice, Ginger, Poria and White Atractylodes Decoction) is the governing formula."

This quotation explains the pathomechanical changes of cold-damp abiding in the house of the kidney.

In a commentary on the above paragraph, the chapter, "Pulse Symptoms and Treatments of Wind-Cold Accumulations and Gatherings in the Five Viscera" in the *Jīn Guì Yào Lüe Xīn Diǎn* ("Heart-Insights Classic of the Essential Prescriptions of the Golden Coffer") notes further:

> "When the kidney contracts cold-damp, and this becomes fixed instead of being eliminated, it causes kidney fixity. Heavy body, coldness in the lower back as if sitting in water, cold pain below the lower back, and heaviness in the abdomen as if carrying five thousand coins are all signs of cold-damp affixed to the kidney and of yáng qì failing to transform. Absence of thirst indicates an absence of heat in the upper body. Uninhibited urination indicates cold in the lower body. Eating and drinking as normal indicates that the stomach is not diseased. Therefore it states that the disease belongs to the lower burner... This disease is not located inside the viscus of the kidney, but in the outer house of the kidney [the lower back]. Therefore, it is treated not by warming the kidney to disperse cold, but by warming earth to overcome water."

This quotation analyzes in detail the pathomechanism of kidney fixity, which consists of cold-damp damaging the kidney and causing spleen yáng depletion.

Cold-damp affixed to the kidney is treated by warming the kidney and strengthening the lower back, and by warming earth to overcome water. The recommended formula is *shèn zhuó sǎn* (Kidney Fixity Powder) from the *Qiān Jīn Yào Fāng* ("A Thousand Gold Pieces Prescriptions").

Shèn Zhuó Sǎn 肾着散 Kidney Fixity Powder
gān cǎo (甘草 Glycyrrhizae Radix, licorice)
bái zhú (白朮 Atractylodis Macrocephalae Rhizoma, white atractylodes)
gān jiāng (干姜 Zingiberis Rhizoma, dried ginger)
fú líng (茯苓 Poria, poria)
ròu guì (肉桂 Cinnamomi Cortex, cinnamon bark)
zé xiè (泽泻 Alismatis Rhizoma, alisma)
niú xī (牛膝 Achyranthis Bidentatae Radix, achyranthes)
dù zhòng (杜仲 Eucommiae Cortex, eucommia)

寒湿着肾

肾主水，可以调节水液代谢。腰为肾之府，为身体转动屈伸的枢纽。如睡卧湿地，冒雨涉水，浴后入房，导致寒湿之邪困扰肾府，且独附着于肾府之域，则可引起寒湿着肾的病机变化，又名“肾着”。寒湿困着于腰府，肾阳被遏，湿性沉重，则腰冷如坐水中，沉重如带五千钱币；寒湿困肾，脾阳亦虚，水液运行失调，游溢肌肤，可见全身浮肿，腰以下为甚，腹大胫肿，身体沉重；上焦无热，故口不渴；寒湿在肾府，膀胱气化未受影响，则小便自利；如膀胱气化失常，则小便不利；肾不暖土，脾虽受伤，但胃纳无妨，则饮食如故。寒湿着肾，则舌淡苔白腻，脉沉迟。如《金匮要略•五脏风寒积聚病脉证并治》描述道：“肾着之病，其人身体重，腰中冷，如坐水中，形如水状，反不渴，小便自利，饮食如故，病属下焦，身劳汗出，衣里冷湿，久久得之，腰以下冷痛，腹重如带五千钱，甘姜苓术汤主之。”说明寒湿留着肾府的病机改变。《金匮要略心典•五脏风寒积聚病脉证并治》尤在泾注解上条时又云：“肾受冷湿，着而不去，则为肾着。身重，腰中冷，如坐水中，腰下冷痛，腹重如带五千钱，皆冷湿着肾，而阳气不化之征也。不渴，上无热也；小便自利，寒在下也；饮食如故，胃无病也，故曰病属下焦。…然其病不在肾之中脏，而在肾之外府，故其治法不在温肾以散寒，而在燠土以胜水。”详细分析了肾着的病机为寒湿伤肾，脾阳亏损。治法为温肾强腰，暖土胜水。方药选用《千金要方》肾着散（甘草、白术、干姜、茯苓、桂心、泽泻、牛膝、杜仲）。

Literature Review of Cold-Damp Affixed to the Kidney

📖 *Dān Xī Xīn Fǎ* (“Dān Xī’s Heart-Approach”), “Lumbar Pain”

> “The lower back is the external indicator of the kidney, and the whole body relies on it for turning, and for opening and closure. All the channels pass through the kidney and net the lumbar spine. As soon as kidney qì is vacuous, whenever the body is drenched with cold and contracts dampness …it manifests in all sorts of lumbar pain piling up in layers… Dampness lumbar pain that feels as if sitting in water is possibly caused by wind, dampness, rain, or dew becoming fixed and by dampness flowing into the kidney channel, causing lumbar pain. It should be treated with *shèn shī tāng* (Dampness-Percolating Decoction) or if this shows no results, with *shèn zhuó tāng* (Kidney Fixity Decoction).”

This quotation also describes how cold-damp affixed to the kidney leads to the pathomechanical change of pain in the lumbar region.

🕮 *Yī Xué Zhèng Zhuàn* ("The Orthodox Tradition of Medicine"), "Lumbar Pain"

"The disease of kidney fixity manifests with heaviness of the body, icy coldness in the lower back, eating and drinking as normal, uninhibited urination, and cold pain and heaviness below the lower back. It is best treated by spreading dampness while simultaneously using warming medicinals."

This quotation describes the pathomechanical changes of cold-damp affixed to the kidney.

🕮 *Biàn Zhèng Lù* ("Records on Pattern Differentiation"), "Impediment Pattern"

"When people with vacuity cold in the lower origin furthermore contract cold-damp, they will suffer from heavy pain in the lower back and kidney and from lack of strength in both feet. People believe that this is a case of kidney impediment, and yet the formation of kidney impediment is not limited to the causes of wind, cold, and dampness. While the kidney is the viscus of cold, originally there is fire in its center. The presence of fire ensures that the water is not cold. As a result, wind, cold, and dampness have no way of entering. If people inadvertently labor excessively, this causes water of earlier heaven to drain out day after day. As water is eliminated, fire follows along and is also eliminated. This causes the origin of engendering qì to ultimately turn into a 'hole for storing ice.' Fire is unable to defeat cold, allowing cold evil to invade. Cold qì directly enters the kidney palace and as evil attracts evil, wind and dampness also arrive as mutual causes. This results in the pathocondition of impediment."

This quotation describes the pathomechanism by which the three evils of wind, cold, and dampness in combination cause trouble by invading the kidney channel and attaching themselves to the kidney's house.

文献评述

《丹溪心法•腰痛》曰："腰者肾之外候，一身所恃以转移阖辟者也。盖诸经皆贯于肾而络于腰脊，肾气一虚，凡冲寒受湿，…种种腰痛，叠见而层出矣。…若湿腰痛，如坐水中，或为风湿雨露所着，湿流入肾经，以致腰痛，宜渗湿汤，不效，宜肾着汤。"也阐述了寒湿着肾引起腰部疼痛的病机变化。

《医学正传•腰痛》曰："肾着为病，其体重，腰冷如冰，饮食如故，小便自利，腰以下冷痛而重，治宜流湿兼用温药。"论述了寒湿着肾的病机变化。

《辨证录•痹证门》曰："人有下元虚寒，复感寒湿，腰肾重痛，两足无力，人以为此肾痹也。而肾痹之成，非尽由於风寒湿也。夫肾虽寒脏，而其中原自有火，有火则水不寒，而风寒湿无从而入。无奈人过于作强，将先天之水，日日奔 泄，水去而火亦随流而去，使生气之原，竟成为藏冰之窟，火不能敌寒，而寒邪侵之矣。寒气直入于肾宫，以邪招邪，而风湿又相因而至，则痹症生矣。"对风寒湿三邪合而为患侵袭肾经，留着肾府的病机变化进行了阐述。

Summary of Cold-Damp Affixed to the Kidney
1. Wind-Damp Affixed to the Kidney
Coldness in the lower back as if sitting in water, heaviness as if carrying five thousand coins.
2. Cold-Damp in the Spleen and Kidney
Generalized puffy swelling that is particularly pronounced below the lower back, abdominal enlargement and swelling of the shins, heavy body.
3. No Detriment to the Urinary Bladder
Uninhibited urination.
4. No Harm to Stomach Intake
Eating and drinking as normal.
5. Cold-Damp Affixed to the Kidney
Pale tongue with white slimy tongue fur, slow sunken pulse.

寒湿着肾
寒湿着腰—腰冷如坐水中，沉重如带五千钱
脾肾寒湿—全身浮肿，腰以下为甚，腹大胫肿，身体沉重
膀胱无损—小便自利
胃纳无妨—饮食如故
寒湿着肾—舌淡苔白腻，脉沉迟

4.3 Cold-Damp Damaging the Bones

The kidney governs the bones and is in charge of joints and movement throughout the entire body. Therefore, the "Treatise of the Arcane Book of the Orchid Chamber of the Spirit Tower" in the *Sù Wèn* ("Plain Questions") states: "The kidney holds the office of labor, whence agility emanates." If cold-damp evil directly invades the kidney channel or if a prior depletion of spleen-earth allows cold-damp to arise internally and damage the kidney viscus, this will invariably affect the physiological function of the kidney to govern the bones. Forming the pathomechanism of cold-damp damaging the bones, the resulting disturbances in skeletal growth, development, and movement manifest in changes like skeletal deformities and crippling.

The chapter, "Needling Divisions, True [Qì] and Evil [Qì]" in the *Líng Shū* ("The Magic Pivot") states:

> "A person who is struck by vacuity evil will be shivering as if splashed with water. [The disease] begins in the downy body hair and erupts through the interstices. Entering deeply, it internally overpowers the bones, resulting in bone impediment."

This quotation expressed basic knowledge about the pathomechanical process of "bone impediment," but did not yet point by name to the pathomechanism of cold-damp damaging the bones.

In the chapter, "Pulse Symptoms and Treatments of Wind Strike Joint Running Disease" in the *Jīn Guì Yù Hán Jīng Èr Zhù* ("Classic of the Golden Coffer and Jade Sheath: Second Annotation"), Zhào Yì-Dé also explained:

> "The formation of dampness responds internally to the spleen. The spleen is earth; because earth restrains kidney water, dampness damages the bones. Now the joints are where the bones press against each other and where the sinews are tied together. Therefore, dampness is likely to abide in the joints and thereby restrain its overcoming phase and rebel against that which it fails to overcome."

This quotation describes how a prior depletion of spleen earth allows cold-damp to arise internally, spread from the spleen to the kidney, and invade the limbs and joints, forming the pathomechanical changes of malfunctioning or deformed joints.

When cold-damp damages the kidney, kidney yáng fails to move and double yīn congeals, causing qì stagnation and blood stasis. This results in pain and heaviness in the large and small joints of the skeleton, inhibited bending and stretching, and swollen joints.

If the condition of cold-damp damaging the bones continues for many days, the pathology of qì can affect the blood. In that case, obstruction of the network vessels and blood stasis further obstruct the nutritional metabolism of the skeleton. This results in deformities in both the large and small joints, but particularly in the small joints.

The kidney foot lesser yīn channel runs diagonally across the sole of the foot, exits below Blazing Valley (*rán gǔ*, KI-2), follows the backside of the inner ankle bone, and separates to enter at the center of the heel. Therefore when cold-damp evil enters lesser yīn and damages the bones, it tends to start in the feet with obstructions in the growth and nutritional metabolism of the bones of the feet and with skeletal deformities there, leading to crippling of both feet and inability to walk.

If the kidney fails to govern the bones and engender marrow, the celestial pillar [neck bone] is deprived of nourishment and the vertebral column becomes curved to the point where the head is carried on the back.

When cold-damp damage to the kidney affects the bones, it results in a fat pale tongue with dark purple margins, and a fine and faint sunken pulse.

The "Treatise on Impediment" in the *Sù Wèn* ("Plain Questions") states: "Kidney impediment manifests in susceptibility to distention, and in the sacrum and coccyx carrying the heel and the spine carrying the head." Wáng Bīng explained thusly in the commentary:

> "The kidney is the gate to the stomach. When the gate is inhibited, stomach qì is unable to convert. This causes susceptibility to distention. The sacrum and coccyx carrying the heel refers to hypertonicity of the feet. The spine carrying the head refers to the body being curled… When qì is insufficient and contracts evil, this causes inability to stretch and bend."

Contraction of evil refers to the contraction of wind, cold, or dampness evil. When damage to the kidney affects the bones, this can lead to skeletal deformities and difficulty to move.

Cold-damp damaging the bones is treated by warming the kidney and dispersing cold, and by eliminating dampness and freeing the network vessels. The recommended formula is *yì shèn juān bì wán* (Kidney Boosting Impediment-Alleviating Pill) from the *Shí Yòng Zhōng Yī Nèi Kē Xué* ("Practical Chinese Internal Medicine") with the addition of *lù róng* (Cervi Cornu Pantotrichum) or *lù jiǎo jiāo* (Cervi Cornus Gelatinum), *chuān wū* (Aconiti Radix), and *zhì mǎ qián zǐ* (prepared Strychni Semen).

Yì Shèn Juān Bì Wán 益肾蠲痹丸 Kidney Boosting Impediment-Alleviating Pill
lù xián cǎo (鹿衔草 Pyrolae Herba, pyrola) *yín yáng huò* (淫羊藿 Epimedii Herba, epimedium) *quán xiē* (全蝎 Scorpio, scorpion) *wú gōng* (蜈蚣 Scolopendra, centipede) *jiāng cán* (僵蚕 Bombyx Batryticatus, silkworm) *fēng fáng* (蜂房 Vespae Nidus, hornet's nest) *zhè chóng* (䗪虫 Eupolyphaga seu Steleophaga, ground beetle) *wū shāo shé* (乌梢蛇 Zaocys, black-striped snake) *qiāng láng* (蜣螂 Catharsius, dung beetle) *shú dì huáng* (熟地黄 Rehmanniae Radix Praeparata, cooked rehmannia) *dāng guī* (当归 Angelicae Sinensis Radix, Chinese angelica) *shēng dì huáng* (生地黄 Rehmanniae Radix, dried rehmannia) *jī xuè téng* (鸡血藤 Spatholobi Caulis, spatholobus) *lǎo guàn cǎo* (老鹳草 Erodii seu Geranii Herba, cranesbill) *xún gǔ fēng* (寻骨风 Aristolochiae Mollissimae Herba, mollissima) *hǔ zhàng* (虎杖 Polygoni Cuspidati Rhizoma, bushy knotweed) Plus: *lù róng* (鹿茸 Cervi Cornu Pantotrichum, velvet deerhorn) or: *lù jiǎo jiāo* (鹿角胶 Cervi Cornus Gelatinum, deerhorn glue) *chuān wū* (川乌 Aconiti Radix, aconite main root) *mǎ qián zǐ* (马钱子 Strychni Semen, nux vomica)

寒湿伤骨

肾主骨，主司人体一身之关节和运动。故《素问•灵兰秘典论》曰："肾者，作强之官，伎巧出焉。"寒湿之邪直接侵犯肾经，或因脾土先亏，寒湿内生，损伤肾脏，必然影响肾主骨的生理功能，导致骨骼生长发育和运动障碍，出现骨骼变形，骨骼残废等寒湿伤骨的病机改变。《灵枢•刺节真邪》云："虚邪之中人也，洒淅动形，起毫毛而发腠理，其入深，内搏于骨，则为骨痹。"对"骨痹"的病机变化过程有了初步的认识，但未指出寒湿伤骨的病机名称。赵义德《金匮玉函经二注•中风历节病脉证并治》又说："湿成则内应于脾。

脾，土也。土克肾水，是以湿伤其骨。关节者，骨之所凑，筋之所束，故湿独善留关节，以克其所胜，侮其不胜”。论述了因脾土先亏，寒湿内生，由脾及肾，侵犯四肢关节，形成关节活动障碍或关节变形的病机变化。寒湿伤肾，肾阳不运，重阴凝结，气滞血瘀，则骨骼大小关节疼痛重着，屈伸不利，关节肿胀；寒湿伤骨日久，病变由气及血，络阻血瘀，骨骼营养代谢进一步受阻，则大小关节俱可变形，尤以小关节为甚；肾足少阴之脉，斜走足心，出于然谷之下，循内踝之后，别入跟中，故寒湿之邪入少阴伤骨，常从足开始，足骨生长及营养代谢受阻，骨骼变形，导致两足残废而不能行走；肾不主骨生髓，天柱骨失养，脊柱弯曲，则以背代头。寒湿伤肾及骨，则舌质淡胖，舌边紫暗，脉沉细而微。如《素问•痹论篇》曰：“肾痹者，善胀，尻以代踵，脊以代头。”王冰注解到：“肾者，胃之关，关不利，则胃气不转，故善胀也。尻以代踵，谓足挛急也。脊以代头，谓身踡屈也。 …气不足而受邪，故不伸展。”受邪即指感受风寒湿邪，伤肾及骨，可导致骨骼变形，难以行动。治法为温肾散寒，除湿通络。方药选用《实用中医内科学》益肾蠲痹丸（鹿衔草、仙灵脾、全蝎、蜈蚣、僵蚕、蜂房、地鳖虫、炙乌梢蛇、炙蜣螂虫、熟地、当归、生地黄、鸡血藤、老鹳草、寻骨风、虎杖）加鹿茸或鹿角胶、川乌、制马前子。

Literature Review of Cold-Damp Damaging the Bones

🕮 *Zhōng Zàng Jīng* (“Central Treasury Classic”), “Discussing the Pulses and Patterns of Vacuity and Repletion, Cold and Heat, Life and Death, and Favorable and Unfavorable Shifts in Kidney Disease”

> “Yīn veil entering the kidney results in bone pain, lumbar pain, and upward pulling nape, spine, and back pain. All these are caused by exerting oneself lifting heavy weights, by sweating during sexual intercourse, by getting exposed to wind during bathing, or by prolonged standing, all of which damage the kidney.”

Sweating and exposure to wind while bathing allows cold-dampness to assail the kidney. It can lead to such pathomechanical changes as bone pain or pain in the vertebral column.

🕮 *Māi Yīn Zhèng Zhì* (“Pulses, Causes, Patterns and Treatment”), “Patterns of the Five Viscera”

> “Kidney: Lumbar and leg pain, inhibition in the large joints, impaired bending of the body, abdominal fullness, glomus and hardness, and night sweating.”

Although his quotation does not explicitly name cold-damage invading the kidney as the disease cause, it nevertheless describes how cold-damp assault leading to inhibition in the joints, lower back, and legs.

🕮 *Zhèng Yīn Mài Zhì* ("Pathoconditions: Causes, Pulses, and Treatments"), "Impediment Conditions: Kidney Impediment"

> "The pathocondition of kidney impediment is the same as bone impediment. It manifests in susceptibility to distention, lumbar pain, seminal emission, frequent change in the color of urine, hypertonicity in the feet with failure to stretch them, and bone disease with failure to rise."

The kidney governs the bones. When kidney impediment persists for a long time, it invariably damages the bones. While this quotation does not discuss the causes of this disease, clearly cold-damp would be among them.

文献评述

《中藏经•论肾脏虚实寒热生死逆顺脉证之法》曰："阴邪入肾，则骨痛，腰痛，上引项脊背疼，此皆举重用力及遇房汗出当风浴水，或久立则伤肾也。"汗出当风浴水，寒湿侵犯于肾，故可导致骨痛、脊柱痛等多种病机变化。

《脉因证治•五脏证》曰："肾：腰腿痛，大关节不利，屈身不便，腹满痞坚，寐汗。"虽未明确指出寒湿犯肾的病因，但对寒湿侵犯导致关节腰腿不利的病机变化进行了描述。

《症因脉治•痹症•肾痹》曰："肾痹之症，即骨痹也。善胀，腰痛，遗精，小便时时变色，足挛不能伸，骨病不能起。"肾主骨，肾痹日久，必然伤骨。虽未谈及病因，寒湿自然包含其中。

Summary of Cold-Damp Damaging the Bones

1. Cold-Damp Congealing

   Heavy fixed pain in the large and small joints of the skeleton, inhibited bending and stretching, swollen joints.

2. Obstruction in the Network Vessels and Blood Stasis

   Deformities in both the large and small joints, but particularly in the small joints.

3. Cold-Damp Damaging the Feet

   Crippling of both feet and inability to walk.

4. Deformity of the Vertebral Column

Spine carrying the head.

5. Cold-Damp Damaging the Kidney

Fat pale tongue with dark purple margins, fine and faint sunken pulse.

寒湿伤骨

寒湿凝结—骨骼大小关节疼痛重着，屈伸不利，关节肿胀

络阻血瘀—大小关节俱可变形，尤以小关节为甚

寒湿伤足—两足残废而不能行走

脊柱变形—以背代头

寒湿伤肾—舌质淡胖，舌边紫暗，脉沉细而微

4.4 Cold-Damp Swelling of the Instep

The foot lesser yīn kidney channel begins underneath the foot and runs upward to the instep. If chronic retention of cold-damp evil damages the kidney channel and this is drawn out and not treated, cold-damp can lie hidden in the instep of the foot. This can induce the pathomechanical change of cold-damp swelling of the instep.

When cold-damp damages the kidney, qì is not transformed; it pours downward along the channels and collects in the instep. This results in puffy swelling of the instep (below the ankle joint).

When cold-damp congeals and impedes the qì dynamic in the entire body, channel qì stops. This results in generalized pain.

When cold-damp has damaged yáng but not yet the fluids, this manifests in bland taste in the mouth with absence of thirst, physical cold and cold limbs.

Cold-damp damaging the kidney manifests in a slimy white tongue fur and a faint weak sunken pulse.

The "Treatise on Points for Water and Heat" in the *Sù Wèn* ("Plain Questions") states:

> "The emperor asked: 'How is it that the kidney can gather water and engender disease?' Qí Bó answered: 'The kidney is the gate of the stomach. When the gate fails to open, it causes water to gather and consequently form related diseases. [Water] spills upward and

> downward into the skin, resulting in puffy swelling. Puffy swelling means that gathering water engenders disease. Its root is in the kidney and its tip in the lung."

This quotation analyzes in detail how cold-damp damage to the kidney causes failure of the gate to open and gathering of water-damp, which results in water swelling.

The chapter, "The Lower Burner" in the *Wēn Bìng Tiáo Biàn* ("Systematized Identification of Warm Diseases") also states:

> "When dampness endures without being treated, it becomes deep-lying in the foot lesser yīn channel, resulting in a white tongue, generalized pain, and puffy swelling in the instep. *Lù fù tāng* (Velvet Deerhorn and Aconite Decoction) governs it."

The commentary to this same text elaborates:

> "This section establishes a treatment method for dampness damaging kidney yáng. Nevertheless, any disease caused by dampness must spring from spleen yáng being devitalized. Therefore the formula includes *cǎo guǒ* (Tsaoko Fructus) and *fú líng* (Poria)."

This quotation clearly points out that this is not a disorder caused by water qì but by cold-damp damaging the spleen and kidney and pouring down to cause swelling and distention in the instep. Since the pathomechanism is caused by cold-damp lying deeply in the lesser yīn, it is thus a case of cold-damp swelling of the instep.

This pathomechanism is treated by warming kidney yáng and dispelling cold-damp. The recommended formula is *lù fù tāng* (Velvet Deerhorn and Aconite Decoction) from the *Wēn Bìng Tiáo Biàn* ("Systematized Identification of Warm Diseases").

Lù Fù Tāng 鹿附汤
Velvet Deerhorn and Aconite Decoction

lù róng (鹿茸 Cervi Cornu Pantotrichum, velvet deerhorn)
fù zǐ (附子 Aconiti Radix Lateralis Praeparata, aconite)
cǎo guǒ (草果 Tsaoko Fructus, tsaoko)
tù sī zǐ (菟丝子 Cuscutae Semen, cuscuta)
fú líng (茯苓 Poria, poria)

寒湿跗肿

足少阴肾经起于足下，向上行于足跗，如寒湿之邪久留伤肾，迁延不治，伏于足跗，可引起寒湿跗肿的病机变化。寒湿伤肾，气化不行，随经下注，停于足跗，则足跗（踝关节以下）浮肿；寒湿凝滞，全身气机阻碍，经气不通，则全身疼痛；寒湿伤阳，津液未伤，则口淡不渴，形寒肢冷。寒湿伤肾，则舌苔白腻，脉沉微弱。如《素问•水热穴论篇》曰："帝曰：肾何以能聚水而生病?岐伯曰：肾者，胃之关也，关门不利，故聚水而从其类也，上下溢于皮肤，故为胕肿。胕肿者，聚水而生病也。其本在肾，其末在肺。"对寒湿伤肾，关门不利，水湿积聚，引起水肿的病机变化进行了详细的分析。《温病条辨•下焦篇》也曰："湿久不治，伏足少阴，舌白，身痛，足跗浮肿，鹿附汤主之。"该书评注指出："为湿伤肾阳者立治法。而湿之为病，必由脾阳不振而乘，故方中有草果、茯苓。"明确指出此非水气为患，而是寒湿损伤脾肾，下注而引起的足跗肿胀，其病机为寒湿伏于少阴，故为寒湿跗肿。治法为温肾阳，祛寒湿。方药选用《温病条辨》鹿附汤（鹿茸、附子、草果、菟丝子、茯苓）。

Literature Review of Cold-Damp Swelling of the Instep

📖 *Lín Zhèng Zhǐ Nán Yī Àn* ("A Clinical Guide with Case Histories"), "Dampness"

> "An 83-year-old patient presented with a white tongue, generalized pain, puffy swelling in the instep, and water spurting out from the Great Ravine (*tài xī,* KI-3) point. These symptoms indicated that dampness evil was deep-lying in the foot lesser yīn channel. It was appropriately treated by warming and steaming yáng qì as the primary goal. Thus I used *lù jiǎo* (Cervi Cornu), *dàn fù zǐ* (Aconiti Radix Lateralis Insalsa), *cǎo guǒ* (Tsaoko Fructus), *tù sī zǐ* (Cuscutae Semen), and *fú líng* (Poria)."

This quotation clearly points out how cold-damp encumbering the instep and damaging yáng qì leads to puffy swelling in the instep.

📖 *Yī Biǎn* ("Lancing Stones of Medicine"), "Dampness Damage"

> "When treating dampness engendered by spleen-earth, observe its concurrent transformations… When it is complicated by dampness, it constitutes cold-damp. Impediment pain is the sign for this disease. The cold-damp is in the upper and lower body, in the center and on the outside, reaching every location in the body… In the lower body, it causes swelling in the foot, lower leg, and instep."

Cold-damp is a yīn evil and can easily reduce spleen and kidney yáng and damage a person internally. Since dampness is by nature heavy and fixed and therefore mostly flows downward, it can easily cause swelling and distention of the instep.

文献评述

《临证指南医案•湿》曰："某，83 岁，舌白身痛、足跗浮肿，以太溪穴水流如注，此湿邪伏于足少阴，当用温蒸阳气为主。鹿茸、淡附子、草果、菟丝子、茯苓。"明确指出了寒湿困于足跗，损伤阳气，导致足跗浮肿的病机变化。

《医碥•伤湿》曰："治脾土所生之湿，则察其兼化。 …挟寒则为寒湿，痹痛者是也。上下中外，无处不到， …在下足胫跗肿。"寒湿为阴邪，易损脾肾之阳，中伤人体，湿性重着，多向下流，故易引起足跗肿胀。

Summary of Cold-Damp Swelling of the Instep
1. Cold-Damp Pouring Downward Puffy swelling of the instep. 2. Cold-Damp Congealing Generalized pain. 3. Cold-Damp Damaging Yáng Bland taste in the mouth with absence of thirst, physical cold and cold limbs. 4. Cold-Damp Damaging the Kidney White slimy tongue fur, faint weak sunken pulse.

寒湿跗肿
寒湿下注—足跗浮肿 寒湿凝滞—身体疼痛 寒湿伤阳—口淡不渴，形寒肢冷 寒湿伤肾—舌苔白腻，脉沉微弱

Chapter Five

Kidney Channel Damp-Heat

The kidney controls urine and stool and governs water. Kidney yáng has the function of transforming qì by steaming and has an important regulating effect on the fluid metabolism.

Damp-heat evil can be externally contracted or result from water-damp steaming inside the body for a long time and transforming into heat, or from a predilection for sweet and fatty foods and/or liquor, which brew and form damp-heat. In either case, the center burner and the spleen and stomach lose their function of upbearing the clear and downbearing the turbid, and damp-heat pours down into the kidney. This can lead to the pathomechanical changes of damp-heat damaging the kidney.

The chapter, "Origin and Development of Dampness Disease" in the *Zá Bìng Yuán Liú Xī Zhú* ("Incisive Light on the Source of Miscellaneous Disease") points out: "In all cases of dampness, reddish urine and thirst mean damp-heat." Although this quotation does not explicitly mention the pathomechanical changes of damp-heat damaging the kidney, it is clear that because the kidney controls urine and stool, and urine is issued by qì transformation in the bladder, damp-heat does in fact result in yellow or reddish urine. Thus damage from damp-heat clearly affects the kidney and bladder.

Damp-heat is by nature sticky and stagnating and can therefore easily impede qì and blood, while at the same time reduce the kidney's function of transforming qì. Therefore, damp-heat in the kidney channel can further evolve into four types of pathomechanisms: damp-heat damaging the lower back, damp-heat strangury-turbidity, damp-heat dribbling urinary block, and damp-heat puffy swelling.

肾经湿热

肾司二便，主水，肾阳有蒸腾气化之功能，对水液代谢具有重要的调节作用。如外感湿热之邪，或体内水湿蕴久化热，或嗜食肥甘酒酪，酿成湿热，中焦脾胃失其升清降浊功能，湿热下注于肾，均可导致湿热伤肾的病机变化。《杂病源流犀烛•湿病源流》指出："凡湿，以尿赤而渴为湿热。"虽未明确提出湿热伤肾的病机变化，但因肾司二便，小便乃膀胱气化所出，湿热导致小便黄赤，必然伤及肾与膀胱。湿热之性粘滞，容易阻碍气血，并可使肾之气化功能受损，故肾经湿热可进一步演化为湿热伤腰、湿热淋浊、湿热癃闭、湿热浮肿等四种病机类型。

5.1 Damp-Heat Damaging the Lower Back

The lower back is the house of the kidney. When damp-heat evil assails the kidney channel, it can directly strike the lumbar region. This can induce the pathomechanical changes of damp-heat damaging the lower back.

The foot greater yáng bladder channel runs along both sides of the vertebral column on the body's backside and stands in an exterior-interior relationship with the lesser yīn kidney channel. Therefore, when damp-heat evil pours down into the kidney channel, it usually also affects the foot greater yáng bladder channel. As a result, the contending dampness and heat assail the lumbar region and gather in greater yáng. This manifests in pain in the lumbar region that is accompanied by a sensation of heat in that location, possibly stretching up into the nape and back or down into the sacrum and coccyx and hip.

The season of misty rain [a particular rainy season characterized by near constant, light rain] is the time when damp-heat is depressed and steams. Late summer is the season of summerheat-damp. Therefore, lumbar pain is aggravated at these times.

When damp-heat evil flows into the joints, it can also manifest in redness and swelling of the joints. Damp-heat steaming internally results in vexation heat and thirst.

When damp-heat evil pours from the kidney into the bladder, qì transformation breaks down. The result is short voidings of reddish urine.

Damp-heat brewing internally results in a slimy yellow tongue fur and a rapid soggy pulse.

The chapter, "Lumbar Pain" in the *Yī Xué Xīn Wù* ("Medical Insights") states: "Heaviness and pain in the lower back, heat effusion in the lumbar region, wilting and lack of strength, and a rapid stringlike pulse mean damp-heat." This quotation clearly points out the pathomechanical changes of damp-heat damaging the lower back.

The chapter, "Damp-Heat Lumbar Pain" in the *Zhèng Yīn Mài Zhì* ("Pathoconditions: Causes, Pulses, and Treatments") further states:

> "The symptoms of damp-heat lumbar pain are internal heat, vexation and dryness, spontaneous sweating and thirst, inhibited voidings of red stool and urine, and aching pain and heaviness. These are the symptoms of damp-heat lumbar pain. … The pulse of damp-heat lumbar pain is mostly sunken and rapid… [and] fine and rapid at the left cubit. This means damp-heat in lesser yīn."

The lower back being the house of the kidney, "damp-heat in lesser yīn" must refer to kidney channel damp-heat. Damp-heat invading the kidney and damaging the lower back results in heavy fixed pain in the lower back, and when it affects the foot greater yáng bladder channel, it causes yellow or reddish urination.

Damp-heat damaging the lower back is treated by clearing heat and disinhibiting dampness, and by soothing the sinews and relieving pain. The recommended formula is *èr miào sǎn* (Mysterious Two Powder) from the *Dān Xī Xīn Fǎ* ("Dān Xī's Heart-Approach") with the addition of *fáng jǐ* (Stephaniae Tetrandrae Radix), *bì xiè* (Dioscoreae Hypoglaucae seu Semptemlobae Rhizoma), *dāng guī* (Angelicae Sinensis Radix), *niú xī* (Achyranthis Bidentatae Radix), *fáng fēng* (Saposhnikoviae Radix), *dú huó* (Angelicae Pubescentis Radix), and *chuān xiōng* (Chuanxiong Rhizoma), or *dāng guī niān tòng tāng* (Chinese Angelica Pain-Assuaging Decoction) from the *Yī Xué Fā Míng* ("Elucidation of Medicine").

Èr Miào Sǎn 二妙散
Mysterious Two Powder

huáng bǎi (黄柏 Phellodendri Cortex, phellodendron)
cāng zhú (苍术 Atractylodis Rhizoma, atractylodes)

Plus:

fáng jǐ (防己 Stephaniae Tetrandrae Radix, fangji)
bì xiè (萆薢 Dioscoreae Hypoglaucae seu Semptemlobae Rhizoma, fish poison yam)
dāng guī (当归 Angelicae Sinensis Radix, Chinese angelica)
niú xī (牛膝 Achyranthis Bidentatae Radix, achyranthes)
fáng fēng (防风 Saposhnikoviae Radix, saposhnikovia)
dú huó (独活 Angelicae Pubescentis Radix, pubescent angelica)
chuān xiōng (川芎 Chuanxiong Rhizoma, chuanxiong)

Dāng Guī Niān Tòng Tāng 当归拈痛汤
Chinese Angelica Pain-Assuaging Decoction

qiāng huó (羌活 Notopterygii Rhizoma et Radix, notopterygium)
rén shēn (人参 Ginseng Radix, ginseng)
kǔ shēn (苦参 Sophorae Flavescentis Radix, flavescent sophora)
shēng má (升麻 Cimicifugae Rhizoma, cimicifuga)
gé gēn (葛根 Puerariae Radix, pueraria)
cāng zhú (苍术 Atractylodis Rhizoma, atractylodes)
huáng qín (黄芩 Scutellariae Radix, scutellaria)
yīn chén (茵陈 Artemisiae Scopariae Herba, virgate wormwood)
fáng fēng (防风 Saposhnikoviae Radix, saposhnikovia)
dāng guī (当归 Angelicae Sinensis Radix, Chinese angelica)
zhī mǔ (知母 Anemarrhenae Rhizoma, anemarrhena)
zé xiè (泽泻 Alismatis Rhizoma, alisma)
zhū líng (猪苓 Polyporus, polyporus)
bái zhú (白术 Atractylodis Macrocephalae Rhizoma, white atractylodes)
zhì gān cǎo (炙甘草 Glycyrrhizae Radix cum Liquido Fricta, mix-fried licorice)

湿热伤腰

腰为肾之府，如湿热之邪侵犯肾经，即可直入腰间，可以导致湿热伤腰的病机变化。足太阳膀胱经循行人体背面脊柱两旁，与少阴肾经相表里，故湿热之邪下流肾经，亦多涉及足太阳膀胱经脉，出现湿热相搏，侵犯腰部，聚于太阳，表现为腰部疼痛，痛处伴有热感，或腰痛上引项背，下及尻髋；梅雨季节为湿热郁蒸之时，长夏为暑湿之季，故腰痛加重；湿热之邪流走关节，又可出现关节红肿；湿热熏蒸于内，则烦热口渴；湿热之邪由肾流注于膀胱，气化失司，则小便短赤。湿热内蕴，则舌苔黄腻，脉濡数。如《医学心悟•腰痛》曰："若腰重疼痛，腰间发热，痿软无力，脉弦数者，湿热也。"明确指出了"湿热伤腰"的病机变化。《症因脉治•湿热腰痛》又曰："湿热腰痛之症，内热烦热，自汗口渴，二便赤涩，酸痛沉重，此湿热腰痛之症也。...湿热腰痛之脉，脉多沉数，...左尺细数，少阴湿热。"腰为肾之府，"少阴湿热"，必为肾经湿热，湿热之邪犯肾伤腰，则为腰痛重着，波及足太阳膀胱经，则表现为小便黄赤等病机改变。治法宜清热利湿，舒筋止痛。方药选用《丹溪心法》二妙散（黄柏、苍术）加防己、萆薢、当归、牛膝、防风、独活、川芎。或选用《医学发明》当归拈痛汤（羌活、人参、苦参、升麻、葛根、苍术、黄芩、茵陈、防风、当归、知母、泽泻、猪苓、白术、炙甘草）。

Literature Review of Damp-Heat Damaging the Kidney

🕮 *Dān Xī Xīn Fǎ* ("Dān Xī's Heart-Approach"), "Lumbar Pain"

> "Lumbar pain primarily indicates damp-heat, kidney vacuity, static blood, contusions and sprains, or the presence of phlegm accumulations... It is further stated that damp-heat lumbar pain is caused by an encounter with heavenly yīn or by prolonged sitting."

This quotation clearly points out the pathomechanical changes of "damp-heat lumbar pain."

🕮 *Xiè Yìng Lú Yī Àn* ("Xiè Yìng-Lú's Case Studies"), "Damp-Heat Lumbar Pain"

> "Damp-heat lumbar pain: Xú Bó-Kūn once walked a long distance home and engaged in excessive drinking, eating, and sexual intercourse. Afterwards, he suffered from lumbar pain, a bent posture, and difficulty walking. Numerous doctors were consulted, all of whom stated that the lower back is the house of the kidney, that sexual taxation had damaged the kidney, and that only supplementing formulas were suitable... Gradually, his condition worsened to include encumbrance and fatigue, inability to turn sides, every afternoon mania in the heart and agitated reflection, slight tidal heat, and extraordinary pain. After a month in bed, he had become practically disabled. When I examined him, I knew that the condition was tied to damp-heat gathering in the lower back and kidney, and that it was inappropriate to apply supplementation... This condition had first been caused by the long walk home, which had harassed the blood in the sinews and bones. Subsequent drunkenness and overeating had disordered construction and defense blood; and following this, sexual taxation had consumed the essence in the hundred

> bones, and the inner orifices had become vacuous. Damp-heat had harassed the body before the blood had stabilized, and had thus been able to exploit the vacuity and enter the body, gathering in the lower back and kidney."

This quotation describes the pathomechanical changes of damp-heat evil gathering in the lower back and kidney.

📖 *Lín Chuáng Zhōng Yī Nèi Kē Xué* ("Clinical Chinese Internal Medicine"), "Lumbar Pain"

> "Damp-heat lumbar pain: When the evil of damp-heat assails the lumbar region and gathers in greater yáng, the result is lumbar pain that is heavy and fixed, accompanied by heat effusion, and reaching to the nape and back. Damp-heat evil can very easily run into the joints, and since heat is a yáng evil, cause redness, swelling, and pain in the limbs and joints, dry mouth and thirst, a slimy yellow tongue fur, and a soggy rapid pulse, which are symptoms of damp-heat."

This quotation clearly describes the pathomechanical changes of damp-heat lumbar pain.

文献评述

《丹溪心法•腰痛》曰："腰痛主湿热、肾虚、瘀血、挫闪、有痰积。 …戴云：湿热腰疼者，遇天阴或久坐而发者是也。"明确提出了"湿热腰痛"的病机变化。

《谢映庐医案•湿热腰痛》曰："湿热腰痛：徐伯昆，长途至家，醉饱房劳之后，患腰痛屈曲难行，延医数手，咸谓腰乃肾府，房劳伤肾，惟补剂相宜， …渐次困倦，转侧不能，每日晡心狂意躁，微有潮热，痛楚异常，卧床一月，几成废人。余诊之，知系湿热聚于腰肾，误在用补。 …此症先因长途扰其筋骨之血，后因醉饱乱其营卫之血，随因房劳耗其百骸之精，内窍空虚，湿热扰乱，血未定静，乘虚而入，聚于腰肾之中。"阐述了湿热之邪聚于腰肾的病因病机变化。

《临床中医内科学•腰痛》曰："湿热腰痛：湿热之邪侵袭腰部，聚于太阳，腰痛重着而热，痛及项背。湿热之邪极易流走关节，热为阳邪，故肢节红肿疼痛，口干口渴。舌苔黄腻、脉濡数为湿热之象。"明确阐述了湿热腰痛的病机变化。

Summary of Damp-Heat Damaging the Lower Back
1. Damp-Heat Damaging the Lower Back Pain in the lumbar region that is accompanied by a sensation of heat there and stretches up to the nape and back and down into the sacrum and coccyx and hip. 2. Damp-Heat Depression and Steaming Lumbar pain that is aggravated during the rainy season. 3. Flowing into the Joints Redness and swelling in the joints. 4. Internal Steaming Vexation heat and thirst. 5. Pouring into the Bladder Short voidings of reddish urine. 6. Damp-Heat Brewing Internally Yellow slimy tongue fur, rapid soggy pulse.

湿热伤腰
湿热伤腰—腰部疼痛，痛处伴有热感，腰痛上引项背，下及尻髋 湿热郁蒸—梅雨季节腰痛加重 流走关节—关节红肿 熏蒸于内—烦热口渴 流注膀胱—小便短赤 湿热内蕴—舌苔黄腻，脉濡数

5.2 Damp-Heat Strangury-Turbidity

The kidney governs water and stands in exterior-interior relationship with the bladder. Thus it has an important regulating effect on engenderment and elimination of urine. If for a variety of reasons damp-heat arises internally or if externally contracted damp-heat evil directly assails and damages the kidney, brewing and binding there instead of dispersing, then qì transformation in the kidney breaks down. The elimination of urine is inhibited, and damp-heat runs into the bladder, causing symptoms like dribbling, roughness, and pain. This manifests in the pathological changes of damp-heat strangury-turbidity.

The term "strangury" first occurred in the *Nèi Jīng* ("The Inner Canon"). The "Great Treatise on the Regular Principles of the Six Origins" in the *Sù Wèn* ("Plain Questions") states: "In this disease, there is heat distention in the center... reddish yellow urine, and in severe cases strangury." This quotation reflects a rudimentary recognition of the manifestations of damp-heat strangury-turbidity.

The chapter, "Pulse Symptoms and Treatments of Dispersion-Thirst, Inhibited Urination, and Strangury" in the *Jīn Guì Yào Lüè* ("Essential Prescriptions of the Golden Coffer") added this description: "The disease of strangury manifests in urine dribbling like millet, bowstring tension in the smaller abdomen, and pain stretching to the center of the umbilicus." Furthermore, the section, "Wind-Cold Accumulations and Gatherings in the Five Viscera" in the same text suggested that this pathomechanism could be blamed on "heat in the lower burner."

The chapter, "Discussing the Treatment of Strangury and Disinhibition" in the *Yán Shì Jì Shēng Fāng* ("Yan's Remedies for Curing All People") states: "Taxation damage in the kidney channel and heat in the kidney itself can result in heat being retained in the bladder; as it flows in, it forms the disease of strangury." This quotation clearly indicates how damp-heat in the kidney channel can flow into the bladder and form the pathomechanical changes of damp-heat strangury-turbidity.

When damp-heat damages the kidney, it can distress the bladder, disorder qì transformation, and obstruct the process of eliminating urine. This results in frequent and urgent urination and roughness and pain in the urethra.

When damp-heat pours downward, it steams urine, resulting in short voidings of reddish and possibly turbid urine.

Heat damages the blood network vessels and makes blood stray outside the vessels. This results in occasional bright red blood in the urine.

When damp-heat swelters for a long period of time, boiling urine, the impurities in the urine can accumulate and form sand and stones. This manifests in occasional elimination of sand and stones, with aching pain in the lower back that stretches to the genitals.

Damp-heat brewing and binding results in a red tongue with a slimy yellow tongue fur, and a slippery rapid pulse.

The chapter, "Expounding Pathoconditions and Formulas: Fire" in the *Gù Shì Yī Jìng* ("Master Gu's Reflections on Medicine") states:

> "Fire in the kidney results in night sweating and seminal emission, and invariably in the emission of heat from the bladder in the form of dribbling and dripping white ooze. These are all symptoms of heat being emitted from the viscus to the bowel. It is treated in the viscus, and the disease of the bowel will disperse on its own."

This quotation describes in depth how strangury-turbidity occurs as a result of kidney channel damp-heat shifting heat into the bladder.

Damp-heat strangury-turbidity is treated by clearing heat and disinhibiting dampness, and by draining the kidney and freeing strangury. The recommended formula is *qīng shèn tāng* (Clear the Kidney Decoction) from the *Yī Xué Zhōng Zhōng Cān Xī Lù* ("Records of Chinese Medicine with Reference to Western Medicine").

Qīng Shèn Tāng 清肾汤 Clear the Kidney Decoction
zhī mǔ (知母 Anemarrhenae Rhizoma, anemarrhena)
huáng bǎi (黄柏 Phellodendri Cortex, phellodendron)
lóng gǔ (龙骨 Mastodi Ossis Fossilia, dragon bone)
mǔ lì (牡蛎 Ostreae Concha, oyster shell)
hǎi piāo xiāo (海螵蛸 Sepiae Endoconcha, cuttlefish bone)
qiàn cǎo (茜草 Rubiae Radix, madder)
bái sháo (白芍 Paeoniae Radix Alba, white peony)
shān yào (山药 Dioscoreae Rhizoma, dioscorea)
zé xiè (泽泻 Alismatis Rhizoma, alisma)

湿热淋浊

肾主水，与膀胱相表里，对小便的生成和排泄有着重要的调节作用。如因多种因素导致湿热内生，或外感湿热之邪直接侵扰伤肾，蕴结不散，导致肾之气化失司，小便排泄不利，湿热流于膀胱，出现淋漓涩痛等症状，表现为湿热淋浊的病机变化。"淋"之名首见于《内经》，《素问•六元正纪大论》曰："其病中热胀， …小便黄赤，甚则淋。"对湿热淋浊的病机表现有了初步的认识。《金匮要略•消渴小便不利淋病脉证并治》进一步描述曰："淋之为病，小便如粟状，小腹弦急，痛引脐中。"且《金匮要略•五脏风寒积聚》中认为其病机责之"热在下焦。"《重订严氏济生方•淋利论治》曰："劳伤肾经，肾脏有热，热留膀胱，流入脬脏，遂成淋病。"明确指出了肾经湿热，流入膀胱，可形成湿热淋浊的病机变化。湿热伤肾，逼迫膀胱，气化失常，小便排泄过程受阻，则尿频、尿急、尿道涩痛；湿热下流，蒸腾尿液，则小便短赤，或浑浊；热伤血络，血逸脉外，则有时小便带血，血色鲜红；湿热熏蒸日久，煎熬尿液，尿中杂质聚积，则可形成砂石，表现为有时排出砂石，腰酸腰痛，引及前阴。湿热蕴结，则舌红苔黄腻，脉滑数。如《顾氏医镜•症方发明•火》曰："如肾有火，盗汗遗精，必遗热于膀胱，则白淫淋沥，此皆脏遗热于腑之症，治在脏而腑病自消也。" 深刻阐述了肾经湿热移热于膀胱发为淋浊的病机变化。治宜清热利湿，泻肾通淋。方药选用《医学衷中参西录》清肾汤（知母、黄柏、生龙骨、生牡蛎、海螵蛸、茜草、生白芍、生山药、泽泻）。

Literature Review of Damp-Heat Strangury-Turbidity

🕮 *Zhū Bìng Yuán Hòu Lùn* ("Origin and Indicators of Disease"), "Symptoms of Strangury"

> "Heat strangury means that there is heat in the triple burner, which contends with qì in the kidney, flows into the womb, and forms strangury. Its symptom is inhibited voidings of reddish urine."

This quotation points out that the pathomechanism of heat strangury is caused by heat in the triple buner contending qì in the kidney and flowing downward into the bladder.

🕮 *Jǐng Yuè Quán Shū* ("Jǐng-Yuè's Complete Compendium"), "Schema of Miscellaneous Patterns: Strangury-Turbidity"

> "Whenever fatty, sweet, alcoholic, acrid, hot, or roasted foods are enjoyed beyond their proper limit, they can all induce turbidity. These are a cause of damp-heat arising internally. In addition, turbidity can arise from seasonal qì in the form of flaming heat and steaming dampness, which invades the organs. This is damp-heat entering from the outside."

This quotation describes succinctly how internal or external damp-heat evil can invade the organs and induce strangury-turbidity.

🕮 *Yī Biǎn* ("Lancing Stones of Medicine"), "Miscellaneous Pathoconditions: Red and White Turbidity"

> "This condition is mostly due to essence that at the time of sexual intercourse has already left its position and is possibly held back forcibly from being discharged or obstructed and stopped in the center.

> The essence that has left its position transforms into vanquished turbidity and flows out from the orifices and extremities. Therefore it resembles pus or eye discharge and smells putrid. In addition, if essence is not discharged [normally], kidney fire is depressed and not dispersed, and vanquished essence exits, clasping depressed fire. This causes swelling of the penis, roughness in the orifices, and pain."

This quotation describes the pathomechanism by which kidney fire, when it is not dispersed, hurries downward into the urethra and forms white turbidity.

文献评述

《诸病源候论•淋病诸候》曰："热淋者，三焦有热，气搏于肾，流入于胞，而成淋也，其状，小便赤涩。"指出热淋的病机是热搏于肾，下流膀胱所致。

《景岳全书•杂证谟•淋浊》曰："凡肥甘酒醴，辛热炙煿之物，用之过当，皆能致浊，此湿热之由内生者也。又有炎热湿蒸，主客时令之气侵及脏腑者，亦能致浊。此湿热之由外入者也。"详细论述了内外湿热之邪进犯脏腑，导致小便淋浊的病机变化。

《医碥•杂症•赤白浊》曰："多由房事时精已离位，或强忍不泄，或被阻中止，离位之精化成败浊，流出窍端，故如脓如眵，其气臭腐。又不泄则肾火郁而不散，败精挟郁火以出，故茎肿窍涩而痛也。"论述肾火不散，下迫溺道，形成白浊的病机。

Summary of Damp-Heat Strangury-Turbidity

1. Damp-Heat Causing Distress
   Urinary frequency and urgency, roughness and pain in the urethra.
2. Damp-Heat Steaming
   Short voidings of reddish and possibly turbid urine.
3. Heat Damaging the Blood Network Vessels
   Occasional bright red blood in the urine.
4. Damp-Heat Boiling
   Occasional elimination of sand and stones, aching pain in the lower back that stretches to the genitals.
5. Damp-Heat Brewing and Binding
   Red tongue with yellow slimy tongue fur, slippery rapid pulse.

湿热淋浊
湿热逼迫—尿频，尿急，尿道涩痛
湿热蒸腾—小便短赤，或浑浊
热伤血络—有时小便带血，血色鲜红
湿热煎熬—有时排出砂石，腰酸腰痛，引及前阴
湿热蕴结—舌红苔黄腻，脉滑数

5.3 Damp-Heat Dribbling Urinary Block

The kidney governs water, regulates the waterways, and stands in exterior-interior relationship with the bladder. The "Treatise of the Arcane Book of the Orchid Chamber of the Spirit Tower" in the *Sù Wèn* ("Plain Questions") states: "The bladder holds the office of regional island (or Regional Rectifier), stores fluid, and by qì transformation lets it out." If damp-heat evil brews and binds in the lower burner, the kidney is unable to regulate the waterways, bladder qì transformation breaks down, the fluid metabolism is disordered, and the formation of urine is without source. This manifests in the pathomechanical changes of damp-heat dribbling urinary block.

Beginning with the *Nèi Jīng* ("The Inner Canon"), we can find numerous descriptions of pathomechanisms related to dribbling urinary block. For example, the "Treatise Explaining the Five Qì" in the *Sù Wèn* ("Plain Questions") already pointed out that "inhibition in the bladder means dribbling block." The "Great Treatise on the Five Normal Rules" in the same text also stated: "Periods of drying up and flowing are what is called opposing yáng... In the disease of dribbling urinary block, evil has damaged the kidney."

This passage notes that the pathomechanical development of dribbling urinary block is closely related to evil qì damaging the kidney. The chapter, "Channel Vessels" in the *Líng Shū* ("The Magic Pivot") also pointed out: "The foot lesser yīn divergent channel diverges from Large Goblet (*dà zhōng*, KI-4). When replete, it results in dribbling urinary block; when vacuous, in lumbar pain." While this quotation did not yet mention the disease evil "damp-heat" directly, the term "repletion evil" naturally includes damp-heat evil.

Following the *Nèi Jīng* ("The Inner Canon"), the chapter, "Various Symptoms of Urinary Disease; Urinary Stoppage" in the *Zhū Bìng Yuán Hòu Lùn* ("Origin and Indicators of Disease") explicitly raised the following point:

> "Urinary stoppage is caused by the presence of heat in both the bladder and the kidney. The kidney governs water, the bladder is the storehouse of the fluids, and these two channels stand in exterior-interior relationship. Water moves into the small intestine and enters the bladder as urine. As soon as the kidney and bladder contract heat, the heat enters the physical bladder, resulting in a great exuberance of hot qì. The resulting binding and roughness causes urinary stoppage."

This quotation thus elaborated in depth on the pathomechanism by which the kidney shifts heat to the bladder, the bladder contracts damp-heat and becomes obstructed and qì transformation is inhibited, resulting in urinary stoppage.

The kidney stands in exterior-interior relationship with the bladder. Heat binding in the kidney leads to breakdown in bladder qì transformation and exhaustion of liquid. The result is urinary dripping and stoppage, in severe cases urinary block, and extremely scanty amounts of urine.

When damp-heat boils and hurries downward, the result is inhibited voidings of reddish yellow urine and the sensation of scorching heat in the urethra.

Binding heat can cause water to collect and thereby stagnate bladder qì transformation. This results in smaller-abdominal distention.

Exuberant heat damaging liquid results in dry mouth with thirst, and dry bound stool. Damp-heat damaging the kidney results in a red tongue with a slimy yellow tongue fur, and a fine rapid pulse.

The chapter, "Urinary Stoppage" in the *Yī Biǎn* ("Lancing Stones of Medicine") explains:

> "Urinary dripping and inability to discharge it, with smaller-abdominal distention and pain is due to blockage in the pathways of qì… Qì in the lower burner is governed by the liver and kidney yīn. When the kidney shifts heat into the bladder, there is no yīn, and yáng lacks that which it can transform."

This quotation indicates that the pathomechanism of heat shifting from the kidney to the bladder and poor qì transformation form the pathomechanism of dribbling urinary block.

This condition is treated by clearing heat and disinhibiting stool and urine, and by enriching the kidney and freeing the gate. The recommended formula is *dì fū zǐ tāng* (Kochiae Decoction) from the *Qiān Jīn Yào Fāng* ("A Thousand Gold Pieces Prescriptions") with the addition of *huáng bǎi* (Phellodendri Cortex), *chē qián zǐ* (Plantaginis Semen), *shí wéi* (Pyrrosiae Folium), and *dà huáng* (Rhei Radix et Rhizoma).

Dì Fū Zǐ Tāng 地肤子汤
Kochiae Decoction

dì fū zǐ (地肤子 Kochiae Fructus, kochia)
qú mài (瞿麦 Dianthi Herba, dianthus)
zhū líng (猪苓 Polyporus, polyporus)
zhǐ shí (枳实 Aurantii Fructus Immaturus, unripe bitter orange)
shēng má (升麻 Cimicifugae Rhizoma, cimicifuga)
hǎi zǎo (海藻 Sargassum, sargassum)
zhī mǔ (知母 Anemarrhenae Rhizoma, anemarrhena)
huáng qín (黄芩 Scutellariae Radix, scutellaria)
dōng kuí zǐ (冬葵子 Malvae Semen, mallow seed)
tōng cǎo (通草 Tetrapanacis Medulla, rice-paper plant pith)

Plus:

huáng bǎi (黄柏 Phellodendri Cortex, phellodendron)
chē qián zǐ (车前子 Plantaginis Semen, plantago seed)
shí wéi (石韦 Pyrrosiae Folium, pyrrosia)
dà huáng (大黄 Rhei Radix et Rhizoma, rhubarb)

湿热癃闭

肾主水，通调水道，与膀胱互为表里。《素问•灵兰秘典论》曰："膀胱者，州都之官，津液藏焉，气化则能出矣。"如湿热之邪蕴结于下焦，肾不能通调水道，膀胱气化失司，水液代谢失常，小便化生无源，则出现湿热癃闭的病机变化。从《内经》起，就有许多与癃闭有关的病机论述。如《素问•宣明五气论》指出："膀胱不利为癃。"《素问•五常政大论》又云："涸流之纪，是谓反阳。 …其病癃闭，邪伤肾也"。指明癃闭的病机发展与邪气伤肾密切相关。《灵枢•经脉》亦指出："足少阴之别，名曰大钟。实则癃闭，虚则腰痛。"虽未直接提及"湿热"病邪，但"实邪"之中，自然包含"湿热"之邪为患。《诸病源候论•小便病诸候•小便不通候》则明确提出："小便不通，由膀胱与肾俱有热故也。肾主水，膀胱为津液之腑，此二经为表里，而水行于小肠，入胞者为小便，肾与膀胱即热，热入于胞，热气大盛，故结涩令小便不通。"对肾移热于膀胱，膀胱湿热阻滞，气化不利，小便不通的病机作了深刻的阐述。肾与膀胱为表里，热结于肾，膀胱气化失职，水津耗竭，则小便点滴不通，甚至闭塞，尿量极少；湿热煎熬、下迫，则小便不利而黄赤，尿道有灼热感；热结水停，膀胱气机滞塞，则小腹胀急；热盛伤津，则口干而渴，大便干结。湿热伤肾，则舌红苔黄腻，脉细数。正如《医碥•小便不通》所说："点滴不出，小腹胀痛，由气道闭塞。 …下焦之气，肝肾主之，肾移热于膀胱，无阴则阳无以化。"指出肾移热于膀胱，气化不行，是形成癃闭的病机。治宜清热利便，滋肾通关。方药选用《千金要方》地肤子汤（地肤子、瞿麦、猪苓、枳实、升麻、海藻、知母，黄芩、冬葵子、通草）加黄柏、车前仁、石苇、大黄。

Literature Review of Damp-Heat Dribbling Urinary Block

📖 *Qiān Jīn Yào Fāng* ("A Thousand Gold Pieces Prescriptions"), "The Bladder: Treatise on the Bladder"

> "It is said that the physical bladder is the indicator of the kidney and bladder. It stores fluids and urine. In cases of heat disease in the viscus, the bladder is dry and urine fails to flow freely and is reddish yellow… By treating kidney heat, you will be able to affect the [symptoms of] dryness and heat in the bladder, reddish yellow urine, and painful stoppage. Use a brew formula with *yú pí* (Ulmi Parvifoliae Cortex (Radicis) to promote flow, lubricate, and discharge heat."

Heat in the viscus refers to kidney heat. When the kidney shifts heat into the bladder, this can lead to reddish yellow urine and dryness, heat, and stoppage. Thus this passage points to the pathomechanism by which damp-heat damage to the kidney can lead to dribbling urinary block.

📖 *Lán Shì Mì Cáng* ("Secret Treasure of the Orchid Chamber"), "Urinary Dribbling and Block"

> "Lack of thirst with stopped urination indicates heat in the blood aspect of the lower burner. For this reason, there is no thirst but great dryness and stopped urination. When heat blocks the lower burner, this refers to the kidney and bladder, which are yīn within yīn. When yīn contracts heat evil, this blocks its flow. As Zhāng Yuán-Sù stated, 'cold in the

chest means obstruction, expiry, and lack of intake; heat in the lower burner means fullness, congestion, and absence of bowel movements.' You must use the method of transforming cold and water employed by the Northern School. Medicinals should all be yīn in qì and flavor to eliminate this heat and discharge the block."

This quotation analyzes in detail how damp-heat brewing and binding in the lower burner can damage the kidney and bladder, forming dribbling urinary block.

🕮 *Xiè Yìng Lú Yī Àn* ("Xiè Yìng-Lú's Case Studies"), "Section on Dribbling Urinary Block: Discussing the Treatment of Urinary Stoppage"

"Whether urine flows freely or not depends completely on whether qì is transformed or not. Nevertheless, the concept of qì transformation is difficult to explain. In cases where damp-heat depression and block prevent qì from being transformed, use the formulas for *wǔ líng sǎn* (Poria Five Powder), *bā zhèng sǎn* (Eight Corrections Powder), *yǔ gōng sǎn* (Water Controller Yǔ Powder), and *zhōu chē (jū) wán* (Boats and Carts Pill), to clear heat and abduct dampness, and thereby transform it."

This quotation also indicates clearly that damp-heat can induce dribbling urinary block.

文献评述

《千金要方•膀胱腑•胞囊论》曰："论曰：胞囊者，肾膀胱候也，贮津液并尿。若脏中热病者，胞涩，小便不通，尿黄赤；…治肾热应胞囊涩热，小便黄赤，苦不通，榆皮通滑泄热煎方。"胞囊，即膀胱。脏中热，即肾热，肾移热于膀胱，可引起小便黄赤、涩热不通，即指湿热伤肾，引起癃闭的病机。

《兰室秘藏•小便淋闭》曰："不渴而小便不通者，热在下焦血分，故不渴而大燥，小便不通也。热闭于下焦者，肾也，膀胱也，乃阴中之阴，阴受热邪，闭塞其流。易上老(指张元素)云，寒在胸中，遏绝不入，热在下焦，填塞不便。须用感北方寒水之化，气味俱阴之药，以除其热，泄其闭塞。"详细分析了湿热蕴结下焦，伤及肾与膀胱，而成癃闭的病机变化。

《谢映庐医案•癃闭门•论治小便不通》曰："小便之通与不通，全在气之化与不化，然而气化二字难言之矣，有因湿热郁闭而气不化者，用五苓、八正、禹功、舟车之剂，清热导湿而化之。"亦明确指出了湿热可导致癃闭的病机改变。

Summary of Damp-Heat Dribbling Urinary Block
1. Exhaustion of Liquid Urinary dripping and stoppage, in severe cases urinary block, extremely scanty amounts of urine. 2. Damp-Heat Hurrying Downward Inhibited discharge of reddish yellow urine, sensation of scorching heat in the urethra. 3. Bladder Qì Stagnation Lesser-abdominal distention. 4. Exuberant Heat Damaging Liquid Dry mouth with thirst, dry bound stool. 5. Damp-Heat Damaging the Kidney Red tongue with yellow slimy tongue fur, fine rapid pulse.

湿热癃闭
水津耗竭—小便点滴不通，甚至闭塞，尿量极少 湿热下迫—小便不利而黄赤，尿道有灼热感 膀胱气滞—小腹胀急 热盛伤津—口干而渴，大便干结 湿热伤肾—舌红苔黄腻，脉细数

5.4 Damp-Heat Puffy Swelling

The kidney opens at the two yīn and is in charge of fluid metabolism. Owing to a constitutional insufficiency of kidney yáng and congenital yáng qì vacuity, kidney qì transformation can be inhibited. This can be further complicated by a contraction of damp-heat evil. Since damp-heat is by nature sticky, stagnating, heavy, and turbid, it impedes the normal movement of the fluids, so that they spill outward instead of following their ordinary pathways. This results in root vacuity and tip repletion, forming the pathomechanism of damp-heat puffy swelling.

The lower back is the house of the kidney. When damp-heat evil encumbers the kidney, it therefore causes lumbar and abdominal pain.

When kidney yáng is insufficient and is furthermore tied up by damp-heat, yáng is unable to outthrust. The result is fear of cold and cold limbs.

Being heavy and turbid, damp-heat impedes the movement of the qì dynamic, and clear qì fails to bear upward. This results in clouded head and tinnitus.

When damp-heat pours into the lower body, it inhibits bladder qì transformation. This results in short inhibited voidings of yellow urine.

Damp-heat can percolate down into the large intestine, impairing large intestinal conveyance. This results in thin sloppy stool.

Yáng vacuity and failure to transform causes damp-heat to collect internally and water qì to spill outward. The result is puffy swelling in the whole body.

Debilitation of kidney yáng results in a pale tongue and fine sunken pulse. Damp-heat brewing internally results in a slimy yellow tongue fur.

The chapter, "Water Swelling" in *Dān Xī Xīn Fǎ* ("Dān Xī's Heart-Approach") states:

> "Conditions with generalized swelling, vexation and thirst, inhibited voidings of reddish urine, and fecal block are ascribed to yáng water... *dà jú pí tāng* (Major Tangerine Peel Decoction) treats an internal attack of damp-heat manifesting in abdominal distention and water swelling, inhibited urination, and efflux diarrhea."

This passage describes how an internal exuberance of damp-heat induces pathomechanical changes like water swelling and inhibited urination.

The "Schema of Miscellaneous Patterns; Discussing the Treatment of Water Swelling" in the *Jǐng Yuè Quán Shū* ("Jǐng-Yuè's Complete Compendium") also points out:

> "Any signs like water swelling indicate disease related to the three viscera of spleen, lung, and kidney. Since water is consummate yīn, its root is in the kidney. ...In all patients with a constitutional exuberance of yáng, there is increased fire in the triple burner. When such a person suffers from water swelling, symptoms invariably include vexation and thirst, and liking for cold, possibly with red face and bound stool, heat effusion with panting and cough, swelling of the head and face, and a slippery replete pulse. These are signs of dampness and heat functioning as mutual causes, in combination with yīn vacuity."

This is a clear description of the process by which damp-heat invading the kidney leads to inhibited movement and transformation of water-damp, and to puffy swelling in the face and eyes.

Patients with the biomedical condition of chronic renal failure tend to manifest with signs of spleen-kidney yáng vacuity like heavy edema in the lower limbs, short voidings of scant urine, and physical cold and cold limbs. If this is complicated by concurrent infection or by causes like hematuria, albuminuria, or retention of nitrogenous substances, the condition can furthermore transform into damp-heat, forming the concurrent pathomechanisms of kidney yáng vacuity and damp-heat water swelling. This constitutes a root vacuity and tip repletion, with repletion as the dominant factor. Therefore, this condition is associated with the pathomechanism of kidney repletion heat.

Damp-heat puffy swelling is treated by warming and supplementing kidney yáng, and by clearing heat and disinhibiting dampness. The recommended formula is *wēn shèn qīng lì tāng* (Warm and Disinhibit the Kidney Decoction) from the *Mì Fāng Qiú Zhēn* ("Secret Recipes for Seeking the Truth").

Wēn Shèn Qīng Lì Tāng 温肾清利汤
Warm and Disinhibit the Kidney Decoction

fù zǐ (附子 Aconiti Radix Lateralis Praeparata, aconite) [cooked]
dà xuè téng (大血藤 Sargentodoxae Caulis, sargentodoxa)
pú gōng yīng (蒲公英 Taraxaci Herba, dandelion)
bài jiàng cǎo (败酱草 Patriniae Herba, patrinia)
zǐ huā dì dīng (紫花地丁 Violae Herba, violet)
nuò mǐ cǎo (糯米草 Oryzae Glutinosae Herba, glutinous rice herb)
shēng dì huáng (生地黄 Rehmanniae Radix, rehmannia)
yīn chén (茵陈 Artemisiae Scopariae Herba, virgate wormwood)
hǎi jīn shā (海金沙 Lygodii Spora, lygodium spore)
yè míng shā (夜明砂 Verspertilionis Faeces, bat's droppings)
gǒu qǐ zǐ (枸杞子 Lycii Fructus, lycium)
jiāng huáng (姜黄 Curcumae Longae Rhizoma, turmeric)
hǔ pò (琥珀 Succinum, amber)

湿热浮肿

肾开窍于二阴，司水液之代谢。如素体肾阳不足，先天之阳气亏虚，肾之气化失利，又复感湿热之邪，湿热之性粘滞重浊，阻碍水液的正常运行，水液不循常道而外溢，导致本虚标实，湿热浮肿的病机变化。腰为肾之府，湿热之邪困于肾，故腰腹疼痛；肾阳不足，又被湿热所缚，阳不外达，则畏寒肢冷；湿热重浊，阻碍气机运行，清气不升，则头眩耳鸣；湿热下注，膀胱气化不利，则小便短黄不利；湿热下渗大肠，大肠传导失司，则大便溏稀；阳虚不化，湿热内停，水气外溢，则全身浮肿。肾阳虚衰，则舌质淡，脉沉细；湿热内蕴，则舌苔黄腻。如《丹溪心法•水肿》曰："若遍身肿烦渴，小便赤涩，大便闭，此属阳水。 …大橘皮汤，治湿热内攻，腹胀水肿，小便不利，大便滑泄。"论述了湿热内盛引起的水肿、小便不利等病机变化。《景岳全书•杂证谟•水肿论治》也指出："凡水肿等证，乃脾肺肾三脏相关之病，盖水为至阴，故其本为肾。 …凡素禀阳盛，三焦多火，而病为水肿，其证必烦渴喜冷，或面赤便结，或热而喘嗽，或头面皆肿，或脉见滑实，此湿热相因，阴虚之证也。"明确论述了湿热犯肾导致水湿运化不利，面目浮肿的病机变化。现代医学慢性肾功能衰竭患者容易出现下肢高度水肿，小便短少，形寒肢冷等脾肾阳虚表现，加之合并感染，或因血尿、蛋白尿、氮质滞留等原因，又易化生湿热，形成肾阳虚兼湿热水肿的病机。此为本虚标实，以实为主，故仍属肾实热的病机。治宜温补肾阳，清热利湿。方药选用《秘方求真》温肾清利汤（熟附片、红藤、蒲公英、败酱草、紫花地丁、糯米草、细生地、茵陈、海金砂、夜明砂、枸杞子、姜黄、琥珀）。

Literature Review of Damp-Heat Puffy Swelling

📖 *Yán Shì Jì Shēng Fāng* ("Yan's Remedies for Curing All People"), "Discussing the Treatment of Water Swelling"

> "In patients of young age, when blood heat engenders sores and this transmutes into swelling and fullness with vexation, thirst, and reduced urination, this constitutes heat swelling. What the *Sù Wèn* ("Plain Questions") calls 'binding in yáng' refers to this condition of swelling in the four limbs."

The same text also states:

> "*Chì xiǎo dòu tāng* (Rice Bean Decoction) treats dual heat of blood and qì in young patients that subsequently engenders scab sores and transmutes into swelling and fullness, possibly with vexation, thirst, and inhibited urination."

What this quotation refers to as "heat swelling" is precisely the condition of damp-heat invading the kidney channel, which manifests in the pathological changes of swelling and fullness in the four limbs.

📖 *Zhèng Yīn Mài Zhì* ("Pathoconditions: Causes, Pulses, and Treatments"), "Externally Contracted Swelling"

> "The symptoms of damp-heat water swelling are generalized heat effusion and yellowing of the eyes, inhibited voidings of reddish urine, distention and oppression in the chest and abdomen, yellow swelling in the four limbs, and thirst and heart vexation. These are the signs of swelling caused by damp-heat."

This quotation clearly points out the pathomechanical changes of damp-heat puffy swelling.

文献评述

《济生方•水肿论治》曰："又有年少，血热生疮，变为肿满，烦渴小便少，此为热肿，素问所谓结阳者肿四肢是也。"又曰："赤小豆汤，治年少血气俱热，遂生疥疮，变为肿满，或烦，或渴，小便不利。"所谓"热肿"，即是湿热为患，侵及肾经，表现为四肢肿满的病机改变。

《症因脉治•外感肿胀》曰："湿热水肿之症，身热目黄，小便赤涩，胸腹胀闷，四肢黄肿，口渴心烦，此湿热作肿。"明确提出了湿热浮肿的病机变化。

Summary of Damp-Heat Puffy Swelling
1. Damp-Heat Encumbering the Lower Back Pain in the lower back and abdomen.
2. Yáng Failing to Outthrust Fear of cold and cold limbs.
3. Clear Qì Failing to Upbear Dizzy head and tinnitus.
4. Damp-Heat Pouring Downward Short inhibited voidings of yellow urine, thin sloppy stool.
5. Water Qì Spilling Out Generalized puffy swelling.
6. Debilitation of Kidney Yáng Pale tongue, fine sunken pulse.
7. Damp-Heat Brewing Internally Yellow slimy tongue fur.

湿热浮肿
湿热困腰—腰腹疼痛
阳不外达—畏寒肢冷
清气不升—头眩耳鸣
湿热下注—小便短黄不利，大便溏稀
水气外溢—全身浮肿
肾阳虚衰—舌质淡，脉沉细
湿热内蕴—舌苔黄腻

Chapter Six

Kidney Channel Repletion Fire

The kidney is the viscus of fire and water. It stores original yáng and is the root of the body's yáng qì. If a patient with a constitutional hyperactivity of kidney yáng contracts wind-heat, yáng can easily transform into fire. Alternatively, yáng evils like fulminant heat or rapid fire can directly attack the liver channel. As a third alternative, in a person who has been ingesting acrid, spicy, and stimulating foods or warm and hot medicinals, internal and external yáng can fan each other. All these can lead to the pathomechanism of kidney channel repletion fire.

The chapter, "Treatment of Vacuity and Repletion in the Kidney and Bladder" in the *Yán Shì Jì Shēng Fāng* ("Yan's Remedies for Curing All People") points out:

> "The kidney is associated with the foot lesser yīn channel... If it is replete, repletion engenders heat. Heat results in a dry tongue with swollen throat, heart vexation with dry throat, intermittent chest and rib-side pain, panting and cough with sweating, smaller-abdominal fullness and distention, hypertonicity of the back and lower back, heaviness of the body and heat in the bones, reddish yellow urine, heat and pain on the underside of the feet, and a tight floating pulse. These are the signs of kidney repletion."

The chapter, the "Origin and Development of Kidney Disease" in the "Section on the Viscera and Bowels" in the *Zá Bìng Yuán Liú Xī Zhú* ("Incisive Light on the Source of Miscellaneous Disease") further points out:

> "The kidney is originally afflicted by diseases of water and fire. In fire disease, dragon fire soars intensely and scorches upward, causing harm. Its symptoms include thirst with dry throat, heart vexation, a sensation in the heart as if it was suspended, shouting and panting, a lacquer-like facial complexion, and coughing and spitting of blood."

This quotation describes the numerous pathomechanical changes resulting from repletion fire brewing in the kidney.

Because of differences in the pathogenic factors and outcome of the pathomechanism of kidney channel repletion fire, we can further differentiate it into the categories of repletion heat brewing in the kidney, kidney heat damaging liquid, and fire toxin congesting the kidney.

肾经实火

肾为水火之脏，藏元阳，为人体阳气之根本。如遇素体肾阳偏亢，稍感风热，则阳易化火，或暴热急火等阳邪直攻肾经，或久服辛辣刺激食物、温热药物，内外两阳相煽，皆可导致肾经实火的病机改变。《济生方•五脏门•肾膀胱虚实论治》指出："夫肾者，足少阴之经，...及其实也，实则生热，热则舌燥咽肿，心烦咽干，胸胁时痛，喘嗽汗出，小腹胀满，腰背拘急，体重骨热，小便赤黄，足下热痛，诊其脉浮紧者，是肾实之候也。"《杂病源流犀烛•脏腑门•肾病源流》又指出："肾家本有水火两病，火病者，龙火腾炽，上烁为害也，其症有口热咽干，烦心，心如悬，喝喝而喘，面如漆柴，咳唾有血等类。"对实火蕴肾引起的多种病机变化进行了阐述。肾经实火，因致病因素及病机转归有异，又分为实热蕴肾、肾热津伤、火毒壅肾等病机类型。

6.1 Repletion Heat Brewing in the Kidney

The kidney stores the ministerial fire, and the liver and kidney are of the same source. The kidney can cause frenetic stirring of ministerial fire in a number of circumstances: Kidney yáng qì can be abnormally exuberant by congenital constitution. Alternatively, great anger can cause liver fire to rise fulminantly and spread to the kidney. Lastly, prolonged use of warming and supplementing formulas can also cause ministerial fire to stir frenetically. As fire gathers in the kidney, a series of symptoms of fire harassing and being disquieted will manifest in the kidney itself and in the locations through which the kidney channel runs. This forms the pathomechanism of repletion heat brewing in the kidney.

The lower back is the house of the kidney. The kidney channel originates at the sole of the foot at Gushing Spring (yǒng quán, KI-1), runs along the inner ankle bone, rises up into the throat, and clasps the root of the tongue. When repletion heat follows the channel to swelter in the sole of the foot, inner ankle bone, and lower back, it can manifest in symptoms like lumbar pain, soreness in the inner ankle bone, and heat on the underside of the feet. When it rises and fumigates the throat, head, and face, this results in dry throat and tongue, thirst with frequent drinking, and sweating with heat effusion.

When fire-heat surges upward, kidney qì ascends counterflow. Consequently, yáng qì is unable to bear downward and warm the lower limbs. This results in cold and discomfort in the calf.

The foot lesser yīn kidney channel stands in exterior-interior relationship with the foot greater yáng bladder channel. When repletion heat brews in the kidney, it can externally invade channel qì in the nape and back, where it runs in the foot greater yáng bladder channel. This results in symptoms like stiffness and pain in the neck and nape and clouding and shaking of the head.

The kidney governs water and is in charge of stool and urine. When heat evil brewing in the kidney damages liquid, the result is yellow or reddish urine.

Repletion heat brewing in the kidney manifests in a red tongue with yellow tongue fur and a sunken rapid pulse.

The "Treatise on Needling Heat" in the *Sù Wèn* ("Plain Questions") states:

> "Kidney heat disease manifests first in lumbar pain and aching shins, bitter thirst with frequent drinking, and generalized heat effusion; heat struggling then results in pain and stiffness in the neck, cold and aching shins, heat on the underside of the feet, and no desire to talk; if the heat counterflows, this results in dizzy head and shaking."

This quotation describes pathomechanical changes like lumbar pain and thirst that result from repletion heat brewing in the kidney.

The treatise "On Wilting" in the *Sù Wèn* ("Plain Questions") further states: "When liver qì is hot, it results in inability to lift the lumbar spine and desiccated bone and reduced marrow, which erupts as bone wilting."

The section, "Lumbar Pain" in "Schema of Miscellaneous Patterns" in the *Jǐng Yuè Quán Shū* ("Jǐng-Yuè's Complete Compendium") points out:

> "In lumbar pain, there are cold and heat patterns… If evil heat amassing in the lower back and kidney is not rooted in vacuity detriment, there must be extreme pain and heat vexation, possibly with great heat with fluid intake, or with hot, inhibited, and stopped urine and stool. In treatment, you must directly attack this fire. *Dà fēn qīng yǐn* (Major Clear-Turbid Separation Beverage) with modifications is suitable for governing this condition."

This quotation discusses in detail how externally contracted repletion heat fire evil can brew and bind in the kidney to cause an internal exuberance of yáng heat, manifesting in the pathomechanical changes of repletion heat brewing in the kidney.

Repletion heat brewing in the kidney is treated by draining the kidney and clearing heat. The recommended formula is *dà fēn qīng yǐn* (Major Clear-Turbid Separation Beverage) from the *Jǐng Yuè Quán Shū* ("Jǐng-Yuè's Complete Compendium").

Dà Fēn Qīng Yǐn 大分清饮 Major Clear-Turbid Separation Beverage
zhī zǐ (栀子 Gardeniae Fructus, gardenia)
fú líng (茯苓 Poria, poria)
zé xiè (泽泻 Alismatis Rhizoma, alisma)
zhū líng (猪苓 Polyporus, polyporus)
mù tōng (木通 Akebiae Trifoliatae Caulis, trifoliate akebia)
chē qián zǐ (车前子 Plantaginis Semen, plantago seed)
zhǐ qiào (ké) (枳壳 Aurantii Fructus, bitter orange)

Alternatively, use *xiè shèn tāng* (Drain the Kidney Decoction) from the *Qiān Jīn Yào Fāng* ("A Thousand Gold Pieces Prescriptions").

Xiè Shèn Tāng 泻肾汤 Drain the Kidney Decoction
máng xiāo (芒硝 Natrii Sulfas, mirabilite)
dà huáng (大黄 Rhei Radix et Rhizoma, rhubarb)
fú líng (茯苓 Poria, poria)
huáng qín (黄芩 Scutellariae Radix, scutellaria)
shēng dì huáng (生地黄 Rehmanniae Radix, dried rehmannia)
shí chāng pú (石菖蒲 Acori Tatarinowii Rhizoma, acorus)
cí shí (磁石 Magnetitum, loadstone)
xuán shēn (玄参 Scrophulariae Radix, scrophularia)
xì xīn (细辛 Asari Herba, asarum)
gān cǎo (甘草 Glycyrrhizae Radix, licorice)

实热蕴肾

肾藏相火，肝肾同源。如因肾之阳气先天偏盛，或因大怒肝火暴升，波及于肾，或久服温补之剂，则容易引起相火妄动，火聚于肾，在肾体和肾经循行部位出现一系列火扰不宁的表现，形成实热蕴肾的病机变化。腰为肾之府，肾经经脉起源于足底涌泉穴，循内踝，上循喉咙，挟舌本。实热循经熏蒸足心、内踝、腰府，则可出现腰痛，内踝酸痛，足底下热等症状；上熏咽喉头面，则咽干舌燥，口渴数饮，汗出发热；火热上冲，肾气上逆，阳气不能下降，下肢失于温煦，则小腿反而寒冷不适；足少阴肾经与足太阳膀胱经相为表里，实热蕴肾，外犯足太阳膀胱经循行之项背经气，则见颈项强痛，头昏头摇等症状；肾主水，司二便，热邪蕴肾伤津，则小便赤黄。实热蕴肾，则舌红苔黄，脉沉数。如《素问•刺热论》曰："肾热病者，先腰痛胻酸，苦渴数饮，身热，热争则项痛而强，胻寒且酸，足下热，不欲言，其逆则项痛员员（指头眩晕）淡淡然（指动摇不安的表现）。"即论述了实热蕴肾引起的腰痛口渴等病机改变。《素问•痿论》又曰："肾气热，则腰脊不举，骨枯而髓减，发为骨痿。"《景岳全书•杂证谟•腰痛》也指出："腰痛有寒热证，…若邪火蓄结腰肾，而本无虚损者，必痛极，必烦热，或大渴引饮，或二便热涩不通，当直攻其火，宜大分清饮加减主之。"详细论述了外感实热火邪，蕴结于肾，阳热内盛，出现实热蕴肾的病机变化。治则为泻肾清热。方药选用《景岳全书》大分清饮（栀子、茯苓、泽泻、猪苓、木通、车前仁、枳壳），或用《千金要方》泻肾汤（芒硝、大黄、茯苓、黄芩、生地黄汁、石菖蒲、磁石、玄参、细辛、甘草）。

Literature Review of Repletion Heat Brewing in the Kidney

📖 *Qiān Jīn Yào Fāng* ("A Thousand Gold Pieces Prescriptions"), "On the Pulse in Kidney Disease: Formula for *Xiè shèn tāng* (Drain the Kidney Decoction)"

> "*Xiè shèn tāng* (Drain the Kidney Decoction) treats kidney repletion heat with smaller-abdominal fullness and distention, pure blackness of the four limbs, deafness, and dreams of the lower back and spine separating and of being submerged in water."

This quotation clearly addresses the pathomechanism of kidney repletion heat by name.

📖 *Tài Píng Shèng Huì Fāng* ("The Great Peace Sagacious Benevolence Formulary"), "Various Kidney-Draining Formulas for Treating Kidney Repletion"

> "The kidney governs water and storage of essence. If it is replete, yáng qì exuberates. If yáng qì exuberates, heat arises. Heat results in a dry tongue with swollen throat, heart vexation with dry throat, rigidity in the back and lower back, heaviness of the body with heat in the bones, reddish or yellow urine, competitiveness and forgetfulness, and heat and pain on the underside of the feet."

This quotation describes the pathomechanical changes of kidney repletion heat due to kidney yáng exuberance.

📖 *Zá Bìng Yuán Liú Xī Zhú* ("Incisive Light on the Source of Miscellaneous Disease"), "Bladder: Yellow or Reddish Urine"

> "Yellow or reddish urine means repletion heat disease. All the viscera and bowels can equally cause this, but the lower burner will aggravate it further."

What this quotation calls the "lower burner" includes pathologies of the kidney. Thus, this quotation elaborates on how repletion heat brewing in the kidney can lead to yellow or reddish urine.

文献评述

《千金要方•肾脏病脉论•泻肾汤方》曰："治肾实热，小腹胀满，四肢正黑，耳聋，梦腰脊离解及伏水等。"明确提出了"肾实热"的病机名称。

《太平圣惠方•治肾实泻肾诸方》曰："夫肾主水而藏于精，若实则阳气盛，若阳气盛则生热。热则舌燥咽肿，心烦嗌干，腰背强急，体重骨热，小便赤黄，好强好忘，足下热疼。" 阐述了肾阳亢盛而导致肾实热的病机变化。

《杂病源流犀烛•膀胱•小便黄赤》曰："小便黄赤，实热病也。凡脏腑皆能为之，而下焦更甚。"所述"下焦"，则包括肾之病变，对实热蕴肾导致小便黄赤的病机变化进行了阐述。

Summary of Repletion Heat Brewing in the Kidney
1. Sweltering along the Channel Lumbar pain, soreness in the inner ankle bone, heat on the underside of the feet. 2. Fire Heat Harassing Upward Dry throat and tongue, thirst with frequent drinking, sweating with heat effusion. 3. Fire Invading Greater Yáng Stiffness and pain in the neck and nape, clouding and shaking of the head. 4. Fire Counterflow and Cold in the Lower Body Cold in the shins. 5. Heat Evil Damaging Liquid Yellow or reddish urine. 6. Repletion Heat Brewing in the Kidney Red tongue with yellow tongue fur, sunken rapid pulse.

实热蕴肾
循经熏蒸—腰痛，内踝酸痛，足底下热 火热上扰—咽干舌燥，口渴数饮，汗出发热 火犯太阳—颈项强痛，头昏头摇 火逆下寒—小腿寒冷 热邪伤津—小便赤黄 实热蕴肾—舌红苔黄，脉沉数

6.2 Kidney Heat Damaging Liquid

The kidney governs water. Water transforms the five humors to moisten the whole body, the viscera and bowels, and the hundred vessels. If evil fire assails the kidney and exuberant heat damages liquid, this can form the pathomechanism of kidney channel exuberant heat with water depletion.

The kidney channel runs through the throat. When kidney fire ascends counterflow and causes damage to liquid and loss of moistening, the result is thirst and dry throat.

When liquid is depleted due to kidney heat, it is unable to descend and moisten the intestinal tract, causing bound stool and qì stagnation. This results in abdominal distention and fullness, and dry bound inhibited stool.

The left-over fluids can percolate out alongside the abiding bound stool, forming the pathomechanism of heat bind with circumfluence. This can further manifest in spontaneous clear-water diarrhea of pure green-blue color.

When kidney heat damages liquid, counterflow fire can harass the heart and thereby deprive the heart spirit of nourishment. This results in fatigued spirit-affect.

Depletion of liquid due to kidney heat manifests in a red tongue with dry yellow tongue fur and a fine rapid pulse.

The chapter, "Pulses and Signs of the Eleven Channels of the Five Viscera and Six Bowels, With the Exception of the Pericardiac Network" in the *Yī Xué Qǐ Yuán* ("The Source of Medicine") explains:

> "Disease engendered by the kidney manifests in heat in the mouth and a dry tongue, a swollen pharynx, qì ascent, dry and painful throat, vexation and pain in the heart, jaundice, intestinal aggregations, wilting reversal, acute pain in the lumbar spine and back, somnolence, heat and pain in the heart of the soles, and aching shins."

This quotation describes how damage to liquid from kidney channel repletion heat causes fire exuberance and water depletion, inducing changes like heat in the mouth and dry tongue, swollen throat, and acute pain in the lumbar spine and back.

The "Treatise on Constipation" in the *Yī Xué Zhèng Zhuàn* ("The Orthodox Tradition of Medicine") also explains:

> "The kidney governs the five humors. Therefore, repletion in the kidney means sufficient fluids and moistened stool, while vacuity in the kidney means exhausted fluids and bound stool. The reason for this is always found in excessive sexual intercourse… As the fire of wanton desire arises in the Life Gate, the resulting fire exuberance and water depletion prevents fluids from being engendered; thereby causing abnormalities in the passageways, which gradually create signs of binding and dryness."

This quotation incisively sets out the pathomechanism by which water depletion from kidney heat can lead to constipation.

Because this condition is rooted in intense heat evil, is caused by heat damaging liquid, and by nature is associated with repletion, the treatment method must focus on emergency precipitation to preserve yīn. The recommended formula is *dà chéng qì tāng* (Major Qì-Coordinating Decoction) from the *Shāng Hán Lùn* ("On Cold Damage").

Dà Chéng Qì Tāng 大承气汤 Major Qì-Coordinating Decoction
dà huáng (大黄 Rhei Radix et Rhizoma, rhubarb)
hòu pò (厚朴 Magnoliae Officinalis Cortex, officinal magnolia bark)
zhǐ shí (枳实 Aurantii Fructus Immaturus, unripe bitter orange)
máng xiāo (芒硝 Natrii Sulfas, mirabilite)

肾热津伤

肾主水，水化五液，滋润全身脏腑百脉。如邪火袭肾，热盛伤津，则可形成肾经热盛水亏的病机变化。肾经循咽喉，肾火上逆，津伤失濡，则口渴，咽干而燥；肾热津亏，不能下润肠道，便结气滞，则腹部胀满，大便燥结不利；残存之津液从宿结大便旁偏渗，形成热结旁流的病机，又可表现为大便自利清水，便色纯青；肾热伤津，逆火扰心，精神失养，则神情疲倦；肾热津亏，则舌红苔燥黄，脉细数。如《医学启源•五脏六腑除心包络十一经脉证法》说："肾生病，口热舌干，咽肿，上气，嗌干及痛，烦心而痛，黄疸，肠澼，痿厥，腰脊背急痛，嗜卧，足心热而痛，胻酸。"对肾经实热伤津，火盛水亏导致口热舌干、咽肿、腰脊背急痛等病机变化进行了论述。《医学正传•秘结论》也说："夫肾主五液，故肾实则津液足而大便滋润，肾虚则津液竭而大便秘结。原其所由，皆房室过度，...淫欲之火起于命门，以致火盛水亏，津液不生，故传道失常，渐成结燥之证。"精辟地阐述了肾热水亏可致大便秘结的病机。由于热邪炽盛为本，因热伤津，性质属实，故治法宜急下存阴。方药选用《伤寒论》大承气汤（大黄、厚朴、枳实、芒硝）。

Literature Review of Kidney Heat Damaging Liquid

📖 *Shāng Hán Lùn* ("On Cold Damage"), "Identifying Pulse Symptoms and Treatments of Lesser Yīn Disease"

> "When in lesser yīn disease there is spontaneous clear-water diarrhea of pure green-blue color, pain below the heart, and a dry mouth, one can precipitate; therefore *dà chéng qì tāng* (Major Qì-Coordinating Decoction) is appropriate."

In his commentary to this passage, Wāng Yǒu-Líng, one of the *Shāng Hán Lùn* commentators, explained:

> "The viscus of lesser yīn is rooted in water. Extreme heat within the channel forces fluid to run downward and makes the kidney dry. The more dryness there is, the more matter inside the intestines hardens. For this reason, you must precipitate to stop the clear water … Therefore, use *dà chéng qì tāng* (Major Qì-Coordinating Decoction) to precipitate repletion heat evil."

This quotation describes the pattern of emergency precipitation in lesser yīn disease: Because the pathomechanism consists of intense kidney heat damaging yīn, it is treated with *chéng qì tāng* (Qì-Coordinating Decoction), by the method of emergency precipitation to preserve yīn.

🕮 *Zá Bìng Yuán Liú Xī Zhú* ("Incisive Light on the Source of Miscellaneous Disease"), "Origin and Development of Constipation"

> "Constipation is a kidney disease. The classic states that 'black water from the north enters through the kidney, which opens at the two yīn' Since the kidney governs the five humors, exuberant fluids result in harmonized stool. If they are reduced by hunger, overeating, or taxation and overwork; or if habitual predilection for acrid, spicy, and rich foods has caused fire evil to stagnate in the blood, this consumes true yīn and depletes the fluids. This causes the pathocondition of constipation."

While this passages emphasizes how kidney yīn depletion causes constipation, the pathomechanism of intense liver fire damaging kidney yīn is of course included in this.

🕮 *Zhèng Yīn Mài Zhì* ("Pathoconditions: Causes, Pulses, and Treatments"), "Internal Damage Wilting: Kidney Heat Wilting and Limpness"

> "The symptoms of kidney heat wilting and limpness are: inability to raise the lumbar bones, sacrum and coccyx carrying the heel [hypertonicity of the feet], spine carrying the head, failure to support the feet on the ground, and bone wilting with inability to get out of bed. These are the symptoms of kidney heat wilting described in the *Nèi Jīng* ("The Inner Canon").
>
> "The causes of kidney heat wilting and limpness are endless thinking, lascivious ideation, too much sexual intercourse, slackness of the ancestral sinew, as well as taxation fatigue due to distant journeys, exposure to great heat and subsequent thirst, quelling of yáng qì internally, water failing to overcome fire, and water being depleted in the lower body. All these result in kidney heat and then bone wilting."

This quotation explains clearly how exuberant heat in the kidney channel and depletion of water can lead to bone wilting.

文献评述

《伤寒论•辨少阴病脉证并治》曰："少阴病，自利清水，色纯青，心下必痛，口干燥者，可下之，宜大承气汤。"伤寒注家之一的汪友苓注释此条时说："少阴之脏本水，经中热极，则迫水液下流而肾燥，愈燥而肠中之物愈坚，故以下利止清水耳。 ...故以大承气汤下实热之邪。"阐述少阴病有急下证，病机为肾热炽盛伤阴，故以承气汤急下存阴作为治疗大法。

《杂病源流犀烛•大便秘结源流》曰："大便秘结，肾病也。经曰北方黑水，入通于肾，开窍于二阴。盖以肾主五液，津液盛则大便调和。若为饥饱劳役所损，或素嗜辛辣厚味，致火邪留滞血中，耗散真阴，津液亏少，故成便秘之症。"此处虽然重点讨论肾阴亏致便秘，然而肾火炽盛，伤及肾阴的病机自然包含在内。

《症因脉治•内伤痿症•肾热痿软》曰："肾热痿软之症，腰骨不举，尻以代踵，脊以代头，足不任地，骨痿不能起于床，此〈内经〉肾热痿弱之症也。肾热痿软之因，思想无穷，意淫于外，入房太甚，宗筋弛纵，又有远行劳倦，逢大热而渴，阳气内伐，水不胜火，水亏于下，则肾热而骨痿"。对肾经热盛水亏导致骨痿的病机变化作了清晰的阐述。

Summary of Kidney Heat Damaging Liquid

1. Kidney Heat Ascending Counterflow

   Thirst, dry throat.

2. Depletion of Liquid due to Kidney Heat

   Abdominal distention and fullness, inhibited stool, dry bound stool.

3. Heat Bind with Circumfluence

   Spontaneous clear-water diarrhea with stool of pure green-blue color.

4. Heat Damaging the Heart Spirit

   Fatigued spirit-affect.

5. Depletion of Liquid due to Kidney Heat

   Red tongue, dry yellow tongue fur, fine rapid pulse.

肾热津伤
肾热上逆—口渴，咽干而燥
肾热津亏—腹部胀满，大便不利，大便燥结
热结旁流—自利清水，便色纯青
热伤心神—神情疲倦
肾热津亏—舌红苔燥黄，脉细数

6.3 Fire Toxin Congesting the Kidney

The house of the kidney is in the lower back, from where it manages stool and urine. The pathomechanism of fire toxin congesting the kidney can have several causes: Warm-heat toxic evil can invade the kidney channel; sore-toxin from the skin or throat can follow the channel and enter the kidney; or damp-heat brewing in the kidney can ferment into toxin.

Fire toxin congesting the kidney impairs qì transformation and disables the distribution of liquid, injures the blood network vessels, and vanquishes blood and qì. This can manifest in voidings of scant yellow or reddish urine, urine containing blood or occasional pus, or anuria, as well as puffy swelling of the face, eyes, and skin.

If fire toxin accumulates in the lower back, it stops the qì dynamic and obstructs the blood flow. This results in scorching heat and stabbing pain in the lumbar region, and possibly generalized soreness in the skeleton.

If fire toxin follows the channels and suffocates the upper body, this results in redness, swelling, heat, and pain in the throat and in heat effusion with vexation and thirst.

Heat toxin can force the blood to move frenetically and spill out of the vessels. This results in tidal reddening of the skin and possibly purple macules and red papules.

Fire toxin congesting the kidney results in a red or crimson tongue, yellow tongue fur, and a rapid surging pulse.

The chapter, "Master Yú Encountering Epidemic Disease; Systematized Identification of Epidemic Patterns" in the *Wēn Rè Jīng Wěi* ("Warp and Weft of Warm Heat") points out:

> "In cases of pain in the joints when leaning, and a feeling in the lower back as if having been clubbed, since both the bones and lower back belong to the kidney channel, this type of pain means that the qì of excess heat has already flowed into the kidney channel. It is suitable to use the formula *qīng wēn bài dú yǐn* (Scourge-Clearing Toxin-Vanquishing Beverage) with increased amounts of *shí gāo* (Gypsum Fibrosum) and *yuán shēn* (Scrophulariae Radix) and the addition of *huáng bǎi* (Phellodendri Cortex). If you inappropriately treat by warming and dispersing, the patient will die before the morning is over."

This quotation describes in detail how scourge epidemic heat toxin assailing the liver channel manifests in pathomechanical changes like lumbar pain and joint pain.

Fire toxin congesting the kidney is treated by draining fire and resolving toxin. The recommended formula is *qīng wēn bài dú yǐn* (Scourge-Clearing Toxin-Vanquishing Beverage) from the *Yì Zhěn Yī Dé* ("A View of Epidemics Characterized by Papules") with modifications.

Qīng Wēn Bài Dú Yǐn 清瘟败毒饮 Scourge-Clearing Toxin-Vanquishing Beverage
shí gāo (石膏 Gypsum Fibrosum, gypsum)
shēng dì huáng (生地黄 Rehmanniae Radix, dried rehmannia)
zhī zǐ (栀子 Gardeniae Fructus, gardenia)
jié gěng (桔梗 Platycodonis Radix, platycodon)
chì sháo (赤芍 Paeoniae Radix Rubra, red peony)
zhú yè (竹叶 bamboo leaf, Lophatheri Folium)
xī jiǎo (犀角 Rhinocerotis Cornu, rhinoceros horn)
mǔ dān pí (牡丹皮 Moutan Cortex, moutan)
xuán shēn (玄参 Scrophulariae Radix, scrophularia)
zhī mǔ (知母 Anemarrhenae Rhizoma, anemarrhena)
huáng lián (黄连 Coptidis Rhizoma, coptis)
huáng qín (黄芩 Scutellariae Radix, scutellaria)
lián qiào (连翘 Forsythiae Fructus, forsythia)
gān cǎo (甘草 Glycyrrhizae Radix, licorice)
huáng bǎi (黄柏 Phellodendri Cortex, phellodendron)

火毒壅肾

肾之府在腰，司二便。如温热毒邪侵犯于肾经，或皮肤咽喉疮毒循经入肾，或湿热蕴肾酿毒，均可导致火毒壅肾的病机变化。火毒壅肾，气化不行，水津失布，血络受损，血气败坏，可见尿少黄赤，尿血或有脓液，或无尿而面目肌肤浮肿；火毒聚集腰府，气机不通，血行阻滞，则腰部灼热刺痛，或一身骨骼酸痛；火毒循经上熏，则咽喉红肿热痛，发热烦渴；热毒迫血妄行，血溢络外，则皮肤潮红，或紫斑红疹。火毒壅肾，则舌红或绛，苔黄，脉洪数。如《温热经纬•余师愚疫病篇•疫证条辨》指出："骨节倾疼，腰如被杖，骨与腰皆肾经所属，其痛若此，是淫热之气，已流于肾经。宜本方（指清瘟败毒饮）增石膏、元参，加黄柏，误用温散，死不终朝矣。"对瘟疫火毒袭肾经，出现腰痛骨节疼痛等病机变化作了深入地阐述。治法宜泻火解毒。方药选用《疫疹一得》清瘟败毒饮加减（石膏、生地、栀子、桔梗、赤芍、竹叶、犀角、丹皮、玄参、知母、黄连、黄芩、连翘、甘草、黄柏）。

Literature Review of Fire Toxin Congesting the Kidney

📖 *Zhū Bìng Yuán Hòu Lùn* ("Origin and Indicators of Disease"), "Various Symptoms of Urinary Disease: Urinary Stoppage"

> "Urinary stoppage is caused by the presence of heat in both the bladder and the kidney… As soon as the kidney and bladder contract heat, the heat enters the physical bladder, resulting in a great exuberance of hot qì. The resulting binding and roughness causes urinary stoppage."

This quotation points out that excessive exuberance of kidney fire can cause urinary congestion and stoppage.

📖 *Jǐng Yuè Quán Shū* (Jǐng-Yuè's Complete Compendium"), "Schema of Miscellaneous Patterns: Dribbling Urinary Block"

> "In most cases of seminal emission or appearance of blood where repletion fire in the liver and kidney is not cleared, clearing the fire will cause fire to flow freely on its own."

This passage expounds that fire toxin congesting the kidney can lead to blood in the urine.

📖 *Yán Shì Jì Shēng Fāng* ("Yan's Remedies for Curing All People"), "Discussing the Treatment of Water Swelling"

> "In patients of young age, when blood heat engenders sores and transmutes into swelling and fullness, with vexation, thirst, and reduced

urination, this constitutes heat swelling. What the *Sù Wèn* ("Plain Questions") calls binding in yáng refers to this swelling in the four limbs."

This quotation discusses that since the kidney governs water, an internal exuberance of fire toxin and disordered qì transformation can cause puffy swelling and inhibited urination because it prevents fluid from following its normal course, causing it to spill out into the skin instead.

文献评述

《诸病源候论•小便病诸候•小便不通》曰："小便不通，由膀胱与肾俱有热故也。…肾与膀胱既热，热入于胞，热气大盛，故结涩令小便不通。"指出肾火太盛，可使小便闭塞不通。

《景岳全书•杂证谟•癃闭》曰："若肝肾实火不清或遗精或见血者，大都清去其火，水必自通。"论述火毒壅肾可导致尿血的病机变化。

《济生方•水肿门•水肿论治》曰："又有年少，血热生疮，变为肿满，烦渴小便少，此为热肿。<素问>所谓结阳者，肿四肢是也。"论述肾主水，火毒内盛，气化失常，水液不循常道，外溢肌肤，可发为浮肿及小便不利等病机改变。

Summary of Fire Toxin Congesting the Kidney

1. Fire Toxin Congesting the Kidney
   - Voidings of scanty yellow or reddish urine, urine containing blood or occasional pus, or anuria, as well as puffy swelling of the face, eyes, and skin.
   - Red or crimson tongue, yellow tongue fur, rapid surging pulse.
2. Fire Toxin Accumulating in the Lower Back
   - Scorching heat and stabbing pain in the lumbar region, possibly generalized soreness in the skeleton.
3. Fire Toxin Attacking the Upper Body
   - Redness, swelling, heat, and pain in the throat; heat effusion with vexation and thirst.
4. Frenetic Movement of the Blood
   - Tidal reddening of the skin, possibly purple macules and red papules.

火毒壅肾
火毒壅肾—尿少黄赤，尿血或有脓液，或无尿而面目肌肤浮肿
火毒积腰—腰部灼热刺痛，或一身骨骼酸痛
火毒上攻—咽喉红肿热痛，发热烦渴
迫血妄行—皮肤潮红，或紫斑红疹
火毒壅肾—舌红或绛，苔黄，脉洪数

Chapter 7

Kidney Channel Static Blood

The kidney is the root of earlier heaven. When enduring illness is not stopped, it will ultimately always return to the kidney. The movement of qì and blood in the kidney channel can be obstructed as a result of a variety of causes.

It is possible that kidney vacuity and non-transformation of water qì cause water-damp to collect and congest the kidney network vessels. Alternatively, damage to the kidney's yáng qì can prevent it from warming and promoting movement. As a result, qì fails to move the blood, causing stasis obstruction in the kidney network vessels. When the kidney's yīn essence is depleted and loses its ability to enrich, blood becomes thick and turbid and impedes the kidney's network vessels. In other cases, internal damage from the seven affects can depress the qì dynamic, causing qì stagnation, blood stasis, and block in the kidney's network vessels.

Beyond these causes, injuries from metal blades or knocks and falls can damage the kidney's network vessels. Additionally, the external evils of wind, cold, dampness, or heat can lodge in the kidney, damage the blood vessels, and stop the flow of blood, causing stasis obstruction in the kidney network vessels. Finally, if pathological substances like damp-heat, phlegm turbidity, or damp turbidity gather in the body over a long period of time, they can also obstruct the movement of qì and blood in the kidney channel.

All these conditions manifest in the pathological changes of kidney channel static blood. Static blood obstructing the kidney is a repletion disease by nature. Depending on differences in the degree of stasis obstruction, we can further differentiate between the two categories of static blood damaging the lower back and static blood accumulating in the kidney.

肾经瘀血

肾为先天之本，久病不已，穷必归肾。或因肾虚水气不化，水湿停留，壅阻肾络；或肾的阳气损伤，失于温煦、推动，气不行血，瘀阻肾络；或肾的阴精亏损，失于滋养，血液稠浊，阻碍肾络；或因七情内伤，气机郁滞，气滞血瘀，闭塞肾络；或金刃跌打，损伤肾络；或风寒湿热，外邪客肾，伤及血脉，血行不通，瘀阻肾络；或湿热、痰浊、湿浊等病理产物，久聚体内，均能导致肾经气血运行受阻，表现为肾经瘀血的病机变化。瘀血阻肾，病性属实，根据瘀阻的程度不同，又分为瘀血伤腰和瘀血积肾两种病机类型。

7.1 Static Blood Damaging the Lower Back

The lower back is the house of the kidney. Knocks and falls, qì damage from fury and anger, and accumulations of pathological substances can all inhibit the flow of blood and qì in the kidney channel. This can manifest in the pathomechanism of static blood damaging the lower back.

When static blood obstructs the kidney channel in the lower back, qì and blood cannot flow freely. This causes lumbar pain that is stabbing, fixed in location, and exacerbated by pressure.

When blood congeals and stagnates in the channels, it damages the sinews. In mild cases, this results in inhibited bending forward and backward; in serious cases, it results in severe pain with inability to turn sides.

Because yáng qì is more exuberant during the day, the movement of blood is forceful and the lumbar pain is still bearable. At night, however, yīn qì is unilaterally exuberant, yáng is weak, and the movement of blood slows down, which aggravates the stasis accumulation of blood. Thus, this situation manifests in lumbar pain that is milder during the day and more severe at night.

Static blood damaging the kidney manifests in a dark purple tongue, possibly with stasis macules or stasis speckles, and a rough pulse.

The chapter, "Various Symptoms of Disease in the Back and lower back; Sudden Lumbar Pain" in the *Zhū Bìng Yuán Hòu Lùn* ("Origin and Indicators of Disease") states:

> "Sudden lumbar pain... refers to sudden pain due to damage to the lower back. This condition is caused by detriment to blood affecting the back and spine. If left untreated for a long period of time, it causes the patient to suffer from reduced breathing and have a colorless facial complexion, because of detriment to the kidney."

This quotation clearly indicates the pathomechanism by which external damage that involves the lower back and kidney leads to static blood and lumbar pain.

The chapter, "Origin and Development of Lumbar and Umbilical Disease" in the *Zá Bìng Yuán Liú Xī Zhú* ("Incisive Light on the Source of Miscellaneous Disease") points out:

> "Pain in the lower back is a disease caused by a vacuity of essential qì and evil settling in. … Kidney vacuity is its root. Wind, cold, dampness, heat, phlegm, rheum, qì stagnation, blood stasis, and wrenching and contusion are its tip.... Pain from dead blood is shifting and moving and feels like being stabbed with an awl or knife, accompanied by black stool, either yellow or black urine, symptoms that are milder during the day and more severe at night, and invariably a scallion-stalk pulse. Pain from wrenching, contusion, and falls is invariably severe. It should be treated with *rǔ xiāng chèn tòng sàn* (Olibanum Pain-Alleviating Powder) with the addition of *quán xiē* (Scorpio) for even faster efficacy. If this fails to show results, it is bound to be a condition of malign blood."

This is a detailed description of the pathomechanism by which static blood damages the kidney and causes lumbar pain. It also suggests that a root vacuity and tip repletion are the essence of this condition.

Static blood damaging the lower back is treated by quickening the blood and transforming stasis, and by rectifying qì and relieving pain. The recommended formula is *hēi niú xù dì yǐn* (Sojae and Achyranthis to Prolong Earth Beverage) from the *Gù Shì Yī Jìng* ("Master Gu's Reflections on Medicine") with the addition of *dān shēn* (Salviae Miltiorrhizae Radix), *rǔ xiāng* (Olibanum), *mò yào* (Myrrha), *táo rén* (Persicae Semen), and *dà huáng* (Rhei Radix et Rhizoma).

Hēi Niú Xù Dì Yǐn 黑牛续地饮
Black Bean and Achyranthes to Prolong Earth Beverage

hēi dòu (黑豆 Sojae Semen Atrum, black soybean)
niú xī (牛膝 Achyranthis Bidentatae Radix, achyranthes)
xù duàn (续断 Dipsaci Radix, dipsacus)
shēng dì huáng (生地黄 Rehmanniae Radix, dried rehmannia)
dāng guī (当归 Angelicae Sinensis Radix, Chinese angelica)
xuán hú (玄胡 Corydalis Rhizoma, corydalis)
mǔ dān pí (牡丹皮 Moutan Cortex, moutan)
chì sháo (赤芍 Paeoniae Radix Rubra, red peony)

Plus:

dān shēn (丹参 Salviae Miltiorrhizae Radix, salvia)
rǔ xiāng (乳香 Olibanum, frankincense)
mò yào (没药 Myrrha, myrrh)
táo rén (桃仁 Persicae Semen, peach kernel)
dà huáng (大黄 Rhei Radix et Rhizoma, rhubarb)

Alternatively, choose *rǔ xiāng chèn tòng sàn* (Olibanum Pain-Alleviating Powder) from the *Zá Bìng Yuán Liú Xī Zhú* ("Incisive Light on the Source of Miscellaneous Disease") with modifications.

Rǔ Xiāng Chèn Tòng Sàn 乳香趁痛散
Olibanum Pain-Alleviating Powder

guī bǎn (龟版 Testudinis Plastrum, tortoise plastron)
chì sháo (赤芍 Paeoniae Radix Rubra, red peony)
rǔ xiāng (乳香 Olibanum, frankincense)
mò yào (没药 Myrrha, myrrh)
dāng guī (当归 Angelicae Sinensis Radix, Chinese angelica)
fáng fēng (防风 Saposhnikoviae Radix, saposhnikovia)
xuè jié (血竭 Daemonoropis Resina, dragon's blood)
ròu guì (肉桂 Cinnamomi Cortex, cinnamon bark)
bái zhǐ (白芷 Angelicae Dahuricae Radix, Dahurian angelica)
niú xī (牛膝 Achyranthis Bidentatae Radix, achyranthes)
tiān má (天麻 Gastrodiae Rhizoma, gastrodia)
qiāng huó (羌活 Notopterygii Rhizoma et Radix, notopterygium)
bīng láng (槟榔 Arecae Semen, areca)
hǔ gǔ (虎骨 Tigris Os, tiger bone)
zì rán tóng (自然铜 Pyritum, pyrite)
bái fù zǐ (白附子 Typhonii Gigantei Rhizoma, giant typhonium rhizome)
cāng ěr zǐ (苍耳子 Xanthii Fructus, xanthium)
bǔ gǔ zhī (补骨脂 Psoraleae Fructus, psoralea)
wǔ jiā pí (五加皮 Acanthopanacis Cortex, acanthopanax)

瘀血伤腰

腰为肾之府，或因跌打损伤，或因恼怒伤气，或因病理产物堆积不去，引起肾经气血流通不畅，可出现瘀血伤腰的病机变化。瘀血阻滞肾经腰府，气血不能畅通，故腰痛如刺，痛有定处，按之痛甚；血脉凝滞，筋脉损伤，故轻则俯仰不便，重则痛剧不能转侧；白天阳气较盛，血行有力，腰痛尚能忍受，夜里阴气偏盛，阳弱运血缓慢，血液瘀积加重，故表现为腰痛日轻夜重。瘀血伤肾，则舌质紫暗，或有瘀斑、瘀点，脉涩。如《诸病源候论•腰背病诸候•既月腰候》曰："既月（音桂，骤然之意）腰者，谓卒然伤损于腰而致痛也，此由损血搏于背脊所为，久不已，令人气息乏少，而无颜色，损肾故也。"明确指出了外伤累及腰肾而引起瘀血腰痛的病机。《杂病源流犀烛•腰脐病源流》指出："腰痛，精气虚而邪客病也。…肾虚其本也，风寒湿热痰饮，气滞血瘀闪挫其标也。…死血痛者，转动如锥刀之刺，大便黑，小便或黄或黑，日轻夜重，脉必芤。闪挫跌扑痛者，痛必甚，宜乳香趁痛散，加全蝎效更速，不效，必有恶血。"亦详细论述了瘀血伤肾而致腰痛的病机，并认为其实质为本虚标实。治法宜活血化瘀，理气止痛。方药选用《顾氏医镜》黑牛续地饮（黑豆、牛膝、续断、生地、当归、玄胡、丹皮、赤芍）加丹参、乳香、没药、桃仁、大黄。或选用《杂病源流犀烛》乳香趁痛散（龟板、赤芍、乳香、没药、当归、防风、血竭、肉桂、白芷、牛膝、天麻、羌活、槟榔、虎骨、自然铜、白附子、苍耳、补骨脂、五加皮）加减。

Literature Review of Static Blood Damaging the Lower Back

📖 *Zhèng Yīn Mài Zhì* ("Pathoconditions: Causes, Pulses, and Treatments"), "Internal Damage Lumbar Pain"

> "The symptoms of internal damage lumbar pain are pain that is milder during the day and more severe at night, fixed in one location, and accompanied by inability to turn sides. …The causes of internal damage lumbar pain are wrenching and contusion, falls, and damage from physical taxation, resulting in lumbar and abdominal pain. …The pulse of internal damage lumbar pain is rough and scallion-stalk at the cubit. This is the diagnosis of static blood."

This quotation describes the disease causes, symptoms, and pulse manifestation of static blood lumbar pain.

📖 *Yī Xué Xīn Wù* ("Medical Insights"), "Lumbar Pain"

> "If wrenching, contusion, or falls have caused stasis accumulation in the body, which manifests in pain as if stabbed with a knife or awl when turning sides, black stool, and a rough or scallion-stalk pulse, this indicates static blood. *Zé lán tāng* (Lycopus Decoction) governs it."

This quotation clearly points out the pathomechanism of static blood lumbar pain caused by external damage.

📖 *Qī Sōng Yán Jí* ("Records of *Qī Sōng-Yán*"), "Lumbar Pain"

> "The condition referred to as lumbar pain … is not a case of repletion in the viscus of the kidney itself, but in the network and blood vessels in both sides of the lower back. It is caused by an invasion of wind, cold, dampness, or heat, or by impairment from injury within the cavity in the lower back, or by dampness, phlegm, or static blood congealing and stopping, causing pain. …In cases of knocks and falls, dead blood accumulates, causing pain during the day and at night and a rapid scallion-stalk pulse. This is righted by quickening blood and transforming stasis."

This quotation discusses how a variety of causes can result in static blood damaging the kidney and subsequent lumbar pain.

文献评述

《症因脉治•内伤腰痛》曰："内伤腰痛之症，日轻夜重，痛定一处，不能转侧。…内伤腰痛之因，挫闪跌扑，劳动损伤，则腰腹作痛。…内伤腰痛之脉，尺脉芤涩，瘀血之诊。"阐述了瘀血腰痛的病因症状及脉象变化。

《医学心悟•腰痛》曰："若因闪挫跌仆，瘀积于内，转侧如刀锥之刺，大便黑色，脉涩，或芤者，瘀血也，泽兰汤主之"。明确指出外伤所致瘀血腰痛的病机。

《七松岩集•腰痛》曰："所谓腰痛者，…非肾家自实，是两腰经络血脉之中，为风寒湿热之所侵，闪肭锉气（指闪扭锉伤）之所碍，腰内空腔之中，为湿痰瘀血凝滞不通而为痛。…如跌打损伤，死血瘀积，日夜作痛，其脉芤数，以活血化瘀为主。"论述多种原因引起瘀血伤肾而致腰痛的病机变化。

Summary of Static Blood Damaging the Lower Back
1. Static Blood Obstruction Lumbar pain as if stabbed, stasis in a fixed location, and pain exacerbated by pressure.
2. Damage to the Sinews In mild cases, inhibited bending forward and backward; in serious cases, severe pain with inability to turn sides.
3. Yīn Exuberance Intensifying the Stasis Lumbar pain that is milder during the day and more severe at night.
4. Static Blood Damaging the Kidney Dark purple tongue, possibly with stasis macules or stasis speckles, rough pulse.

瘀血伤腰
瘀血阻滞—腰痛如刺，瘀有定处，按之则痛甚
损伤筋脉—轻则俯仰不便，重则痛剧不能转侧
阴盛瘀重—腰痛日轻夜重
瘀血伤肾—舌质紫暗，或有瘀斑、瘀点，脉涩

7.2 Static Blood Accumulating in the Kidney

Only when qì and blood move incessantly within the kidney is the kidney able to guarantee that kidney essence is abundant, that kidney qì is exuberant, and that liquid is distributed throughout the body, thereby maintaining the normal physiological functions of the body. If the free flow of kidney qì is inhibited, qì fails to move blood, and qì and blood stagnate, accumulate within the kidney, and surge upward or downward. This can manifest in the pathomechanism of static blood accumulating in the kidney.

When static blood collects in the kidney, qì is unable to penetrate, blood is unable to move, and channel qì is stopped. This manifests in stabbing pain in the lumbar region and abdominal fullness stretching to the back, or aching pain in the lumbar region and abdominal distention.

When the qì that has accumulated in the kidney surges upward and downward and is unable to remain quiet, this manifests in swelling in the lesser abdomen that extends upward to below the heart, is painful upon breathing, and resembles a running piglet in appearance.

Static blood accumulating in the kidney manifests in a dark purple tongue, possibly with stasis macules, and a stringlike or rough pulse.

The term "running piglet" first occurred in the *Nèi Jīng* ("The Inner Canon"). The chapter, "Forms of Disease from Evil Qì in the Viscera and Bowels" in the *Líng Shū* ("The Magic Pivot") states: "When the kidney pulse... is slightly urgent, it means deep reversal, running piglet, loss of use of the legs, and inability to urinate or defecate." Subsequently, this condition was referred to by different names, such as "kidney accumulation running piglet" in the *Nàn Jīng* ("The Classic of Difficult Issues"), "surging mounting" in the *Nèi Jīng* ("The Inner Canon"), and "running piglet qì" in the *Jīn Guì Yào Lüe* ("Essential Prescriptions of the Golden Coffer"). This has blurred and confused the notion of "running piglet" for physicians over the ages.

Essentially, running piglet can be classified as three types: kidney accumulation running piglet, surging mounting running piglet, and running piglet qì. Although their pathomechanisms are not completely identical, what is described here is that of kidney accumulation running piglet.

The "Fifty-Sixth Difficult Issue" in the *Nàn Jīng* ("The Classic of Difficult Issues") states:

> "Accumulation in the kidney is called 'running piglet.' It begins in the lesser abdomen, extends upward to below the heart, resembles a piglet, and surges upward or downward at any time. If the condition endures for a long period of time, it causes the patient to suffer from panting counterflow, bone wilting, and shortage of qì. It is contracted in the summer on *bǐng* and *dīng* days." [the third and fourth days of summer]."

This text sets forth that running piglet is caused by kidney qì vacuity, by phlegm and static blood binding together in the abdominal cavity, and by an inhibited movement of the qì dynamic. Thus, it certainly recognizes the pathomechanism of static blood accumulating in the kidney and erupting as running piglet.

This condition is treated by quickening the blood and dispelling stasis, and by moving qì and relieving pain. The recommended formula is *bēn tún tāng* (Running Piglet Decoction) from the *Zá Bìng Yuán Liú Xī Zhú* ("Incisive Light on the Source of Miscellaneous Disease") adjusted by eliminating *shēng jiāng* (Zingiberis Rhizoma Recens) and *dà zǎo* (Jujubae Fructus) and adding *huái niú xī* (Achyranthis Bidentatae Radix), *tù sī zǐ* (Cuscutae Semen), and *bǔ gǔ zhī* (Psoraleae Fructus).

Bēn Tún Tāng 奔豚汤
Running Piglet Decoction

bàn xià (半夏 Pinelliae Rhizoma, pinellia)
chuān xiōng (川芎 Chuanxiong Rhizoma, chuanxiong)
dāng guī (当归 Angelicae Sinensis Radix, Chinese angelica)
gān lǐ gēn pí (甘李根皮 Pruni Salicinae Radicis Cortex, plum root bark)
gān gēn (干葛 Puerariae Radix, pueraria)
huáng qín (黄芩 Scutellariae Radix, scutellaria)
bái sháo (白芍 Paeoniae Radix Alba, white peony)
shēng jiāng (生姜 Zingiberis Rhizoma Recens, fresh ginger)
dà zǎo (大枣 Jujubae Fructus, jujube)
gān cǎo (甘草 Glycyrrhizae Radix, licorice)

Minus:
shēng jiāng (生姜 Zingiberis Rhizoma Recens, fresh ginger)
dà zǎo (大枣 Jujubae Fructus, jujube)

Plus:
niú xī (牛膝 Achyranthis Bidentatae Radix, achyranthes)
tù sī zǐ (菟丝子 Cuscutae Semen, cuscuta)
bǔ gǔ zhī (补骨脂 Psoraleae Fructus, psoralea)

瘀血积肾

肾脏之中，气血运行不息，才能保证肾精充沛，肾气旺盛，水津四布，维持人体正常生理功能。若肾气不畅，气不行血，气血瘀滞，积于肾中，上下攻冲，则可出现瘀血积肾的病机变化。瘀血停积于肾，气不得走，血不得行，经气不通，则表现为腰部刺痛，腹满引背，或为腰部酸痛，腹部胀大；肾之积气上下攻冲，不得安宁，则表现为肿块发于少腹，上至心下，随呼吸而痛，如豚奔之状。瘀血积肾，则舌质紫暗，或有瘀斑，脉弦或涩。奔豚之名首见于《内经》，《灵枢•邪气脏腑病形篇》曰："肾脉 ...微急，为沉厥、奔豚、足不收、不得前后。"其后，因《难经》之"肾积奔豚"、《内经》之"冲疝"、《金匮》之"奔豚气"等病名的不同，使历代医家对"奔豚"的概念模糊不清，混淆视听。实际上归纳而言，奔豚可分为肾积奔豚、冲疝奔豚、及奔豚气病等三种类型，其病机变化不尽相同，此条所述仅限于肾积奔豚。如《难经•五十六难》曰：“肾之积，名曰奔豚，发于少腹，上至心下，若豚状，或上或下无时，久不已，令人喘逆，骨痿少气，以夏丙丁日得之。”认为是肾气虚衰，痰瘀互结于腹腔内，气机运行不畅所致。对瘀血积肾，发为奔豚的病机有一定的认识。治则为活血祛瘀，行气止痛。方药选用《杂病源流犀烛》奔豚汤（半夏、川芎、当归、甘李根皮、干葛、黄芩、白芍、生姜、大枣、甘草）去生姜、大枣，加怀牛膝、菟丝子、补骨脂。

Literature Review of Static Blood Accumulating in the Kidney

📖 *Jīn Guì Yào Lüe* (“Essential Prescriptions of the Golden Coffer”), “Pulse Symptoms and Treatments of Running Piglet Qì”

> “Kidney accumulation running piglet refers to suffering from accumulation lumps in the lesser abdomen that manifest with pain extending from the diseased region upward to below the heart at the onset of an episode, intermittent surges upward or downward, and accumulation lumps that endure after the episode is over.”

This quotation clearly indicates that kidney accumulation running piglet is caused by static blood accumulation lumps.

📖 *Zhèng Zhì Huì Bǔ* (“Combined Supplements to Patterns and Treatment”), “Accumulations and Gatherings: Names of Accumulations in the Five Viscera”

> “Kidney accumulation, called ‘running piglet,’ begins in the lesser abdomen, rises up to below the heart, and resembles a running piglet in appearance. If not cured for a long time, it causes the patient to suffer from panting counterflow, bone wilting, and shortage of qì.”

This quotation describes the pathomechanism by which static blood in the kidney channel erupts as running piglet.

文献评述

《金匮要略选读•奔豚气病脉证治》曰：“肾积奔豚是少腹素有积块，在发作时，其痛从病部上至心下，或上下无时，发作后积块仍在。”明确指出了肾积奔豚，是由瘀血积块所致。

《证治汇补•积聚•五脏积名》曰："肾积曰奔豚，发于少腹，上至心，如豚奔走状。久不愈，令人喘逆，骨痿少气。"阐述了肾经瘀血，发为奔豚的病机变化。

Summary of Static Blood Accumulating in the Kidney
1. Qì and Blood Stasis in the Kidney Stabbing pain in the lumbar region, abdominal fullness stretching to the back, or aching pain in the lumbar region, and abdominal distention. 2. Surging Attacks of Accumulated Qì Swelling in the lesser abdomen, extending upward to below the heart, resembling a running piglet in appearance, pain upon breathing. 3. Static Blood Accumulating in the Kidney Dark purple tongue, possibly with stasis macules, stringlike or rough pulse.

瘀血积肾
气血瘀肾—腰部刺痛，腹满引背，或为腰部酸痛，腹部胀大 积气攻冲—肿块发于少腹，上至心下，随呼吸而痛，如豚奔之状 瘀血积肾—舌质紫暗，或有瘀斑，脉弦或涩

Chapter Eight

Kidney Channel Phlegm Turbidity

The kidney governs water, and when kidney qì is weak, the fluid metabolism becomes abnormal. As a result, gathering dampness can engender phlegm, or phlegm turbidity can arise internally, both of which can then pour into the kidney. Alternatively, when a body with a constitutional exuberance of internal phlegm-damp in addition contracts external dampness, the two kinds of dampness can combine, pour into the kidney channel, and in heavy accumulation form phlegm. Alternatively, if spleen qì is habitually depleted, phlegm turbidity can arise internally and since upbearing and downbearing are disordered, collect in the kidney channel, forming the pathomechanism of kidney channel phlegm turbidity.

Phlegm is a yīn evil and when it congeals in the kidney channel, it can easily damage yáng qì. This results in cold pain and heaviness in the lumbar region and in pain stretching to the back and rib-side, which are aggravated on rainy overcast days.

If phlegm and dampness binds together and enter the blood before transforming into heat, the result is painful spots where the skin color has not changed and swelling of the lumbar region.

Phlegm brewing in the spleen and stomach impairs movement and transformation by the spleen, which results in torpid food intake, nausea and desire to retch, and diarrhea with thin sloppy stool.

When phlegm turbidity invades the upper body, and clear yáng fails to bear upward, dizzy head and tinnitus result.

Phlegm turbidity obstructing the kidney manifests in a slimy white tongue fur, a fat pale tongue, and a stringlike slippery pulse.

The chapter, "Types of Dampness; Lumbar Pain" in the *Yī Xué Rù Mén* ("The Gateway to Medicine") explains:

> "In cases of damp phlegm streaming into the channels and network vessels, which manifests in pain in the back and rib-side and a slippery pulse, *èr chén tāng* (Two Matured Ingredients Decoction) with the addition of *nán xīng* (Arisaematis Rhizoma), *cāng zhú* (Atractylodis Rhizoma), and *huáng bǎi* (Phellodendri Cortex) is recommended."

The chapter, "Internal Damage Lumbar Pain" in the *Zhèng Yīn Mài Zhì* ("Pathoconditions: Causes, Pulses, and Treatments") also explains:

> "Heaviness and stagnation in the lumbar region and a sensation like from a piece of ice, which is slightly relieved when exposed to heat, but greatly aggravated when exposed to cold, these are the symptoms of pain from phlegm streaming into the lower back."

Both these quotations describe how phlegm turbidity invading the kidney channel and congealing in the lower back leads to lumbar pain.

Kidney channel phlegm turbidity is treated by dispelling dampness and transforming phlegm, and by rectifying qì and quieting the lower back. The recommended formula is *dǎo tán tāng* (Phlegm-Abducting Decoction) from the *Yán Shì Jì Shēng Fāng* ("Yan's Remedies for Curing All People"), with the addition of *xiāng fù* (Cyperi Rhizoma), *tái wū* (Linderae Radix), *cāng zhú* (Atractylodis Rhizoma), and *bái jiè zǐ* (Sinapis Albae Semen).

Dǎo Tán Tāng 导痰汤
Phlegm-Abducting Decoction

bàn xià (半夏 Pinelliae Rhizoma, pinellia)
fú líng (茯苓 Poria, poria)
chén pí (陈皮 Citri Reticulatae Pericarpium, tangerine peel)
nán xīng (南星 Arisaematis Rhizoma, arisaema)
zhǐ shí (枳实 Aurantii Fructus Immaturus, unripe bitter orange)
gān cǎo (甘草 Glycyrrhizae Radix, licorice)

Plus:

xiāng fù (香附 Cyperi Rhizoma, cyperus)
tái wū (台乌 Linderae Radix, lindera)
cāng zhú (苍术 Atractylodis Rhizoma, atractylodes)
bái jiè zǐ (白芥子 Sinapis Albae Semen, white mustard)

Alternatively, use *guī shū wán* (Tortoise Shell and Ailanthus Bark Pill) from the *Yī Xué Rù Mén* ("The Gateway to Medicine"), with the addition of *fáng jǐ* (Stephaniae Tetrandrae Radix), *hǎi fēng téng* (Piperis Kadsurae Caulis), *sāng zhī* (Mori Ramulus), *luò shí téng* (Trachelospermi Caulis), *bái zhú* (Atractylodis Macrocephalae Rhizoma), *bái kòu* (Amomi Fructus Rotundus), and *shā rén* (Amomi Fructus).

Guī Shū Wán 龟樗丸
Tortoise Shell and Ailanthus Bark Pill

guī bǎn (龟版 Testudinis Plastrum, tortoise plastron)
shū bái pí (樗白皮, Ailanthi Altissimae (Radicis) Cortex, ailanthus (root) bark)
cāng ěr zǐ (苍耳子 Xanthii Fructus, xanthium)
huá shí (滑石 Talcum, talcum)
bái sháo (白芍 Paeoniae Radix Alba, white peony)
xiāng fù (香附 Cyperi Rhizoma, cyperus)
Plus:
fáng jǐ (防己 Stephaniae Tetrandrae Radix, fangji)
hǎi fēng téng (海风藤 Piperis Kadsurae Caulis, kadsura pepper stem)
sāng zhī (桑枝 Mori Ramulus, mulberry twig)
luò shí téng (络石藤 Trachelospermi Caulis, star jasmine stem)
bái zhú (白术 Atractylodis Macrocephalae Rhizoma, white atractylodes)
bái dòu kòu (白豆蔻 Amomi Fructus Rotundus, cardamom)
shā rén (砂仁 Amomi Fructus, amomum)

肾经痰浊

肾主水，肾气虚弱，水液代谢异常，可以聚湿生痰，痰浊内生又可流注于肾；或平素痰湿内盛之体，复感外湿，两湿相合，流注肾经，沉积为痰；或脾气素亏，痰浊内生，升降失调，停留肾经，形成肾经痰浊的病机变化。痰为阴邪，凝滞肾经，易伤阳气，则腰部冷痛沉重，痛引背胁，阴雨天加重；痰湿互结，未化热入血，则痛处皮色不变，腰部肿胀；痰蕴脾胃，脾失健运，则纳食呆顿，恶心欲呕，便泄溏稀；痰浊上犯，清阳不升，则头晕耳鸣。痰浊阻腰，则苔白腻，舌淡胖，脉弦滑。如《医学入门•湿类•腰痛》说："湿痰流注经络，背胁疼痛，脉滑者，二陈汤加南星、苍术、黄柏。"《症因脉治•内伤腰痛》也说："腰间重滞，一片如冰，得热减寒，得寒愈甚，此痰注腰痛之症”均论述了痰浊侵犯肾经，凝滞腰府，引起腰痛的病机变化。治法宜祛湿化痰，理气安腰。方药选用《济生方》导痰汤（半夏、茯苓、陈皮、南星、枳实、甘草）加香附、台乌、苍术、白芥子。或用《医学入门》龟樗（樗，音 chu，指臭椿树）丸（龟板、樗白皮、苍术、滑石、白芍、香附）加防己、海风藤、桑枝、络石藤，白术、白蔻、砂仁。

Literature Review of Kidney Channel Phlegm Turbidity

📖 *Dān Xī Xīn Fǎ* ("Dān Xī's Heart-Approach"), "Dizzy Head"

> "Dizziness in the head indicates phlegm complicated by qì vacuity and fire. Make treating phlegm your first priority... Dizziness cannot not arise without there being phlegm, and phlegm simply stirs because of fire. Furthermore, there are cases of damp phlegm and of fire phlegm."

This passage describes how phlegm turbidity can cause the pathological change of dizzy head and vision.

📖 *Jǐng Yuè Quán Shū* ("Jǐng-Yuè's Complete Compendium"), "Schema of Miscellaneous Patterns: Phlegm-Rheum"

> "Although disease in any of the five viscera can equally engender phlegm, invariably it is caused by the spleen and kidney. The spleen governs dampness, and when dampness stirs, it causes phlegm. The kidney governs water, and when water floods, this also causes phlegm. Thus the transformation of phlegm is always found in the spleen, and the root of phlegm is always found in the kidney. For this reason, all phlegm patterns invariably involve these two viscera…
>
> "If there is phlegm in the kidney, it is invariably a case of vacuity. When fire fails to engender earth, this means that fire fails to restrain water. When yáng fails to prevail over yīn, water invariably invades the spleen. All this means that fire within yīn is vacuous. …If there is phlegm in the kidney channel, this is phlegm that is caused by water flooding. It is also invariably a vacuity pattern. In cases of swelling engendering phlegm, this means that water has entered the spleen channel, which is called reverse restraint."

This quotation describes how phlegm turbidity in the kidney channel is completely due to kidney vacuity.

📖 *Yī Xué Xīn Wù* ("Medical Insights"), "Lumbar Pain"

> "Swelling of the lumbar region that feels soggy and soft and not painful when pressure is applied and a slippery pulse indicate phlegm. *Èr chén tāng* (Two Matured Ingredients Decoction) with the addition of *bái zhú* (Atractylodis Macrocephalae Rhizoma), *bì xiè* (Dioscoreae Hypoglaucae

> seu Semptemlobae Rhizoma), *bái jiè zǐ* (Sinapis Albae Semen), *zhú lì* (Bambusae Succus), and *jiāng zhī* (Zingiberis Rhizomatis Succus) governs it."

This quotation indicates how phlegm-turbidity invading the kidney's house leads to swelling in the lumbar region.

文献评述

《丹溪心法•头眩》曰："头眩，痰挟气虚并火，治痰为主，…无痰不作眩，痰因火动，又有湿痰者，有火痰者。"论述了痰浊可致头晕目眩的病机变化。

《景岳全书•杂证谟•痰饮》曰："五脏之病，虽俱能生痰，然无不由乎脾肾。盖脾主湿，湿动则为痰，肾主水，水泛亦为痰，故痰之化无不在脾，而痰之本无不在肾，所以凡是痰证，非此则被，必与二脏有涉。…若肾家之痰，则无非虚耳。盖火不生土者，即火不制水，阳不胜阴者，必水反侵脾，是皆阴中之火虚也；…肾经之痰，水泛为痰者也，无非虚证。有以肿胀而生痰者，此水入脾经，谓之反克。"认为肾经痰浊全由肾虚所致。

《医学心悟•腰痛》曰："腰间肿，按之濡软不痛，脉滑者，痰也，二陈汤加白术、萆薢、白芥子、竹沥、姜汁主之。"指出了痰浊侵犯肾府，导致腰府肿胀的病机变化。

Summary of Kidney Channel Phlegm Turbidity

1. Phlegm Congealing in the Kidney Channel

   Cold pain and heaviness in the lumbar region, pain stretching to the back and rib-side, aggravated symptoms on rainy overcast days.

2. Phlegm Brewing in the Kidney and Spleen

   Torpid food intake, nausea and desire to retch, diarrhea with thin sloppy stool.

3. Phlegm and Dampness Binding Together

   Painful spots where the skin color has not changed, swelling of the lumbar region.

4. Phlegm Turbidity Invading the Upper Body

   Dizzy head and tinnitus.

5. Phlegm Turbidity Obstructing the Lower Back

   Slimy white tongue fur, fat pale tongue, stringlike slippery pulse.

肾经痰浊
痰凝肾经—腰部冷痛沉重，痛引背胁，阴雨天加重
痰蕴脾胃—纳食呆顿，恶心欲呕，便泄溏稀
痰湿互结—痛处皮色不变，腰部肿胀
痰浊上犯—头晕耳鸣
痰浊阻腰—苔白腻，舌淡胖，脉弦滑

Chapter Nine

Kidney Channel Stones

The kidney controls urine and stool, governs water, and is closely related to the fluid metabolism. In case of increased consumption of acrid, hot, fatty, and sweet foods or excessive fondness of liquor, these can brew and form damp-heat, which accumulates in the kidney, streams downward into the bladder, and boils the urine. If this continues for days and months, impurities within the urine can gradually accumulate and form stones. These collect in and obstruct the kidney, resulting in the pathomechanism of kidney channel stones.

When these stones obstruct the kidney, qì and blood are stopped. As a result, we may observe gripping pain within the kidney, or aching lower back as if it were breaking.

An enduring accumulation of stones damages the network vessels in the kidney viscus, which manifests in bloody urine. When stones collect internally and obstruct the urinary tract, this manifests in urinary frequency, urgency, or block.

Damp-heat boiling in the kidney manifests in a dark red tongue, slimy yellow tongue fur, and a rough sunken or slippery rapid pulse.

The chapter, "Symptoms of Strangury; Stone Strangury" in the *Zhū Bìng Yuán Hòu Lùn* ("Origin and Indicators of Disease") states:

> "Stone strangury is strangury with discharge of stones. The kidney governs water, and when water is bound, it transforms into stones, which therefore settle in the kidney. When the kidney is vacuous, this is exploited by heat, and heat results in strangury. This disease manifests in pain in the penis after urination, sudden inability to discharge urine, pain stretching to the lesser abdomen, urgency within the bladder, and discharge of stones from the urinary tract."

This quotation describes how heat evil damaging the kidney leads to stones.

The "Section on Urine; Discussing Treatment of Strangury and Disinhibition" in the *Yán Shì Jì Shēng Fāng* ("Yan's Remedies for Curing All People") also explains:

> "The disease of stone strangury manifests with pain in the penis and sudden inability to discharge urine… Indulgence in improper leisure or forced excessive labor taxes and damages the kidney channel and causes heat in the kidney. The heat lodged in the kidney can flow into the bladder, consequently forming the disease of strangury."

This quotation discusses in detail the formation and progression of kidney channel stones, while also explaining that damp-heat fire toxin is a contributing factor to kidney channel stones.

Kidney channel stones are treated by clearing heat and transforming stones, and by disinhibiting urine and freeing strangury. The recommended formula is *wǔ lín sǎn* (Five Stranguries Powder) from the *Tài Píng Huì Mín Hé Jì Jú Fāng* ("Tài-Píng Imperial Grace Pharmacy Formulas"), or *shí wéi sǎn* (Pyrrosia Powder) from the *Zhèng Zhì Huì Bǔ* ("Combined Supplements to Patterns and Treatment") with the addition of *jīn qián cǎo* (Lysimachiae Herba), *hǎi jīn shā* (Lygodii Spora), *jī nèi jīn* (Galli Gigeriae Endothelium Corneum), *pāo shān jiǎ* (quick fried Manis Squama), *shēng mǔ lì* (Ostreae Concha Cruda), *hǔ pò* (Succinum), and *shí hú* (Dendrobii Herba).

Wǔ Lín Sǎn 五淋汤 Five Stranguries Powder
chì fú líng (赤茯苓 Poria Rubra, red poria)
sháo yào (芍药 Paeoniae Radix, peony)
zhī zǐ (栀子 Gardeniae Fructus, gardenia)
dāng guī (当归 Angelicae Sinensis Radix, Chinese angelica)
gān cǎo (甘草 Glycyrrhizae Radix, licorice)

Shí Wéi Sǎn 石苇散 Pyrrosia Powder
shí wéi (石韦 Pyrrosiae Folium, pyrrosia)
dōng kuí zǐ (冬葵子 Malvae Semen, mallow seed)
qú mài (瞿麦 Dianthi Herba, dianthus)
huá shí (滑石 Talcum, talcum)
chē qián zǐ (车前子 Plantaginis Semen, plantago seed)

Plus:

jīn qián cǎo (金钱草 Lysimachiae Herba, moneywort)
hǎi jīn shā (海金沙 Lygodii Spora, lygodium spore)
jī nèi jīn (鸡内金 Galli Gigeriae Endothelium Corneum, gizzard lining)
chuān shān jiǎ (穿山甲 Manis Squama, pangolin scales)
mǔ lì (牡蛎 Ostreae Concha, oyster shell)
hǔ pò (琥珀 Succinum, amber)
shí hú (石斛 Dendrobii Herba, dendrobium)

肾经砂石

肾司二便，主水，与水液代谢有密切关系。如多食辛热肥甘之品，或嗜酒太过，酿成湿热，蕴积于肾，下流膀胱，煎熬尿液，日积月累，尿中杂质逐渐累积成石，停留阻滞于肾，引起肾经砂石的病机变化。砂石阻塞肾中，气血不通，则可见肾中绞痛，或腰酸如折；砂石积久，损伤肾脏络脉，则可见血尿；砂石内停，阻塞尿路，则出现尿频，尿急或尿闭。肾中湿热煎熬，则舌质暗红，苔黄腻，脉沉涩或滑数。如《诸病源候论•淋病诸候•石淋候》曰："石淋者，淋而出石也。肾主水，水结则化为石，故肾客沙石。肾虚为热所乘，热则成淋。其病之状，小便则茎里痛，尿不能卒出，痛引少腹，膀胱里急，沙石从小便道出。"论述了热邪伤肾，导致砂石的病机变化。《济生方•小便门•淋利论治》也说："石淋为病，茎中痛，溺卒不得出。 …人之有生，将理失宜，役用过度，劳伤肾经，肾藏有热，热留膀胱，流入胞脏，遂成淋病。"详细论述了肾经砂石的生成及病机变化过程，说明了肾经砂石的形成因素为湿热火毒。治当清热化石，利尿通淋。方药选用《和剂局方》五淋汤（赤茯苓、赤芍药、山栀子、当归、甘草），或选用《证治汇补》石苇散（石苇、冬葵子、瞿麦、滑石、车前子）加金钱草、海金砂、鸡内金、炮山甲，生牡蛎、琥珀、石斛。

Literature Review of Kidney Channel Stones

📖 *Dān Xī Xīn Fǎ* ("Dān Xī's Heart-Approach"), "Strangury"

"There are five types of strangury, all of which are ascribed to heat. [Treat by] resolving heat and disinhibiting urine. …The reason for the occurrence of all types of strangury is kidney vacuity and engenderment of heat in the bladder. When water and fire fail to interact, heart and kidney qì are depressed. This perverts yīn and yáng and causes the clear and turbid to interfere with each other and amass in the lower burner. Therefore, we see urgency in the bladder and abdomen, and discharge of unctuous blood and stones from the urinary tract."

In this discussion of stone strangury, which also includes the pathomechanical changes of kidney channel stones, the text finds the fundamental pathomechanism to be kidney vacuity and engenderment of heat in the bladder, describing a root vacuity and tip repletion.

🕮 *Jǐng Yuè Quán Shū* ("Jǐng-Yuè's Complete Compendium"), "Schema of Miscellaneous Patterns: Strangury-Turbidity"

> "Stone strangury manifests in pain in the penis, discharge of stone-like matter in the urine, and inability to freely discharge urine… Generally speaking, these signs are mostly caused by non-interaction of the heart and kidney, accumulated heat toxin, or sexual taxation after getting soaked, consumption of dry and hot foods, and a binding depression of the seven affects. This is Master Yán's theory. The fact that the beginning of strangury is invariably caused by severe heat is beyond discussion."

This quotation describes how damp-heat leads to the pathomechanical changes of kidney channel stones.

文献评述

《丹溪心法•淋》曰："淋有五，皆属于热，解热利小便。 …诸淋所发，皆肾虚而膀胱生热也。水火不交，心肾气郁，遂使阴阳乖戾，清浊相干，蓄在下焦，故膀胱里急，膏血砂石从小便道而出焉。"对"石淋"，也包括了肾经砂石的病机变化进行了阐述，认为基本病机为"肾虚而膀胱生热"，属本虚标实。

《景岳全书•杂证谟•淋浊》曰："石淋，茎中痛，溺如砂石，不得卒出。 …大抵此证，多出心肾不交，积蕴热毒，或酒后房劳，服食燥热，七情郁结所致。此严氏之说。固已尽之，然淋之初病，则无不由乎热剧，无容辨矣。"论述了湿热导致肾经砂石的病机变化。

Summary of Kidney Channel Stones

1. Stoppage of Qì and Blood
   Gripping pain within the kidney, or aching in the lower back as if it was breaking.
2. Damage to the Blood Network Vessels
   Bloody urine.
3. Obstruction of the Urinary Tract
   Urinary frequency, urgency, or block.
4. Kidney Channel Stones
   Dark red tongue, slimy yellow tongue fur, rough sunken or rapid slippery pulse.

肾经砂石

气血不通—肾中绞痛，或腰酸如折

损伤血络—血尿

阻塞尿路—尿频，尿急或尿闭

肾经砂石—舌质暗红，苔黄腻，脉沉涩或滑数

Chapter Ten

Kidney Channel Qì Stagnation

The kidney is the root of earlier heaven and stores the body's original qì. The qì of the kidney region is stirring qì; it values flowing smoothly and without inhibition. Nevertheless, fury and anger can damage the liver and result in a binding depression of liver qì, which can then affect the kidney. Alternatively, great fright and sudden fear or an invasion and harassment by external evils can disorder the free flow of the qì dynamic in the kidney. This manifests in the pathomechanism of kidney channel qì stagnation.

When qì stagnates in the kidney channel and is unable to flow freely, qì obstruction in the lower back and rib-side results in distention and pain in the lumbar region linking to the abdomen, as well as distention and pain in the abdomen and rib-side and a sensation like traveling influx of qì that is now gathering, now dispersing.

The kidney governs the bones and is in charge of movement and walking. When qì stagnates in the kidney channel, essential qì cannot endure the wear and tear of movement. This results in inability to stand or walk for any duration.

Qì stagnation in the kidney channel can disorder qì transformation and prevent distribution of fluids. The result is short voidings of scant urine.

When kidney qì fails to move, water qì inundates the skin. This manifests in mild puffy swelling of the face and eyes.

Kidney channel qì stagnation manifests in a thin white tongue fur and a stringlike replete sunken pulse.

The chapter, "Discussing the Pulses and Patterns of Vacuity and Repletion, Cold and Heat, Life and Death, and Favorable and Unfavorable Shifts in Kidney Disease" in the *Zhōng Zàng Jīng* ("Central Treasury Canon") points out: "Kidney distention results in abdominal pain and fullness stretching to the back, a morose state of mind, and impediment in the lower back." What this quotation calls "kidney distention" refers to depression and obstruction of the qì dynamic in the kidney channel that manifests in distention and pain in the back and lower back.

The chapter, "Types of Dampness; Lumbar Pain" in the *Yī Xué Rù Mén* ("The Gateway to Medicine") also explains: "Deep depression, swelling, and inability to stretch in the lumbar region causes vacuity emaciation, a black facial complexion, and inability to stand for a long time or walk far." It further explains:

> "When anxiety and thought damage the spleen, the result is stoppage of stomach qì, lumbar pain linking to distention and fullness in the abdomen and rib-side, and internal impediment and numbness. Treat this condition with *chén xiāng jiàng qì tāng* (Aquilaria Qì-Downbearing Decoction) or *mù xiāng yún qì san* (Costusroot Qì-Evening Powder). … The ancestral sinew gathers in the genitals, and the liver is tied to the kidney. If anger damages the liver, it causes slackening of the various sinews and lumbar pain linking to the rib-side. Treat this condition with *wǔ mò yǐn zǐ* (Five Milled Ingredients Drink) and *tiáo gān sǎn* (Liver-Regulating Powder)."

This is a very detailed description of the pathomechanism by which anxiety and thought, depressed anger, and damage from the seven affects can depress the qì dynamic and cause stoppage of qì in the kidney channel, leading to lumbar and rib-side pain.

Kidney channel qì stagnation is treated by moving and disinhibiting qì, and by coursing the lower back and relieving pain. The recommended formula is *wǔ mò yǐn zǐ* (Five Milled Ingredients Drink) from the *Yī Fāng Jí Jiě* ("Medical Formulas Gathered and Explained") with the addition of *xiāng fù* (Cyperi Rhizoma), *xù duàn* (Dipsaci Radix), *dù zhòng* (Eucommiae Cortex), and *xuán hú* (Corydalis Rhizoma), or *chén xiāng sǎn* (Aquilaria Powder) from the *Jīn Guì Yì* ("The Wings of the Golden Coffer") with the addition of *gǒu qǐ zǐ* (Lycii Fructus) and *sāng shèn* (Mori Fructus).

Wǔ Mò Yǐn Zǐ 五磨饮子
Five Milled Ingredients Drink

chén xiāng (沉香 Aquilariae Lignum Resinatum, aquilaria)
tái wū (台乌 Linderae Radix, lindera)
bīng láng (槟榔 Arecae Semen, areca)
zhǐ shí (枳实 Aurantii Fructus Immaturus, unripe bitter orange)
mù xiāng (木香 Aucklandiae Radix, costusroot)

Plus:

xiāng fù (香附 Cyperi Rhizoma, cyperus)
xù duàn (续断 Dipsaci Radix, dipsacus)
dù zhòng (杜仲 Eucommiae Cortex, eucommia)
xuán hú (玄胡 Corydalis Rhizoma, corydalis)

Chén Xiāng Sǎn 沉香散
Aquilaria Powder

chén xiāng (沉香 Aquilariae Lignum Resinatum, aquilaria)
shí wéi (石韦 Pyrrosiae Folium, pyrrosia)
huá shí (滑石 Talcum, talcum)
dāng guī (当归 Angelicae Sinensis Radix, Chinese angelica)
jú pí (橘皮 Citri Reticulatae Pericarpium, tangerine peel)
bái sháo (白芍 Paeoniae Radix Alba, white peony)
dōng kuí zǐ (冬葵子 Malvae Semen, mallow seed)
wáng bù liú xíng (王不留行 Vaccariae Semen, vaccaria)
gān cǎo (甘草 Glycyrrhizae Radix, licorice)

Plus:

gǒu qǐ zǐ (枸杞子 Lycii Fructus, lycium)
sāng shèn (桑椹 Mori Fructus, mulberry)

肾经气滞

肾为先天之本，藏人身之元气。肾间之气为动气，贵于顺畅。如因恼怒伤肝，肝气郁结，肝病及肾，或大惊卒恐，或外邪侵扰，扰乱肾之气机通畅，则可出现肾经气滞的病机变化。肾经气滞，气行不畅，腰胁气阻，则腰部胀痛连腹，及胁腹胀痛，似有气走注，忽聚忽散；肾主骨，司运动行走，肾经气滞，精气不赖运动的损耗，则不能久立行走；肾经气滞，气化失常，水津不布，则小便短少；肾气不行，水气泛溢于肌肤，则可见面目轻度浮肿。肾经气滞，则舌苔薄白，脉沉弦实。如《中藏经•论肾脏虚实寒热生死逆顺脉证之法》指出："肾胀，则腹痛满引背，怏怏然，腰痹痛。"其中"肾胀"，是指肾经气机郁滞，阻塞不畅，故可引起现腰背胀痛。《医学入门•湿类•腰痛》也说："腰间郁郁膨胀不伸，令人虚羸面黑，不能久立远行。"又说："忧思伤脾，则胃气不行，腰痛连腹胁胀满，内痹不仁，沉香降气汤、木香匀气散。 ...宗筋聚于阴器，肝者，肾之同系也。怒伤肝，则诸筋纵弛，腰痛连胁，聚香饮子、调肝散。"最为详细论述了忧思郁怒，七情损伤，气机郁滞，肝肾经气不通，引起腰胁疼痛的病机变化。治法为行气利气，疏腰止痛。方药选用《医方集解》五磨饮子（沉香、台乌、槟榔、枳实、木香）加香附、续断、杜仲、玄胡，或选《金匮翼》沉香散（沉香、石苇、滑石、当归、橘皮、白芍、冬葵子、王不留行、甘草）加枸杞、桑椹。

Literature Review of Kidney Channel Qì Stagnation

📖 *Jǐng Yuè Quán Shū* ("Jǐng-Yuè's Complete Compendium"), "Lumbar Pain"

> "In patterns of lumbar pain… when there is depressed anger and pain, this is qì stagnation."

The lower back is the house of the kidney. When fury and anger damage the liver and liver depression accumulates and extends to qì depression in the kidney channel, the pathomechanism of lumbar pain after fury and anger can arise.

📖 *Zhèng Yīn Mài Zhì* ("Pathoconditions: Causes, Pulses, and Treatments"), "Internal Damage Lumbar Pain"

> "The condition of internal damage lumbar pain … manifests in qì distention in the rib-side that is greatly aggravated by anger. This is a condition of anger depression bind. … Binding depression of the seven affects, fury and anger, or anxiety and thought result in lumbar and rib-side pain."

This quotation describes how affect-mind binding depression results in lumbar pain.

📖 *Yī Xué Xīn Wù* ("Medical Insights"), "Lumbar Pain"

> "Traveling influx stabbing pain, now gathering now dispersing, and an urgent stringlike pulse mean qì stagnation. *Jú hé wán* (Tangerine Pit Pill) governs it."

This quotation discusses how qì depression can lead to pain in the lumbar region that is now gathering, now dispersing.

文献评述

《景岳全书•腰痛》曰："腰痛证，…郁怒而痛者气之滞也。"腰为肾之府，恼怒伤肝，肝郁而累及肾经气郁，故出现恼怒而腰痛的病机变化。

《症因脉治•内伤腰痛》曰"内伤腰痛之症，… 胁肋气胀，遇怒愈甚，此怒气郁结之症。 …七情恼怒，忧思郁结，则腰胁疼痛。"论述情志郁结引起腰痛的病机变化。

《医学心悟•腰痛》曰："走注刺痛，忽聚忽散，脉弦急者，气滞也，橘核丸主之。"对气郁可引起腰部疼痛，忽聚忽散的病机变化进行了论述。

Summary of Kidney Channel Qì Stagnation

1. Inhibition of Kidney Qì

   Distention and pain in the lumbar region linking to the abdomen, distention and pain in the rib-side and abdomen, a sensation like traveling influx of qì, now gathering now dispersing.

2. Failure to Manage Movement

   Inability to stand or walk for a long time.

3. Disordered Qì Transformation

   Short voidings of scant urine.

4. Inundation by Fluids

   Mild puffy swelling of the face and eyes.

5. Kidney Channel Qì Stagnation

   Thin white tongue fur, stringlike replete sunken pulse.

肾经气滞

肾气不畅—腰部胀痛连腹，胁腹胀痛，似有气走注，忽聚忽散

不司运动—不能久立行走

气化失常—小便短少

水液泛溢—面目轻度浮肿

肾经气滞—舌苔薄白，脉沉弦实

Part Two

Pathomechanisms of Kidney Vacuity

肾虚的病机

Kidney Vacuity

The kidney is the root of earlier heaven. It governs the storage of essential qì and houses original yīn and yáng. Essential qì, original yīn, and original yáng within the kidney should be full and overflowing. They should be stored and internally safeguarded, and should not discharge or leak to ensure the normal performance of vital activities. Essential qì in the kidney is the motivating force that maintains the normal physiological functions in the body. Because it can easily be consumed, physicians constantly attend its insufficiency and are unconcerned about its superabundance.

Disease of the kidney viscus, whether it is a disease of this viscus itself or one that is due to the passage and transmutation of diseases from other bowels and viscera, can equally reduce essential qì within the kidney. Pathomechanisms of the kidney mostly involve depletion of the kidney's yīn, yáng, essence, and qì. Therefore, the ancients generally considered that the kidney suffered predominantly from vacuity.

Already in the Spring and Autumn period (770-476 BCE), the *Huáng Dì Nèi Jīng* ("The Yellow Emperor's Inner Canon") clearly recognized the existence of the pathomechanism of kidney vacuity. For example, the "General Treatise on Vacuity and Repletion" in the *Sù Wèn* ("Plain Questions") states: "When essential qì is despoliated, there is vacuity." The kidney is the viscus that stores essence, and the place from which original qì springs. Despoliation of essential qì thus refers to damage to essence qì within the kidney.

The chapter, "Forms of Disease from Evil Qì in the Viscera and Bowels" in the *Líng Shū* ("The Magic Pivot") also states: "If people exert themselves lifting heavy weights, engage in excessive sexual intercourse, or sweat while bathing, this damages the kidney." Kidney damage invariably leads to kidney vacuity. While this source did not explicitly mention the term "kidney vacuity," it nevertheless implicity described the pathomechanism of kidney vacuity.

The chapter, "The Spirit" in the *Líng Shū* ("The Magic Pivot") states: "Kidney qì vacuity results in reversal." Kidney qì vacuity is one aspect of kidney vacuity. This text therefore indirectly refers to the pathomechanism of kidney vacuity.

During the Hàn period, Huá-Tuó first elaborated on the manifestations of "vacuity in the kidney viscus." Thus, the chapter, "Discussing the Pulses and Patterns of Vacuity and Repletion, Cold and Heat, Life and Death, and Favorable and Unfavorable Shifts in Kidney Disease" in the *Zhōng Zàng Jīng* ("Central Treasury Canon") states: "Vacuity results in dreams of boats and drowning people and of being submerged in water, and of that which a person fears." This source analyzed the pathomechanical changes of kidney vacuity from the perspective of yīn and yáng, vacuity and repletion, and cold and heat.

In the Jìn period, Wáng Shū-Hé first mentioned the term kidney vacuity. As he stated in the chapter, "Normal Pulses in Front and Back of Shén-Mén and Qì-Kǒu" in the *Mài Jīng* ("The Pulse Canon"):

> "Kidney vacuity: The cubit pulse behind Spirit Gate (shén mén, HT-7) on the left hand will indicate yīn vacuity. This is the foot lesser yīn channel. Such a patient suffers from oppression in the heart, lower-body heaviness, and swelling in the feet that does not tolerate pressure."

In "Discussion on the Kidney; Various Kidney-Supplementing Formulas for Treating Kidney Vacuity" in the *Tài Píng Shèng Huì Fāng* ("The Great Peace Sagacious Benevolence Formulary"), the Sòng dynasty author Wáng Huái-Yǐn stated:

> "The kidney is ascribed to the foot lesser yīn channel. On the left is the kidney; on the right is the life gate. The kidney and the life gate together are the abode of the spirit essence and the location where original qì is tied. If the kidney is vacuous, the result is cutting pain in the back and lower back, inability to bend the head forward and backward, small and weak feet and lower legs, increased aversion to wind and cold, reversal cold of the extremities, shortage of qì in breathing, vexing pain in the joints, binding pain in the umbilical region, a soot-black facial complexion, vacuity ringing in both ears, desiccated flesh and bones, frequent uncontrolled urination, and a fine rapid floating pulse. These are the symptoms of kidney vacuity."

This quotation comprehensively describes the manifestations of the pathomechanism of kidney vacuity.

The pathomechanism of kidney vacuity is mostly due to a variety of causative factors like earlier heaven constitutional insufficiency, weakening in old age, excessive sexual taxation, excessive fright and fear, lack of or inappropriate treatment, and enduring illness affecting the kidney, all of which can directly damage kidney yīn, essence, yáng, and qì. Because detriment leads to depletion, a complex situation arises that is can easily deplete further and that is difficult to recover. For this reason, the pathomechanism of kidney vacuity is further divided into six broad categories: debilitation of kidney yáng, kidney yīn depletion, insufficiency of kidney essence, kidney qì vacuity, dual vacuity of kidney yīn and yáng, and kidney vacuity verging on desertion.

肾虚介绍

肾为先天之本，主藏精气，内舍元阴元阳。肾中精气及元阴元阳，宜满宜溢，蛰藏内守，不宜泄漏，才能充分发挥生理效应，保障生命活动正常进行。肾中精气是维持人体生命活动的原动力，容易耗伤，因此常恐其不足，而不虑其有余。若肾脏患病，无论是本脏自病，或是由于其它脏腑的传变，均易耗损肾中精气。肾脏病机，多涉及肾中阴、阳、精、气的亏损，故前人一般认为肾病多虚。早在春秋时代，《黄帝内经》对肾虚病机已有了一定的认识。如《素问•通评虚实论》曰："精气夺则虚。"肾为藏精之脏，元气始发之地，精气夺，即指肾中精气的损伤。《灵枢•邪气脏腑病形》又曰："有所用力举重，若入房过度，汗出浴水，则伤肾。"伤肾必然导致肾虚，虽未直接提出肾虚的名称，但已隐含对肾虚病机的论述。《灵枢•本神》曰："肾气虚则厥。"肾气虚为肾虚的内容之一，间接提出肾虚病机的名称。汉代华佗开始阐述"肾脏虚"的表现。如《中藏经•论肾脏虚实寒热生死逆顺脉证之法》曰："虚则梦舟溺人，得其时，梦伏水中，若有所畏。"从阴阳虚实寒热分析了肾脏虚的病机变化。晋代王叔和首次提出肾虚的名称，如《脉经•平人迎神门气口前后脉》指出："肾虚：左手尺中神门以后脉阴虚者，足少阴经也。病苦心中闷，下重，足肿不可以按地。"宋代王怀隐《太平圣惠方•肾脏论•治肾虚补肾诸方》曰："夫肾脏者，足少阴之经也。左则为肾，右为命门。肾与命门者，神精之所舍，元气之所系也。若肾虚则腰背切痛，不能俛仰，足胫小弱，多恶风寒，手足厥冷，呼吸少气，骨节烦疼，脐腹结痛，面色黧黑，两耳虚鸣，肌骨干枯，小便滑数，诊其脉浮细而数者，肾虚之候也。” 全面地阐述了“肾虚”的病机表现。肾虚的病机多由先天禀赋不足，年老体弱，房劳过度，过度惊恐，失治误治，久病及肾等多种因素造成，直接导致肾中阴、精、阳、气之耗伤，出现因损致亏，易亏难复的复杂状况。故肾虚病机又多分为肾阳虚衰、肾阴亏损、肾精不足、肾气虚弱、肾阴阳两虚、肾虚欲脱等六大类型。

Chapter One

Debilitation of Kidney Yáng

The kidney stores original yáng and is the root of the entire body's yáng qì. It is called the fire of the life gate. Kidney yáng has the important physiological functions of warming, steaming, transforming qì, and promoting movement. Insufficiency of earlier heaven and a constitutional vacuity of yáng, debility in old age, excessive sexual taxation, inappropriate use of cold bitter medicinals, enduring illness, or the passage and transmutation of disease from other bowels and viscera can all cause an insufficiency of kidney yáng. The resulting loss of warming, steaming, qì-transforming, and other functions leads to a possible reduction of functions in the entire body, and consequently to the pathomechanism of debilitation of kidney yáng.

Early on, the *Huáng Dì Nèi Jīng* ("The Yellow Emperor's Inner Canon") discussed the rudiments of debilitation of kidney yáng. Thus, the "Treatise on Reversal" in the *Sù Wèn* ("Plain Questions") states: "Debilitation of yáng qì in the lower body results in cold reversal." Since yáng debilitation in the lower body refers to kidney yáng, cold reversal is thus tied to yáng vacuity.

In the Hàn period, Zhāng Zhòng-Jǐng formulated the famous formulas for *shèn qì wán* (Kidney Qì Pill) and *zhēn wǔ tāng* (True Warrior Decoction) as treatments for the pathomechanical changes of kidney yáng vacuity in the *Shāng Hán Lùn* ("On Cold Damage"), thereby advancing the development of the pathomechanism of kidney yáng vacuity.

In the Suí period, Cháo Yuán-Fāng put forth the notion of "kidney qì vacuity cold." As the chapter, "Symptoms of Vacuity Taxation" in the *Zhū Bìng Yuán Hòu Lùn* ("Origin and Indicators of Disease") states, "Taxation damage to the kidney is the reason for kidney qì vacuity cold."

In the Táng dynasty, Sūn Sī-Miǎo also referred to "kidney vacuity cold" in the *Qiān Jīn Yào Fāng* ("A Thousand Gold Pieces Prescriptions"). Both these texts thus discussed to some depth the pathomechanism of debilitation of kidney yáng.

The Sòng dynasty author Yán Yòng-Hé initially proposed the concept of "debilitation of true yáng." In the chapter, "Supplementing and Boosting" in the *Yán Shì Jì Shēng Fāng* ("Yan's Remedies for Curing All People"), he stated: "If people in the course of their life are not good at conserving and nourishing, they will suffer from excessive vacuity taxation and debilitation of true yáng." This passage expounds that debilitation of kidney yáng is caused by taxation fatigue.

The "Record on Seeking Rightness; Treatise on True Yīn" in the *Lèi Jīng Fù Yì* ("Wings to the Classified Canon") by the Míng period author, Zhāng Jǐng-Yuè, further stated:

> "*Yòu guī wán* (Right-Restoring [Life Gate] Pill) treats insufficiency of original yáng, whether from constitutional debilitation of earlier heaven or excessive taxation damage, both of which cause a debilitation of life gate fire that prevents it from engendering earth. The result is spleen-stomach vacuity cold, low intake of food and drink, possibly with nausea, vomiting, and swelling, or stomach reflux and congestion, or fear of cold, or increased pain in the umbilical region, or loose stool and frequent diarrhea, or spontaneous urination, vacuity strangury, and cold mounting, or if cold invades the ravines and valleys, impediment pain in the limb joints, or if cold is in the lower burner, puffy swelling from water evil."

This quotation discusses in detail how a debilitation of kidney yáng can further induce numerous dysfunctions in other organs.

In the Qīng period, Jiāng Hán-Tūn stated as follows in the "Kidney Section" of the *Bǐ Huā Yī Jìng* ("Bǐ-Huā's Medical Mirror"):

> "Cold in the kidney means kidney vacuity. The pulse at the left and right cubit positions is invariably sunken and slow. The symptoms of this condition are debilitation of the life gate fire, no desire for food, cockcrow diarrhea [diarrhea during the period from 1-3 am], bowed head, lying in a curled position and reversal cold, and running piglet."

This is a rather comprehensive summary of the clinical manifestations of debilitation of kidney yáng.

In more recent times, the famous physician Pú Fǔ-Zhōu described with precision the manifestations of the pathomechanism of kidney yáng vacuity. In the chapter, "Seeking the Root in Pattern Identification" in the *Pú Fǔ Zhōu Yī Liáo Jīng Yàn* ("Pú Fǔ-Zhōu's Medical Experience"), he stated: "Vacuity of kidney yáng results in yáng wilting [impotence], sweating of the lower body, aching lower back and weak legs, fear of cold, and enuresis."

Debilitation of kidney yáng can lead to all kinds of functional disorders in numerous aspects of the organism. The following types of pathomechanisms can arise: Impaired warming, lower back deprived of nourishment, emptiness of the sea of marrow, decline in reproductive functions, indiscriminate flooding of fluids, failure of fire to warm earth, incessant urination, impaired absorption due to yáng vacuity, yáng floating upward, yáng repelled to the outside, surging counterflow qì ascent, and thoroughfare-controlling vessel disharmony.

肾阳虚衰

肾藏元阳，为全身阳气的根本，称为命门之火。肾阳具有温煦、蒸腾、气化、推动等重要生理功能。若先天不足，素体阳虚，或年老体衰，或房劳过度，或过用苦寒，久病或其它脏腑疾病的传变，均可导致肾阳不足，失其温煦、蒸腾、气化等功能，导致全身机能减退，引起肾阳虚衰的病机变化。《黄帝内经》已有肾阳虚衰的初步论述。如《素问•厥论》曰："阳气衰于下，则为寒厥。"阳衰于下即指肾阳，寒厥系指阳虚。汉代张仲景《伤寒杂病论》针对肾阳虚的病机变化制定了著名的肾气丸、真武汤，是对肾阳虚病机的进一步发展。隋代巢元方提出"肾气虚冷"的概念，如《诸病源候论•虚劳候》曰："劳伤于肾，肾气虚冷故也。"唐代孙思邈在《千金要方》中又称为"肾虚寒"，都是对肾阳虚衰病机的深入论述。宋代严用和则首次提出"真阳虚衰"的病机概念，如《济生方•补益》曰："人之有生，不善摄养，虚劳过度，真阳虚衰。"论述了因劳倦而致肾阳虚衰的病机改变。明代张景岳《类经附翼•求正录•真阴论》又曰："右归丸治元阳不足，或先天禀衰，或劳伤过度，以致命门火衰，不能生土，而为脾胃虚寒，饮食少进，或呕恶膨胀，或反胃隔塞，或怯寒畏冷，或脐腹多痛，或大便不实，泻利频作，或小水自遗，虚淋寒疝，或以寒侵溪谷，而为肢节痹痛，或以寒在下焦，而为水邪浮肿。"详细论述了肾阳虚衰可进一步导致多个脏腑器官功能失调的病机变化。清代江涵暾《笔花医镜•肾部》曰："肾之寒，肾之虚也，脉左右尺必迟沉，其症为命门火衰，为不欲食，为鸡鸣泄泻，为天柱倒，为踡卧厥冷，为奔豚。"较为全面的总结了肾阳虚衰的临床表现。近代著名医家蒲辅周对肾阳虚病机的表现作了准确的描述，他在《蒲辅周医疗经验•辨证求本》中曰："肾阳虚，则阳痿，下汗出，腰酸脚弱，畏寒，遗尿。"肾阳虚衰，可引起机体多方面的功能失调，出现温煦失职、腰府失养、髓海空虚、生殖减退、水液泛滥、火不暖土、水泉不止、阳虚失纳、阳浮于上、格阳于外、冲气上逆、冲任不调等多种病机类型。

1.1 Impaired Warming

The kidney is the root of earlier heaven, and kidney yáng constitutes original yáng. It has the function of warming the viscera, bowels, and blood vessels in the entire body, and of agitating the normal performance of all vital activities. Constitutional vacuity, enduring illness in old age, excessive sexual taxation, or excessive use of cold bitter medicinals all tend to damage kidney yáng. When kidney yáng is insufficient, yáng fails to restrain yīn, which results in exuberant yīn internal cold. This can induce the pathomechanism of impaired warming.

When kidney yáng is depleted, it is unable to warm the five viscera, six bowels, four limbs, and hundred bones. Generation of heat is insufficient, and yáng qì has difficulty reaching the lower limbs in particular. The result is fear of cold and cold limbs, especially in the lower limbs.

If yáng qì is unable to propel qì and blood to luxuriate the upper body, they are unable to nourish the face, eyes, and tongue. This results in a bright white facial complexion and a pale white tongue.

An insufficiency of kidney yáng can impair the movement of qì and blood and cause the blood vessels to become cold and congeal. This manifests in a soot-black facial complexion.

When kidney yáng is insufficient, the lower back and joints are deprived of nourishment, which results in cold aching lower back and knees.

A vacuity of kidney yáng prevents it from warming, stimulating, and promoting movement, thereby reducing organ functions. The result is listlessness of the essence-spirit, clouded head, and tinnitus.

When kidney yáng is unable to warm defensive yáng, defensive yáng is not secure, which results in spontaneous sweating, aversion to wind, and a tendency to suffer from recurring bouts of the common cold.

When kidney yáng is depleted, the elimination of stool and urine breaks down, resulting in long voidings of clear urine and thin sloppy stool.

Debilitation of kidney yáng manifests in a pale tongue with white fur and a slow and weak sunken pulse.

The chapter, "Discussing the Treatment of Kidney-Bladder Vacuity and Repletion" in the *Yán Shì Jì Shēng Fāng* ("Yan's Remedies for Curing All People") states:

> "Regarding their vacuity, vacuity causes cold to arise, and cold causes cutting pain in the back and lower back, inability to bend forward and backward, aching and weakness of the feet and lower legs, increased aversion to wind and cold, reversal cold of the extremities, shortage of qì in breathing, vexing pain in the joints, binding pain in the umbilical region, a soot-black facial complexion, vacuity ringing in both ears, desiccated flesh and bones, frequent uncontrolled urination, and a fine rapid floating pulse. These are the symptoms of kidney vacuity."

This quotation describes the numerous pathological changes resulting from a vacuity of kidney yáng and impaired warming.

Impaired warming is treated by warming and supplementing kidney yáng. Recommended formulas are *shí bǔ wán* (Ten Supplements Pill) from the *Yán Shì Jì Shēng Fāng* ("Yan's Remedies for Curing All People") or *hé jiān dì huáng yǐn zǐ* ([Liú] Hé-Jiān's Rehmannia Drink) from the *Xuān Míng Lùn Fāng* ("An Elucidation of Formulas") with modifications.

Shí Bǔ Wán 十补丸 Ten Supplements Pill
shú dì huáng (熟地黄 Rehmanniae Radix Praeparata, cooked rehmannia)
shān yào (山药 Dioscoreae Rhizoma, dioscorea)
shān zhū yú (山茱萸 Corni Fructus, cornus)
zé xiè (泽泻 Alismatis Rhizoma, alisma)
fú líng (茯苓 Poria, poria)
mǔ dān pí (牡丹皮 Moutan Cortex, moutan)
ròu guì (肉桂 Cinnamomi Cortex, cinnamon bark)
fù zǐ (附子 Aconiti Radix Lateralis Praeparata, aconite)
wǔ wèi zǐ (五味子 Schisandrae Fructus, schisandra)
lù róng (鹿茸 Cervi Cornu Pantotrichum, velvet deerhorn)

Hé Jiān Dì Huáng Yǐn Zǐ 河间地黄饮子
[Liú] Hé-Jiān's Rehmannia Drink

fù zǐ (附子 Aconiti Radix Lateralis Praeparata, aconite)
guì zhī (桂枝 Cinnamomi Ramulus, cinnamon twig)
bái sháo (白芍 Paeoniae Radix Alba, white peony)
ròu cōng róng (肉苁蓉 Cistanches Herba, cistanche)
bā jǐ tiān (巴戟天 Morindae Officinalis Radix, morinda) [from Hangzhou]
shēng dì huáng (生地黄 Rehmanniae Radix, rehmannia)
wǔ wèi zǐ (五味子 Schisandrae Fructus, schisandra) [Northern, stir-fried]
shān zhū yú (山茱萸 Corni Fructus, cornus)
chuān bèi mǔ (川贝母 Fritillariae Cirrhosae Bulbus, Sìchuān fritillaria)
dù zhòng (杜仲 Eucommiae Cortex, eucommia)
xù duàn (续断 Dipsaci Radix, dipsacus)
nuò mǐ cǎo (糯米草 Oryzae Glutinosae Herba, glutinous rice herb)
hǎi jīn shā (海金沙 Lygodii Spora, lygodium spore)
yè míng shā (夜明砂 Verspertilionis Faeces, bat's droppings)

温煦失职

肾为先天之本，肾阳为元阳，具有温煦全身脏腑器官血脉，鼓动各项生命活动正常进行的作用。如素体虚弱，或年老久病，或房劳过度，或过用苦寒，均易损伤肾阳。肾阳不足，阳不制阴，阴盛内寒，可引起温煦失职的病机变化。肾阳亏虚，不能温煦五脏六腑，四肢百骸，产热不足，下肢阳气更难到达，则畏寒肢冷，下肢尤甚;阳气不能推动气血上荣，不能充养面目舌体，则面色㿠白，舌体淡白; 肾阳不足，气血失运，血脉寒凝，又可见面色黧黑; 肾阳不足，腰府骨节失养，则腰膝酸冷; 肾阳虚，失于温煦、激发、推动，脏腑功能衰退，则精神萎靡，头昏耳鸣; 肾阳不能温暖卫阳，卫阳失固，则自汗恶风，容易反复感冒; 肾阳亏虚，二便失司，则小便清长，大便溏稀。肾阳虚衰，则舌淡苔白，脉沉迟而弱。如《重订严氏济生方•肾膀胱虚实论治》曰：“方其虚也，虚则生寒，寒则腰背切痛，不能俯仰，足胫酸弱，多恶风寒，手足厥冷，呼吸少气，骨节烦疼，脐腹结痛，面色黧黑，两耳虚鸣，肌骨干枯，小便滑数，诊其脉浮细而数者，是肾虚之候也。”描述了肾阳虚，温煦失职可导致的多种病机改变。治法宜温补肾阳。方药可选《济生方》十补丸（熟地黄、怀山药、山萸肉、泽泻、茯苓、丹皮、肉桂、附子、五味子、鹿茸），或选《宣明论方》河间地黄饮子（熟附片、桂枝、生白芍、肉苁蓉、杭巴戟、细生地、炒北五味、山萸肉、川贝、杜仲、川续断、糯米草、海金砂、夜明砂）加减。

Literature Review of Impaired Warming

🕮 *Sù Wèn* ("Plain Questions"), "On Reversal"

> "When yáng qì is debilitated, it is unable to percolate into and luxuriate the channels and network vessels. Yáng qì decreases daily, until only yīn qì remains. For this reason, the hands and feet suffer from cold."

Yáng vacuity results in yīn exuberance, and yīn exuberance results in cold. Therefore the hands and feet feel cold.

🕮 *Qiān Jīn Yào Fāng* ("A Thousand Gold Pieces Prescriptions"), "On the Pulse in Kidney Disease"

> "Yīn vacuity at the yīn aspect of the cubit pulse behind Spirit Gate (*shén mén,* HT-7) on the right hand disease of the foot lesser yīn channel. The patient suffers from smallness and weakness of the feet and lower legs, aversion to cold, a regularly interrupted pulse that occasionally fails to arrive, coldness in the feet, upper body heaviness and lower body lightness, and walking without pressing on the ground… This is called kidney vacuity cold."

This quotation describes in detail how debilitation of kidney yáng manifests in clinic.

文献评述

《素问•厥论》曰："阳气衰，不能渗营其经络，阳气日损，阴气独在，故手足为之寒也"。阳虚则阴盛，阴盛则寒，故手足发冷。

《千金要方•肾脏病脉论》曰："右手尺中神门以后脉阴虚者，足少阴经也。病苦足胫小弱，恶寒，脉代绝，时不至，足寒，上重下轻，行不按地，…名曰肾虚寒也。"对肾阳虚衰病机的临床表现进行了较详细的描述。

Summary of Impaired Warming

1. Insufficient Creation of Heat
   Fear of cold and cold limbs, especially in the lower limbs.
2. Impaired Nourishment of Qì and Blood
   Bright white facial complexion, pale white tongue.
3. Cold Congealing in the Blood Vessels
   Soot-black facial complexion.
4. Lower Back Deprived of Nourishment
   Cold aching lower back and knees.
5. Reduced Organ Functions
   Listlessness of the essence-spirit, clouded head, tinnitus.
6. Insecurity of Defensive Yáng
   Spontaenous sweating, aversion to wind, tendency to suffer from recurring contractions of the common cold.
7. Breakdown of Urination and Defecation
   Long voidings of clear urine, thin sloppy stool.
8. Debilitation of Kidney Yáng
   Pale tongue with white fur, slow and weak sunken pulse.

温煦失职

产热不足—畏寒肢冷，下肢尤甚

气血失养—面色㿠白，舌体淡白

血脉寒凝—面色黧黑

腰府失养—腰膝酸冷

脏腑衰退—精神萎靡，头昏耳鸣

卫阳失固—自汗恶风，容易反复感冒

二便失司—小便清长，大便溏稀

肾阳虚衰—舌淡苔白，脉沉迟而弱

1.2 Lower Back Deprived of Nourishment

The "Treatise of the Arcane Book of the Orchid Chamber of the Spirit Tower" in the *Sù Wèn* ("Plain Questions") states: "The lower back holds the office of labor, whence agility emanates." The lower back is the external indicator of the kidney and the pivot of the human body. To labor and apply strength, a person must be able to stretch and bend and to stand and walk. These functions are always related to the kidney. Debilitation of kidney yáng and failure to warm the lower back can cause the pathomechanism of the lower back being deprived of nourishment.

When kidney yáng is vacuous, it can cause congealing cold qì stagnation and tension and stoppage of the sinews. Cold and pain in the back and lower back causes inability to bend and stretch, which persists continuously and is exacerbated by exposure to cold and relieved by exposure to warmth.

The kidney channel runs through the lesser abdomen. Since cold governs contracture and tautness, a vacuity of kidney yáng can result in lumbar pain stretching to the lesser abdomen and hypertonicity.

When kidney yáng is vacuous, it loses its ability to warm. This results in frequent fear of cold and lack of warmth in the hands and feet.

As a result of kidney yáng vacuity and inability to warm, qì and blood fail to luxuriate. This results in a pale white facial complexion, and in shortage of qì and lack of strength.

When kidney yáng vacuity causes a disturbance of qì transformation, the result is long voidings of clear urine or urinary block.

Debilitation of kidney yáng manifests in a pale tongue with white tongue fur and a moderate forceless sunken pulse.

The chapter, "Lumbar Pain" in the *Qiān Jīn Yào Fāng* ("A Thousand Gold Pieces Prescriptions") states: "There are five kinds of lumbar pain: The first is called lesser yīn, which refers to the kidney. In the tenth month, the yáng qì of all the myriad things is debilitated. Therefore, they suffer lumbar pain." The foot lesser yīn homes to the kidney, and debilitation of yáng qì in the tenth month indicates a debilitation of kidney yáng. Thus, this quotation indicates that vacuity of kidney yáng and loss of nourishment in the lower back can lead to lumbar disease.

The chapter, "Internal Damage Lumbar Pain" in the *Zhèng Yīn Mài Zhì* ("Pathoconditions: Causes, Pulses, and Treatments") also states: "Insufficiency of earlier heaven and depletion of true yáng result in yáng vacuity and lumbar pain." It further states: "Frequent fear of cold and lack of warmth in the hands and feet whenever encountering cold, which is immediately followed by lumbar and back pain, are signs that true fire is insufficient and yáng vacuous." These quotations both elaborate on the pathomechanism and clinical manifestations of lumbar pain that results from debilitation of kidney yáng and the lower back deprived of nourishment.

When the lower back is deprived of nourishment, it is treated by warming the kidney and assisting yáng, and by invigorating the lower back and relieving pain. The recommended formula is *hé chē bā wèi wán* (Eight-Ingredient Placenta Pill) from the *Yòu Yòu Jí Chéng* ("A Compendium of Pediatrics") with the addition of *dù zhòng* (Eucommiae Cortex) and *huái niú xī* (Achyranthis Bidentatae Radix).

Hé Chē Bā Wèi Wán 河车八味丸 Eight-Ingredient Placenta Pill
zǐ hé chē (紫河车 Hominis Placenta, placenta)
lù róng (鹿茸 Cervi Cornu Pantotrichum, velvet deerhorn)
ròu guì (肉桂 Cinnamomi Cortex, cinnamon bark)
fù zǐ (附子 Aconiti Radix Lateralis Praeparata, aconite)
mǔ dān pí (牡丹皮 Moutan Cortex, moutan)
fú líng (茯苓 Poria, poria)
shān yào (山药 Dioscoreae Rhizoma, dioscorea)
zé xiè (泽泻 Alismatis Rhizoma, alisma)
mài dōng (麦冬 Ophiopogonis Radix, ophiopogon)
wǔ wèi zǐ (五味子 Schisandrae Fructus, schisandra)
dà zǎo (大枣 Jujubae Fructus, jujube)
Plus:
dù zhòng (杜仲 Eucommiae Cortex, eucommia)
niú xī (牛膝 Achyranthis Bidentatae Radix, achyranthes)

腰府失养

《素问•灵兰秘典论》曰："腰者作强之官，伎巧出焉。"腰为肾之外候，人之枢纽，作强用力，能伸能屈，能立能坐，无不与肾相关。

肾阳虚衰，不能温煦腰府，则可引起腰府失养的病机。肾阳虚，腰府筋脉失养，寒凝气滞，筋脉拘急不通，则腰背冷痛，不得屈伸，绵绵不已，遇寒加重，得温可减; 肾的经脉循行少腹，肾阳虚，寒主收引，则腰痛引少腹拘急; 肾阳虚失于温煦，则时常怕冷，手足不温; 肾阳虚，不能温煦，气血失荣，则面色淡 白，少气乏力; 肾阳虚，气化失调，则小便清长或尿闭。肾阳虚衰，则舌质谈，苔白，脉沉缓无力。如《千金要方•腰痛》云："凡腰痛有五，一曰少阴，少阴肾也，十月万物阳气皆衰，是以腰痛。"足少阴属肾，十月阳气衰，即指肾阳虚衰，提出肾阳虚，腰府失养，可致腰病。《症因脉治•内伤腰痛》也云："先天不足，真阳亏损，则为阳虚腰痛。"又云："时常怕冷，手足不温，凡遇寒冷，腰背即痛，此真火不足，阳虚之症。"均阐述肾阳虚衰，腰府失养，可致腰痛的病机和表现。治宜温肾助阳，强腰止痛。方药选《幼幼集成》河车八味丸（紫河车、鹿茸、肉桂、附子、丹皮、茯苓、山药、泽泻、麦冬、五味子、大枣）加杜仲、怀牛膝。

Literature Review of Lower Back Deprived of Nourishment

🕮 *Sù Wèn* ("Plain Questions"), "Treatise on the Essential Subtleties of the Pulse"

> "The lower back is the house of the kidney. If the patient is unable to turn or rock the lower back, it means that the kidney is exhausted."

This quotation points out that impaired movement of the lower back because of pain and other factors is related to vacuity detriment in the kidney, which also includes damage to the kidney's yáng qì.

🕮 *Shèng Jì Zǒng Lù* ("Sages' Salvation Records"), "Section on Lumbar Pain"

> "Discussion: There are five kinds of lumbar pain: the first one is insufficiency of yáng qì. This refers to debilitation of foot lesser yīn kidney qì, which causes a person to suffer from lumbar pain."

This quotation succinctly remarks that debilitation of kidney yáng and lower back deprived of nourishment can lead to the pathomechanism of lumbar pain.

📖 *Zá Bìng Yuán Liú Xī Zhú* ("Incisive Light on the Source of Miscellaneous Disease"), "The Origin and Development of Lumbar and Umbilical Disease"

> "Damage from sexual taxation is the cause of yáng qì vacuity and inability to move. This leads to lumbar pain."

This quotation notes how sexual taxation causes damage to the kidney, vacuity of kidney yáng, and lower back deprived of nourishment, which can lead to lumbar pain.

文献评述

《素问•脉要精微论》曰："腰者肾之府，转摇不能，肾将惫矣。"指出腰府因疼痛等因素而活动障碍，与肾脏虚损有关，其中包含肾的阳气损伤。

《圣济总录•腰痛门》曰："论曰：腰痛有五：一阳气不足，足少阴肾气衰，令人腰痛。"明确提出肾阳虚衰，腰府失养，可致腰痛的病机。

《杂病源流犀烛•腰脐病源流》曰："因伤房劳，阳气虚弱，不能运动，以致腰痛。"论述房劳伤肾，肾阳虚，腰府失养，可致腰痛。

Summary of Lower Back Deprived of Nourishment

1. Congealing Cold Qì Stagnation

   Cold pain in the back and lower back, inability to bend and stretch, which persists continuously and is exacerbated by exposure to cold and relieved by exposure to warmth.

2. Cold Governing Contracture and Tautness

   Lumbar pain stretching to the lesser abdomen and hypertonicity.

3. Impaired Warming

   Frequent fear of cold, lack of warmth in the hands and feet.

4. Qì and Blood Failing to Luxuriate

   Pale white facial complexion, shortage of qì and lack of strength.

5. Disturbance of Qì Transformation

   Long voidings of clear urine or urinary block.

6. Debilitation of Kidney Yáng

   Pale tongue with white tongue fur, moderate forceless sunken pulse.

腰府失养
寒凝气滞—腰背冷痛，不得屈伸，绵绵不已，遇寒加重，得温可减
寒主收引—腰痛引少腹拘急
失于温煦—时常怕冷，手足不温
气血失荣—面色淡 白，少气乏力
气化失调—小便清长或尿闭
肾阳虚衰—舌质谈，苔白，脉沉缓无力

1.3 Emptiness of the Sea of Marrow

The kidney stores essence and engenders marrow, which flows to the brain. Therefore, the treatise "On Seas" in the *Líng Shū* ("The Magic Pivot") states: "The brain is the sea of marrow." Essence is yīn, and essence, qì, yīn, and yáng in the kidney grow and develop in interdependence. Kidney essence is able to engender marrow and nourish the brain, and kidney yáng and life fire are able to warm the brain marrow. For this reason, the pathomechanism of emptiness of the sea of marrow can directly be caused by an insufficiency of essential qì, as well as by an insufficiency of kidney yáng or a debilitation of life gate fire. Any of these can damage kidney yáng and weaken its ability to warm and stimulate. Since it is consequently unable to promote the ascent of kidney essence to nourish the brain, the pathomechanism of emptiness of the sea of marrow arises, manifesting in dizzy head and black vision, tinnitus and deafness, abstraction of the spirit-affect, and forgetfulness.

When kidney yáng is insufficient, it is unable to warm, nourish, and fill the lower back. The result is aching lower back and limpness in the lower legs with pain that causes inability to bend and stretch.

When kidney yáng fails to warm, secure, and contain because of being vacuous, the result is physical cold, fear of cold, and enuresis.

Debilitation of kidney yáng manifests in a pale tongue with white fur and a faint, fine, and forceless cubit pulse.

The treatise "On Seas" in the *Líng Shū* ("The Magic Pivot") states: "Superabundance in the sea of marrow results in lightness, vigor, and strength, and abililty to extend oneself beyond one's limit. Insufficiency in the sea of marrow results in spinning head and ringing ears, aching of the lower limbs, veiling dizziness, loss of vision, and sluggishness, fatigue, and lying down." This quotation is the earliest reference to the pathomechanical changes of sea of marrow deprived of nourishment. Though it does not discuss the causes leading to this pathomechanism, it makes clear that debilitation of kidney yáng can influence engenderment in the sea of marrow, therefore depriving the sea of marrow of nourishment.

The chapter, "The Brain" in "Collected References to Miscellaneous Pathoconditions" in the *Yī Shù* ("Account of Medicine") states:

> "Excessive thought causes the symptoms of heart fire scorching the brain, such as dizzy head, flowery vision, and tinnitus, as well as damage to the marrow. Marrow is originally engendered from essence and passes to the governing vessel in the lower body. When the life fire provides warmth and nourishment, marrow is boosted and filled. Through overindulgence of desires, however, the life gate is damaged. As a result, the life gate fire fails to warm the upper body and pours downward. In such circumstances, how could the brain marrow restrict the give-and-take of the life gate and not get worn out?"

This quotation explicitly describes how debilitation of the life gate fire, impaired warming and nourishing, and emptiness of the sea of marrow lead to dizzy head, flowery vision, and tinnitus.

Emptiness of the sea of marrow is treated by warming yáng and supplementing the kidney, and by replenishing essence and boosting marrow. The recommended formula is *lù róng wán* (Velvet Deerhorn Pill) from the *Yán Shì Jì Shēng Fāng* ("Yan's Remedies for Curing All People"), with the addition of *huáng jīng* (Polygonati Rhizoma) and *hú táo ròu* (Juglandis Semen).

Lù Róng Wán 鹿茸丸
Velvet Deerhorn Pill

lù róng (鹿茸 Cervi Cornu Pantotrichum, velvet deerhorn)
niú xī (牛膝 Achyranthis Bidentatae Radix, achyranthes)
wǔ wèi zǐ (五味子 Schisandrae Fructus, schisandra)
shí hú (石斛 Dendrobii Herba, dendrobium)
tù sī zǐ (菟丝子 Cuscutae Semen, cuscuta)
dù zhòng (杜仲 Eucommiae Cortex, eucommia)
bā jǐ tiān (巴戟天 Morindae Officinalis Radix, morinda)
shān yào (山药 Dioscoreae Rhizoma, dioscorea)
yáng qǐ shí (阳起石 Actinolitum, actinolite)
fù zǐ (附子 Aconiti Radix Lateralis Praeparata, aconite)

chuān liàn zǐ (川楝子 Toosendan Fructus, toosendan)
cí shí (磁石 Magnetitum, loadstone)
guān guì (官桂 Cinnamomi Cortex Tubiformis, quilled cinnamon)
zé xiè (泽泻 Alismatis Rhizoma, alisma)

Plus:

huáng jīng (黄精 Polygonati Rhizoma, polygonatum)
hé táo rén (胡桃仁 Juglandis Semen, walnut)

髓海空虚

肾藏精，生髓，通于脑。故《灵枢•海论》曰："脑为髓之海。"精属阴，肾中精气阴阳，互根互长，相互影响。肾精能生髓养脑，肾阳命火能温煦脑髓，故髓海空虚的病机变化，既可因肾精气不足所致，也可因肾阳不足、命门火衰引起。如各种原因导致肾阳损伤，肾阳温煦、激发功能减弱，不能推动肾精上养于脑，则会形成髓海空虚的病机，见到头晕眼黑，耳鸣耳聋，神情恍惚，健忘遗事的表现; 肾阳不足，不能温养充填腰府，则腰酸胫软，疼痛不可屈伸; 肾阳虚，失于温煦固摄，则形寒怕冷，小便遗溺。肾阳虚衰，则舌淡苔白，尺脉微细无力。如《灵枢•海论》曰："髓海有余，则轻劲多力，自过其度; 髓海不足，则脑转耳鸣，胫痠眩冒，目无所见，懈怠安卧。"最早指出了髓海失养的病机变化，虽未论及引起髓海失养的原因，但肾阳虚衰，可以影响髓海的生成，故亦可成为髓海失养的病因。《医述•杂证汇参•脑》曰："过思则心火烁脑，头眩、眼花、耳鸣之象立见，而髓伤矣。髓本精生，下通督脉，命火温养则髓益充。纵欲者伤其命门，不但无以上温，而且索其下注，脑髓几何，能禁命门之取给而不敝乎?"明确论述命门火衰，失于温养，髓海空虚，引起头昏眼花耳鸣的病机变化。治法宜温阳补肾，填精益髓。方药选用《重订严氏济生方》鹿茸丸（鹿茸、川牛膝、五味子、石斛、菟丝子、杜仲、川巴戟、山药、阳起石、附子、川楝子、磁石、官桂、泽泻）加黄精、胡桃肉。

Literature Review of Emptiness of the Sea of Marrow

📖 *Sù Wèn* ("Plain Questions"), "Engenderment of the Five Viscera"

> "Headache indicates vacuity below and repletion above. It occurs in the foot lesser yīn and greater yáng channels; in severe cases, it enters the kidney."

This quotation points out that kidney vacuity can lead to changes related to the pathomechanism of head deprived of nourishment, such as headache. While this text did not posit the disease cause of kidney yáng vacuity, it provided a theoretical foundation for the recognition of the pathomechanism of kidney yáng vacuity and emptiness of the sea of marrow.

📖 *Jǐng Yuè Quán Shū* ("Jǐng-Yuè's Complete Compendium"), "Schema of Miscellaneous Patterns: Dizziness"

> "Patterns of dizziness manifest in heavy-headedness, black vision, or in spinning of the brain marrow that is preventing the person from moving. Searching the reason for why it is called repletion, people only say that heavy-headedness means repletion in the upper body. They are unaware that the head is really no heavier than on previous days, and that it is only the inability to prevail over its heaviness that is worse than in previous days. The fact that upper-body strength is unable to prevail means yáng vacuity. How could this be repletion in the upper body? Moreover, how could this mean that qì fails to return to its origin and that all qì flees counterflow?"

This quotation differentiates and analyzes the pathomechanism of dizziness caused by yáng vacuity (which includes kidney yáng vacuity).

📖 *Yī Biǎn* ("Lancing Stones of Medicine"), "Miscellaneous Pathoconditions: Ears"

> "Deafness means that something is covering, congesting, and stopping flow in the ears... When lower burner qì moves counterflow and causes vacuity, this can mean either that yīn vacuity fire flames upward or that yáng vacuity fire floats upward."

Yáng vacuity fire floating refers to a vacuity of kidney yáng with yīn exuberating in the lower body and yáng floating to the upper body. Thus this quotation explains how a vacuity of kidney yáng and sea of marrow deprived of nourishment can lead to deafness.

📖 *Yī Lín Gǎi Cuò* ("Correction of Errors in Medical Classics"), "Theories on Brain Marrow"

> "Here is the reason why the spirit and memory are located in the brain: Food and drink engender qì and blood and grow flesh; the clear essence transforms into marrow. This rises upward through the spine and enters the brain, where it is called brain marrow... The reason why children don't have memory is that their brain marrow is not yet full; the reason why people of advanced age do not have memory is that their brain marrow is gradually emptied."

The brain governs the activities of the essence-spirit. The reason for people's lack of memory and forgetfulness is that the sea of marrow is insufficient. In people of advanced age, kidney essence and kidney yáng are easily debilitated, and they therefore tend to suffer from reduced memory.

文献评述

《素问•五脏生成篇》曰："头痛巅疾，下虚上实，过在足少阴、巨阳，甚则入肾。"点出了肾虚可致头痛巅疾等头部失养的病机变化，虽未提出肾阳虚的病因，但对肾阳虚而髓海虚的病机认识给予了理论铺垫。

《景岳全书•杂证谟•眩晕》曰："夫眩晕之证，或为头重，或为眼黑，或为脑髓旋转不可以动，求其言实之由，不过为头重者为上实，而不知头本不重于往日，而唯不胜其重者，乃甚于往日耳，上力不胜，阳之虚也，岂上实乎?又何气不归元，及诸气逆奔之有?"对阳虚（包括肾阳虚）而致眩晕的病机进行了辨别和分析。

《医碥•杂症•耳》曰："耳聋，耳有所蔽塞不通。…下焦气逆为虚，或为阴虚火上炎，或为阳虚火上浮。"阳虚火浮，即指肾阳虚，阴盛于下，阳浮于上，说明肾阳虚，髓海失养，可致耳聋。

《医林改错•脑髓说》曰："灵机记性在脑者，因饮食生气血，长肌肉，精汁之清者，化而为髓，由脊骨上行入脑，名脑髓。…所以小儿无记性者，脑髓未满；高年无记性者，脑髓渐空。"脑主精神活动，人无记性而健忘，是由髓海不足，老年人肾精肾阳容易衰退，故易记忆减退。

Summary of Emptiness of the Sea of Marrow

1. Inability to Nourish the Brain
   Dizzy head and black vision, tinnitus and deafness, abstraction of the spirit-affect, forgetfulness.
2. Inability to Nourish the Lower Back
   Aching lower back and limpness in the lower legs, pain that causes inability to bend and stretch.
3. Impaired Warming
   Physical cold and fear of cold, enuresis.
4. Debilitation of Kidney Yáng
   Pale tongue with white fur, faint, fine, and forceless cubit pulse.

髓海空虛
不能养脑—头晕眼黑，耳鸣耳聋，神情恍惚，健忘遗事
不能养腰—腰酸胫软，疼痛不可屈伸
温煦失职—形寒怕冷，小便遗溺
肾阳虚衰—舌淡苔白，尺脉微细无力

1.4 Decline in Reproductive Functions

The kidney is the root of earlier heaven and governs birth, growth, development, and reproduction. It is only when kidney yáng is plentiful and life fire exuberant that the kidney is able to invigorate the body's mechanism for multiplying ceaselessly and allow for the normal performance of reproductive functions and for the thriving and prospering of later generations. Insufficiency of original yáng, constitutional debilitation of earlier heaven, damage from taxation fatigue, or excessive sexual taxation can all cause a debilitation of life gate fire. As a result, the pathomechanism of decrease in reproductive functions arises.

When kidney yáng is unable to warm the yáng wilt of the ancestral sinew, and essence-blood loses its fullness, the result is yáng wilt and failure to rise, or possibly rising but without hardness, scant or cold semen, or sterility.

When kidney yáng is debilitated and therefore unable to stimulate and excite, the result is reduced sexual functions, indifference, and inability to sustain arousal for a long period of time.

When kidney yáng is vacuous, it is unable to contain semen. The result is premature ejaculation, seminal efflux, and white turbidity.

When in women the life gate fire is debilitated, it is unable to warm the uterus. This results in uterine cold infertility.

Debilitation of the life gate fire manifests in a pale tongue with white fur and a weak sunken pulse.

The "Schema of Miscellaneous Patterns; Yáng Wilt" in the *Jǐng Yuè Quán Shū* ("Jǐng-Yuè's Complete Compendium") states:

> "Yáng wilt and failure to rise in men is mostly caused by debilitation of the life gate fire and by essential qì vacuity cold… To treat debilitation of the life gate fire and essential qì vacuity cold that result in yáng wilt, use formulas like *yòu guī wán* (Right-Restoring [Life Gate] Pill), *zàn yù dān* (Procreation Elixir), or *shí kè ān shèn wán* (Carved in Stone Kidney-Quieting Pill) to govern it."

This quotation indicates that debilitation of kidney yáng and essential qì vacuity cold can lead to disturbances of male sexual function.

The chapter, "Yīn Wilt" in the *Yī Biǎn* ("Lancing Stones of Medicine") also points out: "When yáng is stirred, it rises; when yīn is stirred, it wilts… Firstly, excessive wear and dissipation makes the life gate fire vacuous… For fire vacuity, use *guì fù bā wèi wán* (Cinnamon Bark and Aconite Eight-Ingredient Pill)." This quotation clearly describes how debilitation of the life gate fire leads to yīn wilt.

Decrease in reproductive functions is treated by warming the kidney and invigorating yáng, and by supplementing and boosting essence-blood. Recommended formulas are *yòu guī wán* (Right-Restoring [Life Gate] Pill) from the *Jǐng Yuè Quán Shū* ("Jǐng-Yuè's Complete Compendium") with modifications, or *zàn yù dān* (Procreation Elixir) from the same text, also with modifications.

Yòu Guī Wán 右归丸 Right-Restoring [Life Gate] Pill
shú dì huáng (熟地黄 Rehmanniae Radix Praeparata, cooked rehmannia)
shān yào (山药 Dioscoreae Rhizoma, dioscorea)
shān zhū yú (山茱萸 Corni Fructus, cornus)
gǒu qǐ zǐ (枸杞子 Lycii Fructus, lycium)
dù zhòng (杜仲 Eucommiae Cortex, eucommia)
tù sī zǐ (菟丝子 Cuscutae Semen, cuscuta)
lù jiǎo jiāo (鹿角胶 Cervi Cornus Gelatinum, deerhorn glue)
dāng guī (当归 Angelicae Sinensis Radix, Chinese angelica)
ròu guì (肉桂 Cinnamomi Cortex, cinnamon bark)
fù zǐ (附子 Aconiti Radix Lateralis Praeparata, aconite)

Zàn Yù Dān 赞育丹 Procreation Elixir
shú dì huáng (熟地黄 Rehmanniae Radix Praeparata, cooked rehmannia)
bái zhú (白术 Atractylodis Macrocephalae Rhizoma, white atractylodes)
dāng guī (当归 Angelicae Sinensis Radix, Chinese angelica)
gǒu qǐ zǐ (枸杞子 Lycii Fructus, lycium)
dù zhòng (杜仲 Eucommiae Cortex, eucommia)
xiān máo (仙茅 Curculiginis Rhizoma, curculigo)
bā jǐ tiān (巴戟天 Morindae Officinalis Radix, morinda)

shān zhū yú (山茱萸 Corni Fructus, cornus)
yín yáng huò (淫羊藿 Epimedii Herba, epimedium)
ròu cōng róng (肉苁蓉 Cistanches Herba, cistanche)
jiǔ zǐ (韭子 Allii Tuberosi Semen, Chinese leek seed)
shé chuáng zǐ (蛇床子 Cnidii Fructus, cnidium seed)
fù zǐ (附子 Aconiti Radix Lateralis Praeparata, aconite)
ròu guì (肉桂 Cinnamomi Cortex, cinnamon bark)

生殖减退

肾为先天之本，主生长发育及生殖。肾阳充足，命火旺盛，才能壮其生生不息之机，令生殖功能正常，繁衍后代。如遇元阳不足，或先天禀赋衰减，或劳倦损伤，或房事过度，导致命门火衰，则可形成生殖功能减退的病机变化。肾阳不能温煦宗筋，精血失充，则阳痿不起，或举而不坚，或精少、精冷，不育；肾阳虚衰，不能激发、冲动，则性功能减弱，淡漠，不能持久；肾阳虚，不能收摄精液，则早泄，滑精白浊；命门火衰，不能温暖胞宫，则会引起女子宫寒不孕。命门火衰，则舌淡苔白，脉沉弱。如《景岳全书•杂证谟•阳痿》曰：“凡男子阳痿不起，多由命门火衰，精气虚冷。…命门火衰，精气虚寒而阳痿者，宜右归丸、赞育丹、石刻安肾丸之类主之。”指出了肾阳虚衰，精气虚寒而致男子性功能障碍的病机变化。《医碥•阴痿》也指出：“阳动则举，阴动则痿。…一则耗散过度，命门火虚也。…火虚者，附桂八味丸”。明确了命门火衰而致阳痿的病机。治法宜温肾壮阳，补益精血。方药选用《景岳全书》右归丸（熟地黄、怀山药、山萸肉、枸杞子、杜仲、菟丝子、鹿角胶、当归、肉桂、附子）加减，或选《景岳全书》赞育丹（熟地、白术、当归、枸杞、杜仲、仙茅、巴戟、山茱萸、淫羊藿、肉苁蓉、韭子、蛇床子、附子、肉桂）加减。

Literature Review of Decrease in Reproductive Functions

📖 *Yī Guàn* (“Thorough Knowledge of Medicine”), “On Dream Emission and Seminal Efflux”

“For the treatment of debilitation of the life gate fire, desertion and fall of original essence, and non-closure of the jade gate, urgently use *bā wèi wán* (Eight-Ingredient Pill) or *jīn suǒ zhèng yuán dān* (Golden Lock Origin-Righting Elixir) to invigorate true yáng and let it be moistened by yīn essence instead of being discharged. This is the general idea behind these formulas."

This quotation indicates that debilitation of the life gate fire leads to a decrease in reproductive functions.

📖 *Zá Bìng Yuán Liú Xī Zhú* ("Incisive Light on the Source of Miscellaneous Disease"), "Internal Damage: The Origin and Development of Damage from Sexual Desire"

"Harm from sexual desire… either manifests as yáng vacuity desertion of essence and premature ejaculation before intercourse, or ejaculation at the beginning of intercourse, leakage, and failure to retain. *Qiàn shí wán* (Euryales Pill) and *suǒ yáng dān* (Cynomorii Elixir) are recommended… For cases of slight vacuity of kidney yáng, which manifests in efflux from the essence gate, spontaneous and night sweating, and frequent dreams of intercourse with ghosts, *zhū shèn wán* (Suis Renes Powder) is recommended."

This quotation indicates the pathomechanical changes of debilitation of kidney yáng and insecurity of the essence gate.

📖 *Zhōng Yī Lín Zhèng Bèi Yào* ("Essential Notes of Clinical Chinese Medicine"), "Yáng Wilting"

"In male patients who have not yet reached the age where their sexual desire declines, if their penis fails to rise or rises but fails to harden or to endure, it is called 'yáng wilting.' It is mostly caused by damage at a young age, debilitation of the life gate fire, and essential qì vacuity cold. As Zhāng Jǐng-Yuè said, 'it is fire debilitation seven or eight out of ten'."

This quotation describes in detail the pathomechanism of kidney yáng debilitation and decreased sexual functions.

文献评述

《医贯•梦遗并滑精论》曰："有命门火衰，元精脱陷，玉关不闭者，急用八味丸，用金锁正元丹，以壮真阳，使之涵乎阴精而不泄，此其大略也。"指出了命门火衰而致生殖减退的病机改变。

《杂病源流犀烛•内伤•色欲伤源流》曰："色欲之为害，...其或阳虚精脱，未交先泄，或乍交即泄，滑泂不禁欤。宜芡实丸、锁阳丹。...其或肾阳虚微，精关滑泄，自汗盗汗，夜多梦与鬼交欤，宜猪肾丸。"指出了肾阳虚衰，精关不固的病机变化。

《中医临证备要•阳痿》曰："男子未到性欲衰退时期，阴茎不举，或举而不坚不久，称为'阳痿'，多因少年斫伤，命门火衰，精气虚寒，张景岳所谓：'火衰者十之七八'。"详细论述肾阳虚衰，性功能减退的病机变化。

Summary of Decrease in Reproductive Functions
1. Loss of Warmth in the Ancestral Sinew
Yáng wilt and failure to rise, or rising but without hardness, scant or cold semen, sterility.
3. Inability to be Stimulated
Reduced sexual function, indifference, inability to sustain arousal for a long period of time.
3. Inability to Contain Semen
Premature ejaculation, seminal efflux and white turbidity.
4. Inability to Warm the Uterus
Uterine cold infertility.
5. Debilitation of the Life Gate Fire
Pale tongue with white fur, weak sunken pulse.

生殖减退
宗筋失温—阳痿不起，或举而不坚，或精少、精冷，不育
不能激发—性功能减弱，淡漠，不能持久
不能收摄—早泄，滑精白浊
不能暖宫—女子宫寒而不孕
命门火衰—舌淡苔白，脉沉弱

1.5 Indiscriminate Flooding of Fluids

The kidney is the water viscus and has the function of managing and regulating the fluid metabolism. Kidney yáng has the functions of transforming qì by steaming, upbearing the clear and downbearing the turbid, and regulating the waterways. All these are essential for maintaining balance in the fluid metabolism. Damage to the kidney from cold-damp can lead to irregularities in the fluid metabolism. In addition, debilitation of kidney yáng can also lead to indiscriminate flooding of fluids. When kidney yáng is debilitated, yáng qì is unable to effectively carry out qì transformation by steaming or promote the movement of the fluids. This causes the fluids to collect; instead of following their normal course, they flood and spill everywhere. As a result, the pathomechanism of debilitation of kidney yáng and flooding of water qì arises.

When kidney yáng is debilitated, qì transformation by steaming fails, and water qì is not transformed, but inundates the entire body, causing puffy swelling in the whole body.

The lower back is the house of the kidney. Because it belongs to yīn in the lower body, yáng qì does not easily reach it. In addition, water-qì has a tendency to flow downward. When kidney yáng vacuity causes indiscriminate flooding of water qì, this manifests in water swelling that is particularly pronounced below the lower back and pits when pressure is applied, and counterflow cold in the lower limbs.

When water qì floods and flows into the skin, it is unable to move down into the bladder, and qì transformation lacks its source. This manifests in inhibited urination.

When the fluids collect in the four limbs and inhibit the free movement of qì and blood, this results in heaviness and pain in the four limbs.

Water qì that is not discharged, but soaks into the scrotum results in cold sweating of the scrotum.

When water qì ascends counterflow and harasses the clear orifices, this results in dizzy head and vision.

When water qì collects internally, and yīn cold exuberates internally, fire fails to warm earth, and splenic movement and transformation is impaired. This results in an enlarged abdomen, swelling of the umbilicus, abdominal pain, and diarrhea.

Water qì can rise upward to attack and intimidate the heart, debilitating heart yáng and disquieting the heart spirit. The result is heart palpitations, fearful throbbing, oppression in the chest, and shortness of breath.

When water-cold rises and shoots into the lung, it impairs the lung's diffusion and downbearing. This results in cough, panting, and ejection of phlegm.

Yáng vacuity with water collecting manifests in a pale tender-soft enlarged tongue, glossy white tongue fur, and faint sunken pulse.

The chapter, "Pulse Symptoms and Treatments of Water Qì Disease" in the *Jīn Guì Yào Lüè* ("Essential Prescriptions of the Golden Coffer") states:

> "Kidney water manifests in an enlarged abdomen, swelling of the umbilicus and lumbar pain, inability to urinate, dampness below the genitals like the sweaty nose of an ox, counterflow cold of the feet, and paradoxical thinness of the face."

This quotation describes the pathomechanical changes resulting from debilitation of kidney yáng and water invading and doing harm.

The chapter, "Swelling and Distention" in the *Yī Biǎn* ("Lancing Stones of Medicine") also states:

> "Disease in the water aspect is predominantly a yīn pattern. Why is this? In spite of the fact that water and qì are identical in type, when yáng exuberates, qì transforms and water turns into essence; but when yáng is debilitated, qì is unable to transform, and essence turns into water. For this reason, all cases of water disease are rooted in the blood and qì within the body, but whether it is evil or right all depends on whether or not there is transformation. Water that cannot be transformed is due to vacuity of qì. How could this not be a situation of lack of yáng within yīn? Thus such diseases of water swelling may be predominantly ascribed to yáng vacuity. Water is governed by the kidney, and qì is governed by the lung. When water steeps in the lower body and qì is exhausted in the upper body, this causes swelling and fullness in the lower body and rapid panting in the upper body. The root and tip are both diseased, and such conditions are extremely critical."

This quotation analyzes in detail the problem of indiscriminate flooding of water qì due to debilitation of kidney yáng.

Indiscriminate flooding of fluids is treated by invigorating the kidney and supplementing fire, and by warming yáng and disinhibiting water. Recommended formulas are *zhēn wǔ tāng* (True Warrior Decoction) from the *Shāng Hán Lùn* ("On Cold Damage") or *jì shēng shèn qì wán* (Life Saver Kidney Qì Pill) from the *Yán Shì Jì Shēng Fāng* ("Yan's Remedies for Curing All People") with modifications.

Zhēn Wǔ Tāng 真武汤
True Warrior Decoction

fù zǐ (附子 Aconiti Radix Lateralis Praeparata, aconite)
bái zhú (白朮 Atractylodis Macrocephalae Rhizoma, white atractylodes)
fú líng (茯苓 Poria, poria)
bái sháo (白芍 Paeoniae Radix Alba, white peony)
shēng jiāng (生姜 Zingiberis Rhizoma Recens, fresh ginger)

Jì Shēng Shèn Qì Wán 济生肾气丸|
Life Saver Kidney Qì Pill

fù zǐ (附子 Aconiti Radix Lateralis Praeparata, aconite)
fú líng (茯苓 Poria, poria)
zé xiè (泽泻 Alismatis Rhizoma, alisma)
shān zhū yú (山茱萸 Corni Fructus, cornus)
shān yào (山药 Dioscoreae Rhizoma, dioscorea)
chē qián zǐ (车前子 Plantaginis Semen, plantago seed)
mǔ dān pí (牡丹皮 Moutan Cortex, moutan)
guān guì (官桂 Cinnamomi Cortex Tubiformis, quilled cinnamon)
niú xī (牛膝 Achyranthis Bidentatae Radix, achyranthes)
shú dì huáng (熟地黄 Rehmanniae Radix Praeparata, cooked rehmannia)

水气泛滥

肾为水脏，有主持和调节水液代谢的作用。肾阳的蒸腾气化，升清降浊，通调水道，对维持水液代谢的平衡具有十分重要的意义。不但寒湿伤肾可致水液代谢失常，肾阳虚衰亦可致水液泛滥。肾阳虚衰，阳气不能有效的蒸腾气化及推动水液运行，导致水液停聚，不循常道，四处泛溢，则可形成肾阳虚衰，水气泛溢的病机变化。肾阳虚衰，蒸腾气化无权，水气不化，泛滥全身，则全身浮肿; 腰为肾之府，腰以下属阴，阳气不易到达，水气容易下流，肾阳虚水气泛滥者，水肿腰以下尤甚，按之凹陷不起，下肢逆冷; 水气泛溢，流于肌肤，不能下输膀胱，气化无源，则出现小便不利; 水液停聚于四肢，气血运行不畅，则四肢沉重疼痛; 水气不得泄，浸渍于阴囊，则阴囊冷汗; 水气上逆，扰乱清空，则为头目眩晕; 水气内停，阴寒内盛，火不暖土，脾失健运，则腹大脐肿，腹痛下利; 水气上犯凌心，心阳虚衰，心神不宁，则心悸怔忡，胸闷气短; 水寒上逆射肺，肺失宣降，则咳嗽气喘，吐痰。阳虚水停，则舌淡胖嫩，苔白滑，脉沉微。如《金匮要略•水气病脉证并治》曰：“肾水者，其腹大，脐肿腰痛，不得溺，阴下湿如牛鼻上汗，其足逆冷，面反瘦。”对肾阳虚衰，水犯为害的病机变化进行了论述。《医述•肿胀》也曰：“若病在水分，则多为阴证。何也?盖水之与气虽为同类，但阳旺则气化，而水即为精，阳衰则气不化，而精即为水。故凡病水者，本即身中之血气，但其为邪为正，总在化与不化耳。水不能化，因气之虚，岂非阴中无阳乎?此水肿之病，所以多属阳虚也。然水主于肾，气主于肺，水渍于下，而气竭于上，所以下为肿满，上为喘急，标本俱病，危斯极矣。"详细分析了肾阳虚衰，水气泛滥为患的病机变化。治法以壮肾补火，温阳利水为主。方药宜选用《伤寒论》真武汤（附子、白术、茯苓、白芍、生姜）=，或选《济生方》济生肾气丸（附子、茯苓、泽泻、山茱萸、山药、车前子、丹皮、官桂、牛膝、熟地黄）加减。

Literature Review of Indiscriminate Flooding of Fluids

🕮 *Shāng Hán Lùn* ("On Cold Damage"), "Identifying Pulse Symptoms and Treatments of Lesser Yīn Disease"

> "When lesser yīn disease persists for two to three days without ceasing and on the fourth or fifth day manifests with abdominal pain, inhibited urination, heaviness and pain in the four limbs, and spontaneous diarrhea, this means water qì. If such a patient presents with cough, inhibited urination, diarrhea, or retching, *zhēn wǔ tāng* (True Warrior Decoction) governs it."

This quotation describes the numerous pathological changes such as inhibited urination that result from a vacuity of kidney yáng, poor qì transformation, and water qì collecting internally.

🕮 *Yán Shì Jì Shēng Fāng* ("Yan's Remedies for Curing All People"), "Section on Water Swelling"

> "The disease of water swelling is always caused by timidity and scantness of true yáng, by taxation damage to the spleen and stomach, and by coldness of the spleen and stomach resulting in accumulating cold transforming water. The spleen is earth, and the kidney is water. The kidney has the ability to contain water, and the spleen has the ability to house water. When kidney water does not flow, the spleen's abode becomes congested. This causes panting exhalations and cough in the upper body and swelling of the feet, knees, and skin in the lower body, puffy face and abdominal distention, inhibited urination, possible swelling of the external kidney [the testicles], and in severe cases, flooding and rupture of the flesh, and water flowing from the feet and lower legs, which in most cases cannot be stemmed."

This quotation comprehensively describes the pathomechanical changes of water qì flooding indiscriminately due to debilitation of kidney yáng and spleen failing to move and transform.

文献评述

《伤寒论•辨少阴病脉证并治》曰："少阴病，二三日不已，至四五日，腹痛，小便不利，四肢沉重疼痛，自下利者，此为有水气。其人或咳，或小便利，或下利，或呕者，真武汤主之。"描述了肾阳虚，气化不行，水气内停而引起小便不利等诸多病机变化。

《重订严氏济生方•水肿门》曰："水肿为病，皆由真阳怯少，劳伤脾胃，脾胃既寒，积寒化水。盖脾者土也，肾者水也，肾能摄水，脾能舍水，肾水不流，脾舍堙塞，是以上为喘呼咳嗽，下为足膝肤肿，面浮腹胀，小便不利，外肾或肿，甚则肌肉崩溃，足胫流水，多致不救。"全面论述了肾阳虚衰，脾失健运，水气泛滥的病机变化。

《血证论•脏腑病机论》曰："肾者水脏，水中含阳，...如阳气不足者，则水泛为痰，凌心冲肺，发为水肿，腹痛奔豚，下利厥冷，亡阳大汗，元气暴脱。"论述了肾阳亏虚，水气犯滥的病机变化.

Summary of Indiscriminate Flooding of Fluids

1. Indiscriminate Flooding All Over the Body
   Generalized puffy swelling particularly pronounced below the lower back that pits when pressure is applied; lower limb counterflow cold.
2. Poor Qì Transformation
   Inhibited urination.
3. Steeping into the Scrotum
   Cold sweating of the scrotum.
4. Collecting in the Four Limbs
   Heaviness and pain in the four limbs.
5. Water Qì Counterflow Ascent
   Dizzy head and vision.
6. Spleen Failing to Move and Transform
   Enlarged abdomen and swelling in the umbilicus, abdominal pain and diarrhea.
7. Water Qì Intimidating the Heart
   Heart palpitations and fearful throbbing, oppression in the chest and shortness of breath.
8. Water-Cold Invading the Lung
   Cough and panting, ejection of phlegm.
9. Yáng Vacuity and Water Collecting
   Pale tender-soft enlarged tongue, glossy white tongue fur, faint sunken pulse.

水气泛滥
泛滥全身—全身浮肿，腰以下肿甚，按之凹陷不起，下肢逆冷
气化不行—小便不利
浸渍阴囊—阴囊冷汗
停聚四肢—四肢沉重疼痛
水气上逆—头目眩晕
脾失健运—腹大脐肿，腹痛下利
水气凌心—心悸怔忡，胸闷气短
水寒犯肺—咳嗽气喘，吐痰
阳虚水停—舌淡胖嫩，苔白滑，脉沉微

1.6 Fire Failing to Warm Earth

There is a store of yáng qì within the kidney. This kidney yáng, also called original yáng, true yáng, or true fire, is the root of all yáng qì in the body. It has the function of promoting movement in and warming the bowels and viscera, channels and network vessels, and tissues organs. The life gate is connected to kidney qì. As the "Record of Transmitting Loyalty" in the *Jǐng Yuè Quán Shū* ("Jǐng-Yuè's Complete Compendium") explains: "The life gate is the root of the body's original qì... Without it, yáng qì of the five viscera lacks the ability to effuse." The spleen is associated with earth and is in charge of movement and transformation. Spleen qì, besides depending on the harmonizing effect between itself and the other viscera and bowels, further relies on the steaming and warming action of kidney yáng so as to carry out its normal movement and transformation functions. If kidney yáng is insufficient and the life gate fire is debilitated, fire fails to warm earth. This can manifest in the pathomechanism of devitalized spleen yáng and spleen failing to move and transform.

The "Treatise on Reversal" in the *Sù Wèn* ("Plain Questions") points out: "In reverse flow of lesser yīn, there is vacuity fullness, retching, and clear diarrhea." Lesser yīn homes to the kidney. When kidney yáng vacuity impairs the spleen's ability to move and transform, this can lead to abdominal distention, vomiting and retching, and diarrhea.

When the life gate fire is debilitated fire fails to warm earth. As a result, the spleen fails to move and transform, and large amounts of fluid and undigested food flow downward. This can manifest in incessant diarrhea and non-transformation of food.

After the midnight watch, at the transition between the second and third nightwatch when the roosters crow [around 5 am], clear yáng begins to bear upward. If a patient at that time suffers from kidney yáng vacuity and debilitation of the life gate fire, which weakens yáng qì in the body further, clear yáng lacks support and instead falls downward. The result is fifth watch diarrhea.

Debilitation of the life gate fire deprives the lower back of warmth and nourishment. This results in limp aching lower back and knees.

When yáng is vacuous, it fails to drum up movement and is unable to arouse the heart spirit. The result is listlessness of the essence-spirit.

If splenic movement is further weakened to the point where it is unable to engender the essence of grain and water and supply nourishment for the entire body, emaciation results.

Debilitation of the life gate fire and yáng qì vacuity manifest in a pale tender-soft enlarged tongue, glossy white tongue fur, and a slow forceless sunken pulse.

The chapter, "Supplementing and Boosting" in the *Yán Shì Jì Shēng Fāng* ("Yan's Remedies for Curing All People") states:

> "If people in the course of their life are not good at conserving and nourishing, they will suffer from excessive vacuity taxation and debilitation of true yáng. Fire fails to warm and is unable to ascend and steam spleen-earth. Harmonious flow is not distributed and moved to the central regions. This causes lack of intake of food and drink… This is all related to debilitation of true yáng that is preventing it from ascending and steaming spleen-earth."

This quotation explicitly describes the special characteristics of the pathomechanism by which fire failing to engender earth can lead to disorders in splenic movement.

The "Treatise on Diarrhea and Fecal Stoppage" in the *Yī Guàn* ("Thorough Knowledge of Medicine") also explains:

> "The classic states, 'the kidney governs stool and urine,' 'the kidney is in charge of opening and closing,' and 'the kidney opens at the two yīn.' These quotations show that the kidney not only governs urine, but also wields power over the ability to open and close in defecation. If the kidney is debilitated, the fire in the life gate is extinguished, which

> means that water rules alone. This causes such a person to suffer from frequent incessant water diarrhea, which pours down each morning just before dawn, invariably with two or three bouts of throughflux diarrhea."

This quotation describes incisively how debilitation of life gate fire and failure of fire to warm earth leads to diarrhea and dysentery, especially fifth-watch diarrhea.

Failure of fire to warm earth is treated by warming the kidney and supplementing fire, and by warming the spleen and fortifying movement. The recommended formulas are *fù zǐ lǐ zhōng tāng* (Aconite Center-Rectifying Decoction) from the *Tài Píng Huì Mín Hé Jì Jú Fāng* ("Tài-Píng Imperial Grace Pharmacy Formulas") or *sì shén wán* (Four Spirits Pill) from the *Zhèng Zhì Zhǔn Shéng* ("The Level-Line of Pattern Identification and Treatment") with modifications.

Fù Zǐ Lǐ Zhōng Tāng 附子理中汤 Aconite Center-Rectifying Decoction
fù zǐ (附子 Aconiti Radix Lateralis Praeparata, aconite)
gān jiāng (干姜 Zingiberis Rhizoma, dried ginger)
rén shēn (人参 Ginseng Radix, ginseng)
bái zhú (白术 Atractylodis Macrocephalae Rhizoma, white atractylodes)
zhì gān cǎo (炙甘草 Glycyrrhizae Radix cum Liquido Fricta, mix-fried licorice)

Sì Shén Wán 四神丸 Four Spirits Pill
ròu dòu kòu (肉豆蔻 Myristicae Semen, nutmeg)
wú zhū yú (吴茱萸 Evodiae Fructus, evodia)
wǔ wèi zǐ (五味子 Schisandrae Fructus, schisandra)
bǔ gǔ zhī (补骨脂 Psoraleae Fructus, psoralea)

火不暖土

肾中藏有阳气，肾阳又称元阳、真阳、真火，是人体阳气的根本，对脏腑、经络、组织、器官起着推动、温煦作用。命门与肾气相通，《景岳全书•传忠录》说：“命门为元气之根本，…五脏之阳气非此不能发。"脾属土，主司运化。脾气健运，除取决于自身和其它脏腑的协调作用外，更依赖于肾阳的蒸腾温煦，才能完成正常的运化功能。如肾阳不足，命门火衰，火不暖土，则可出现脾阳不振，脾失健运的病机变化。如《素问•厥论篇》指出："少阴厥逆，虚满呕变，下泄清。"少阴属肾，肾阳虚，脾失健运，则可引起腹胀、呕吐、泄泻。若命门火衰，火不暖土，脾失健运，大量水液和未被腐熟的水谷下流，则会出现下利不止，完谷不化; 夜半之后，寅卯之交，鸡鸣之时，清阳初升，若再遇肾阳虚，命门火衰，人体阳气更弱，清阳不得支助，反而下陷，则为五更泻利; 命门火衰，腰府失于温养，则腰膝酸软; 阳虚失于鼓动，不能振奋心神，则精神萎靡。若脾运进一步减弱，不能化生水谷精微，营养全身，则形体消瘦。命门火衰，阳气虚弱，则舌淡胖嫩，苔白滑，脉沉迟无力。如《济生方•补益》曰："人之有生，不善摄养，虚劳过度，真阳虚衰，坎火不温，不能上蒸脾土，冲和失布，中州不运，是致饮食不进，...此皆真火虚衰，不能上蒸脾土而然"。明确论述了火不生土可致脾运失常的病机特征。《医贯•泻利并大便不通论》也说："经曰：'肾主大小便。'又曰：'肾司开阖。'又曰：'肾开窍于二阴。'可见肾不但主小便，而大便之能开而复能闭者，肾操权也。今肾既虚衰，则命门之火熄矣。火熄则水独治，故令人多水泻不止，其泻每在五更天将明时，必洞泻二三次。"精辟地阐述了命门火衰，火不暖土，引起腹泻下利和五更泻的病机变化。治法以温肾补火，暖脾健运为主。方药选用《太平惠民和剂局方》附子理中汤(附子、干姜、人参、白术、炙甘草)，或选用《证治准绳》四神丸(肉豆蔻、吴茱萸、五味子、补骨脂)加减。

Literature Review of Fire Failing to Warm Earth

📖 *Zhèng Zhì Zhǔn Shéng* ("The Level-Line of Pattern Identification and Treatment"), "Miscellaneous Patterns: Diarrhea"

"Dài states: 'For daily throughflux diarrhea right before dawn, if the patient has taken diarrhea-stopping medicine without any effect, drink *wǔ wèi wán* (Schisandrae Pill) in rice liquid, or use *běi wǔ wèi jiān yǐn* (Prepared Schisandrae Chinensis Beverage). In spite of the fact that the patient has cut down on food and drink and has for the most part fasted, there is no problem during the day or before midnight, but towards the time of dawn, the diarrhea recurs. This disease is located in the kidney aspect. Drink in water *èr shén wán* (Two Spirits Pill) as well as *jiāo pò wán* (Zanthoxylum and Officinal Magnolia Bark Pill), or alternatively *píng wèi sǎn* (Stomach-Calming Powder) and then *xiǎo huí xiāng wán*

> (Foeniculi Pill). *Èr shén wán* (Two Spirits Pill) in combination with *wǔ wèi zǐ sǎn* (Schisandra Powder) is called *sì shén wán* (Four Spirits Pill) and is particularly wondrous for treating diarrhea.'"

This quotation discusses the pathomechanical changes and treatment method for debilitation of life gate fire and spleen failing to move and transform.

📖 *Yī Shù* ("Account of Medicine") "Collected References to Miscellaneous Pathoconditions: Diarrhea"

> "Kidney diarrhea occurs always in the five nightwatches or right at dawn, with several bouts of through-flux diarrhea, sometimes lasting for months or years without stopping, or temporarily recovering and then relapsing, sometimes with pain and sometimes not. The kidney is the gate of the stomach and opens at the two yīn. Opening and closing in urination and defecation are all governed by the kidney. When kidney yáng is insufficient, the life gate fire is debilitated and yīn cold exuberates alone. For this reason, the time period after the first and second night watches [after 3 am] when yáng qì is not yet restored and yīn qì is at its most exuberant, makes such a person suffer from incessant through-flux diarrhea."

This quotation analyzes the reason why debilitation of kidney yáng and failure to warm spleen earth can form "fifth-watch diarrhea." It reflects a thorough understanding of the pathomechanism of fire failing to engender earth.

文献评述

《证治准绳•杂证•泄泻》曰："戴云：有每日五更初洞泻，服止泻药并无效，米饮下五味丸，或专以北五味煎饮。虽节省饮食，大段忌口，但得日间上半夜无事，近五更其泻复作。此病在肾分，水饮下二神丸及椒朴丸，或平胃散下小茴香丸。二神丸合五味子散，名为四神丸，治泻尤妙。"论述了命门火衰，脾失健运的病机变化及治法。

《医述•杂证汇参•泻》曰："肾泄，每于五更或天明时即洞泄数次，有经月连年弗止者，或暂愈而复作者，或痛或不痛者。盖肾为胃关，开窍于二阴，二便开闭，皆肾所主。肾阳不足，则命门火衰，而阴寒独盛，故于子丑之后，阳气未复，阴气盛极之时，即令人洞泄不止也。"分析了肾阳虚衰，不温脾土可成"五更泻"的原理，对火不生土的病机变化有较深的认识。

Summary of Fire Failing to Warm Earth
1. Impaired Warming and Movement of Earth Incessant diarrhea, non-transformation of food. 2. Debilitation of Life Fire Fifth watch diarrhea. 3. Loss of Warmth and Nourishment in the Lower Back Limp aching lower back and knees. 4. Devitalized Yáng Qì Listlessness of the essence-spirit. 5. Loss of Nourishment from Grain and Water Emaciation. 6. Debilitation of the Life Gate Fire Pale tender-soft enlarged tongue, glossy white tongue fur, slow forceless sunken pulse.

火不暖土
土失温运—下利不止，完谷不化 命火衰微—五更泻利 腰失温养—腰膝酸软 阳气不振—精神萎靡 水谷失养—形体消瘦 命门火衰—舌淡胖嫩，苔白滑，脉沉迟无力

1.7 Incessant Urination

The kidney opens at the ears, but also opens at the two yīn. Kidney yáng is in charge of qì transformation and of warming and steaming. Thereby, it is able to transform the fluids into urine and transport them downward into the bladder. The kidney stands in exterior-interior relationship with the bladder. Because kidney yáng is in charge of qì transformation, it is also able to control the opening and closing of the bladder and the elimination of urine. If the life gate fire is debilitated and kidney yáng becomes insufficient, it lacks strength to secure and contain the bladder. This can lead to the pathomechanical changes of incessant urination.

When kidney yáng is insufficient and kidney qì insecure, the bladder fails to retain. This results in urinary incontinence or frequent urination with urine of a white color and profuse amounts.

At night, yīn cold is unilaterally exuberant and kidney yáng has even more difficulty with receiving and containing. As a result, such a person suffers from frequent and profuse urination at night.

In children, incomplete development of kidney yáng and vacuity cold in the bladder can prevent the bladder gate from closing tightly at night. This results in bedwetting.

The lower back is the house of the kidney. When fire is debilitated and deprived of nourishment, the result is cold aching lower back and knees.

When kidney yáng is vacuous, yáng qì fails to reach the entire body and the four limbs. The result is fear of cold and cold limbs.

Debilitation of kidney yáng manifests in a pale white tongue, glossy white tongue fur, and faint sunken pulse.

The chapter, "Various Symptoms of Urinary Disease; Urinary Incontinence" in the *Zhū Bìng Yuán Hòu Lùn* ("Origin and Indicators of Disease") states:

> "Urinary incontinence means that kidney qì is vacuous and that the lower burner has contracted cold. The kidney governs water, and its qì penetrates downward to the genitals. When the kidney is vacuous and the lower burner is cold, they are unable to warm and control the fluids. This is the cause of urinary incontinence."

This quotation clearly points out that the pathomechanism of incessant urination is caused by vacuity of kidney yáng and impaired retention in the bladder.

The chapter, "Enuresis" in the "Schema of Miscellaneous Patterns" in the *Jǐng Yuè Quán Shū* ("Jǐng-Yuè's Complete Compendium") also states:

> "Enuresis patterns include spontaneous emission, which means loss of urine during sleep, as well as incontinence, which means that the qì gate is insecure, causing frequent urination and inability to retain urine… Speaking of cases where urine is excessively uninhibited, they are all ascribed to vacuity cold. How could there be heat patterns among them? …When yáng qì in the liver and kidney is vanquished, the bladder fails to store, and urine flows incessantly. The blame for this is found in the life gate… All cases of enuresis during sleep are invariably due to vacuity cold in the lower origin, which is causing insecurity."

This quotation indicates precisely how insufficiency of the life gate and insecurity of the bladder cause the pathomechanical change of urinary incontinence.

Incessant urination is treated by warming and supplementing the kidney and life gate while securing and astringing urine. Recommended formulas are *gǒng tí wán* (Dyke-Strengthening Pill) from the *Jǐng Yuè Quán Shū* ("Jǐng-Yuè's Complete Compendium"), *suō quán wán* (Stream-Reducing Pill) from the *Fù Rén Dà Quán Liáng Fāng* ("Compendium of Good Remedies for Women"), or *gù pāo wán* (Bladder-Securing Pill) from the *Quán Shēng Zhǐ Mí Fāng* ("Pathfinder Remedies for the Entire Life"), used with modifications.

Gǒng Tí Wán 巩堤丸 Dyke-Strengthening Pill
shú dì huáng (熟地黄 Rehmanniae Radix Praeparata, cooked rehmannia) *tù sī zǐ* (菟丝子 Cuscutae Semen, cuscuta) *bái zhú* (白朮 Atractylodis Macrocephalae Rhizoma, white atractylodes) *wǔ wèi zǐ* (五味子 Schisandrae Fructus, schisandra) *yì zhì rén* (益智仁 Alpiniae Oxyphyllae Fructus, alpinia) *pó gù zhī* (婆固脂 Psoraleae Fructus, psoralea) *fù zǐ* (附子 Aconiti Radix Lateralis Praeparata, aconite) *fú líng* (茯苓 Poria, poria) *jiǔ zǐ* (韭子 Allii Tuberosi Semen, Chinese leek seed)

Suō Quán Wán 缩泉丸 Stream-Reducing Pill
shān yào (山药 Dioscoreae Rhizoma, dioscorea) *wū yào* (乌药 Linderae Radix, lindera) *yì zhì rén* (益智仁 Alpiniae Oxyphyllae Fructus, alpinia)

Gù Pāo Wán 固脬丸 Bladder-Securing Pill
tù sī zǐ (菟丝子 Cuscutae Semen, cuscuta) *xiǎo huí xiāng* (小茴香 Foeniculi Fructus, fennel) *fù zǐ* (附子 Aconiti Radix Lateralis Praeparata, aconite) *sāng piāo xiāo* (桑螵蛸 Mantidis Ootheca, mantis egg-case) *róng yán* (戎盐 Halitum, halite)

水泉不止

肾开窍于耳，也开窍于前后二阴。肾阳主司气化，温煦蒸腾，能使水液变成尿液，下输膀胱。肾与膀胱互为表里，肾阳主司气化，又可控制膀胱的开合和尿液排泄。如命门火衰，肾阳不足，对膀胱的固摄约束无力，可导致水泉不止的病机变化。肾阳不足，肾气不固，膀胱失约，则小便失禁，或小便频数，色白量多; 夜晚阴寒偏盛，肾阳更难收摄，则夜尿频多; 小儿肾阳发育不全，膀胱虚冷，夜间胞门不秘，则为小儿尿床; 腰为肾府，火衰失养，则腰膝酸冷; 肾阳虚，阳气不达全身四肢，则畏寒肢冷。肾阳虚衰，则舌淡白，苔白滑，脉沉微。如《诸病源候论•小便病诸候•小便不禁候》曰：“小便不禁者，肾气虚，下焦受冷也。肾主水，其气下通于阴，肾虚下焦冷，不能温制其水液，故小便不禁也”明确指出水泉不止的病机是肾阳虚，膀胱失约。《景岳全书•杂证谟•遗溺》也曰：“遗溺一证，有自遗者，以睡中而遗失也，有不禁者，以气门不固，而频数不能禁也。...以小水太利者为言，皆属虚寒，何有热证。...肝肾阳气亏败，则膀胱不藏，而水泉不止，此其咎在命门。...凡睡中遗溺者，此必下元虚寒，所以不固。”明确指出了命门不足，膀胱不固，小便失禁的病机变化。治法以温补肾命，固涩水泉为原则。方药选用《景岳全书》巩堤丸（熟地黄、菟丝子、白术、北五味子、益智仁、破故纸、附子、茯苓、家韭子），或用选《妇人大全良方》缩泉丸（怀山药、乌药、益智仁），或选《全生指迷方》固脬丸（制菟丝子、茴香、附子、桑螵蛸、戎盐）加减运用。

Literature Review of Incessant Urination

📖 *Yī Guàn* (“Thorough Knowledge of Medicine”), “Enuresis and Urinary Incontinence”

> “Discharge of urine without awareness thereof constitutes enuresis; being aware but unable to control urination constitutes incontinence… It is mostly caused by vacuity cold in the lung and kidney and by qì being unable to contain. *Bǔ zhōng yì qì tāng* (Center-Supplementing Qì-Boosting Decoction) together with *shèn qì wán* (Kidney Qì Pill) will generally treat the upper body vacuity by supplementing qì and the lower body vacuity by stemming desertion.”

This quotation indicates the pathomechanism by which kidney yáng vacuity and lack of strength in securing and containing lead to incessant urination.

📖 *Zhèng Zhì Huì Bǔ* ("Combined Supplements to Patterns and Treatment"), "Enuresis: Enuresis During Sleep"

> "Enuresis during sleep is a vacuity pattern. For this reason, infants, in whom bladder qì is not yet secure, and old people, who suffer from insufficiency of the lower origin, are both affected by this problem."

This quotation describes the pathomechanism by which kidney yáng vacuity and inability to secure and contain can lead to enuresis during sleep.

📖 *Zhāng Shì Yī Tōng* ("Zhang's Clear View of Medicine"), "Urinary Incontinence"

> "Urinary incontinence and strangury with inhibition and pain mean that true yáng is not secure and percolating downwards. Use *gù pāo wán* (Bladder-Securing Pill). If the condition fails to respond, use a modified version of *sāng piāo xiāo sǎn* (Mantis Egg-Case Powder)."

This quotation succinctly points out how insecurity of kidney yáng and debilitation of the life gate fire can lead to incessant urination.

📖 *Yī Fǎ Yuán Tōng* ("Medical Methods to Free the Garden"), "Incessant Urination"

> "When people with an enduring illness or habitual insufficiency suddenly manifest with frequent voidings of urine, about ten a day, that are clear, long, and profuse, this means absence of fire in the lower origin. This must quickly be treated by returning yáng and by promoting absorption of kidney qì. Be sure you do not recklessly act to disinhibit water."

This quotation describes the pathomechanism by which kidney yáng, when debilitated, loses its ability to contain and absorb, resulting in frequent and profuse urination.

文献评述

《医贯•遗尿、小便不禁》曰："不知而出为遗，知而不能忍为不禁。…多由肺肾虚寒，气不能摄，补中益气汤送肾气丸，大抵上虚补气，下虚固脱。"指出了肾阳虚固摄无力而致小泉不止的病机变化。

《证治汇补•遗溺•睡中遗尿》曰："睡则遗尿，此为虚症，所以婴儿脬气未固，老人下元不足，皆有此患。"论述肾阳虚不能固摄，能致睡中遗尿的病机。

《张氏医通•小便不禁》曰："小便不禁而淋沥涩痛者，此真阳不固而下渗也，固脬丸。不应，用加减桑螵蛸散。"明确提出了肾阳不固，命门火衰而致水泉不止的病机变化。

《医法园通•小便不止》曰："久病与素秉不足之人，忽见小便日数十次，每来清长而多，此是下元无火也，急宜回阳，收纳肾气，切不可妄行利水。"论述肾阳虚衰，失于摄纳，小便频多的病机。

Summary of Incessant Urination
1. Loss of Retention in the Bladder Urinary incontinence, or frequent urination with urine of a white color and profuse amounts.
2. Yīn Exuberance at Night Frequent urination at night.
3. Bladder Vacuity Cold Child bedwetting.
4. Fire Debilitation and Loss of Nourishment Cold aching lower back and knees.
5. Yáng Qì Failing to Outthrust Fear of cold and cold limbs.
6. Debilitation of Kidney Yáng Pale white tongue, glossy white tongue fur, faint sunken pulse.

水泉不止
膀胱失约—小便失禁，或小便频数，色白量多
夜晚阴盛—夜尿频多
膀胱虚冷—小儿尿床
火衰失养—腰膝酸冷
阳气不达—畏寒肢冷
肾阳虚衰—舌淡白，苔白滑，脉沉微

1.8 Impaired Absorption due to Yáng Vacuity

The lung is the governor of qì, and the kidney is the root of qì. The kidney governs the absorption of qì, and the lung governs the exhalation of qì. When yīn and yáng intermingle, inhalation and exhalation are balanced and harmonized. If the lung is vacuous for a long period of time, this is ultimately bound to return to the kidney, making kidney yáng insufficient and preventing it from containing and absorbing. Yīn and yáng fail to intermingle, above and below do not assist each other, and kidney yáng is unable to absorb qì and return it to the origin. As a result, the pathomechanism of impaired absorption due to yáng vacuity arises.

When kidney yáng is exhausted, yáng becomes vacuous and unable to absorb, and lung qì ascends counterflow. As a result, we observe hasty panting that is prolonged and recurrent, exhalation more than inhalation, which is exacerbated by movement, and inability to maintain continuous breathing.

When kidney yáng is exhausted, warming becomes deficient, and the movement of qì and blood is impaired. The result is physical cold and cold limbs, and a green-blue facial complexion and purple lips.

Vacuity of kidney yáng can disturb qì transformation and disorder the fluid metabolism. The result is coughing with profuse clear white phlegm, possibly with increased urination at night and puffy face and swollen limbs.

When kidney yáng is debilitated, yáng qì fails to nourish the essence-spirit. This results in fatigued and feeble spirit.

When yáng qì is unable to secure external defense, the interstices of the flesh lose their seal. This results in intermittent spontaneous sweating.

When yáng is vacuous in the body, the lower back and the knees are deprived of nourishment. The result is emaciation and lack of luster in the body, and limp aching lower back and knees.

Exhaustion of kidney yáng manifests in a pale white or moist black tongue fur, and a fine faint or weak sunken pulse.

The chapter, "Miscellaneous Pathoconditions; Panting and Wheezing" in the *Yī Biǎn* ("Lancing Stones of Medicine") states:

> "Vacuity panting can come from yáng vacuity… When the true origin is consumed, life gate fire spontaneously surges upward or downward. Such people appear free from disease on normal days, but they experience panting. When diagnosing their pulse, it will be rapid, large, and vacuous, or possibly faint and feeble… If kidney fire is vacuous, the qì of yīn cold in the lower burner forces floating yáng to stray upward and cause panting. The external signs for this condition are a red face with upcast yáng, vexation and agitation, and a floating, large, and rapid pulse. The onset of death is not far away. If you employ

> medicinals to assist the origin with settling and downbearing, there is still hope for the patient's life. Nevertheless, you cannot use drastic medicinals, but should initiate treatment with *bā wèi wán* (Eight-Ingredient Pill) and *hēi xí dān* (Galenite Elixir)."

This quotation describes the pathomechanism and tongue and pulse signs of panting counterflow that is caused by debilitation of kidney yáng, failure to contain and absorb, and upward surging of vacuity fire.

The chapter, "Panting" in the *Xuè Zhèng Lùn* ("On Blood Patterns") also states:

> "Kidney vacuity panting is due to the fact that the source of qì lies in the kidney... In cases of non-transformation of urine with simultaneous lumbar pain, yáng within the kidney is unable to transform qì. *Shèn qì wán* (Kidney Qì Pill) is the suitable treatment. *Shēn fù tāng* (Ginseng and Aconite Decoction) with the addition of *wǔ wèi zǐ* (Schisandrae Fructus) and *fú líng* (Poria) is also possible."

This quotation clearly points out that kidney yáng vacuity and failure to contain and absorb can lead to panting.

Impaired absorption due to yáng vacuity is treated by warming the kidney and invigorating yáng, and by promoting qì absorption and calming panting. The recommended formula is *shèn qì wán* (Kidney Qì Pill) from the *Jīn Guì Yào Lüè* ("Essential Prescriptions of the Golden Coffer") in combination with *hēi xí dān* (Galenite Elixir) from the *Tài Píng Huì Mín Hé Jì Jú Fāng* (Tài-Píng Imperial Grace Pharmacy Formulas), with the addition of *hé táo ròu* (Juglandis Semen) and *zǐ hé chē* (Hominis Placenta).

Shèn Qì Wán 肾气丸

Kidney Qì Pill

---

shú dì huáng (熟地黄 Rehmanniae Radix Praeparata, cooked rehmannia)

shān zhū yú (山茱萸 Corni Fructus, cornus)

shān yào (山药 Dioscoreae Rhizoma, dioscorea)

zé xiè (泽泻 Alismatis Rhizoma, alisma)

fú líng (茯苓 Poria, poria)

mǔ dān pí (牡丹皮 Moutan Cortex, moutan)

guì zhī (桂枝 Cinnamomi Ramulus, cinnamon twig)

fù zǐ (附子 Aconiti Radix Lateralis Praeparata, aconite)

With:

Hēi Xí Dān 黑锡丹 Galenite Elixir
hēi xí (黑锡 Galenitum, galenite)
liú huáng (硫黄 Sulphur, sulfur)
ròu guì (肉桂 Cinnamomi Cortex, cinnamon bark)
fù zǐ (附子 Aconiti Radix Lateralis Praeparata, aconite)
bǔ gǔ zhī (补骨脂 Psoraleae Fructus, psoralea)
hú lú bā (胡芦巴 Trigonellae Semen, fenugreek)
yáng qǐ shí (阳起石 Actinolitum, actinolite)
chén xiāng (沉香 Aquilariae Lignum Resinatum, aquilaria)
mù xiāng (木香 Aucklandiae Radix, costusroot)
xiǎo huí xiāng (小茴香 Foeniculi Fructus, fennel)
ròu dòu kòu (肉豆蔻 Myristicae Semen, nutmeg)
Plus:
hé táo ròu (胡桃肉 Juglandis Semen, walnut)
zǐ hé chē (紫河车 Hominis Placenta, placenta)

阳虚失纳

肺为气之主，肾为气之根，肾主纳气，肺主呼气，阴阳相交，则呼吸调和。若肺虚日久，穷必归肾，肾阳不足，失于摄纳，阴阳不交，上下不济，肾阳不能纳气归原，则可形成阳虚失纳的病机。肾阳衰惫，阳虚失纳，肺气上逆，则见喘促日久，反复发作，呼多吸少，动则尤甚，气不得续; 肾阳衰惫，温煦不及，气血失运，则形寒肢冷，面青唇紫; 肾阳虚，气化失调，水液代谢失常，则咳痰清稀量多色白，或夜尿多，或面浮肢肿; 肾阳虚衰，阳气不养精神，则神疲乏力; 阳气不能卫外为固，肌腠失密，则时自汗出; 阳虚形体腰膝失养，则形瘦无华，腰膝酸软。肾阳衰惫，则舌苔淡白或黑润，脉微细或沉弱。如《医碥•杂症•喘哮》曰："虚喘，有出于阳虚者。...乃真元耗损，命门之火自下上冲也。其人平居若无病，但觉喘乏，察其脉，数大而虚，或微而无力者是也。...若肾火虚者，下焦阴寒之气，逼其浮阳上越作喘。外证面赤戴阳，烦躁，脉浮大而数，去死不远。用助元接真镇坠之药，尚可问生。然不可峻骤，且先以八味丸、黑锡丹。"论述肾阳虚衰，不能摄纳，虚火上冲，形成喘逆的病机和舌脉症状。《血证论•喘息》亦云："肾虚喘息者，以气之根源于肾。…若小水不化，兼腰痛者，乃是肾中之阳不能化气，宜肾气丸治之，参附汤加五味、茯苓亦可。”明确提出肾阳虚不能摄纳，可致喘息。治宜温肾壮阳，纳气定喘。方药选用《金匮要略》肾气丸合《和剂局方》黑锡丹（黑锡、硫磺、肉桂、附子、补骨脂、胡芦巴、阳起石、沉香、木香、茴香、肉豆蔻）加黑桃肉、紫河车.

Literature Review of Impaired Absorption due to Yáng Vacuity

🕮 *Yī Xué Rù Mén* ("The Gateway to Medicine"), "Internal Damage: Panting"

> "Kidney cold and failure of original qì to absorb: In cases of vacuity cold in the lower origin and inability of kidney qì to return to the origin, use *jiǔ wèi ān shèn wán* (Nine-Ingredient Kidney-Quieting Pill) and *bā wèi wán* (Eight-Ingredient Pill). For severe conditions, use *hēi xí dān* (Galenite Elixir) to settle and downbear it."

This quotation indicates the treatment method for panting that is caused by kidney yáng vacuity cold and failure of original qì to absorb.

🕮 *Zhèng Zhì Zhǔn Shéng* ("The Level-Line of Pattern Identification and Treatment"), "Miscellaneous Diseases: Panting"

> "When the true origin is consumed, panting arises from the upward flight of kidney qì. When true yáng is exhausted, kidney qì is unable to return to the origin. Historically in order to treat this people have used metal and stones to settle and downbear and to assist yáng by joining the true. Nevertheless, you cannot use drastic or galloping medicinals and should initiate treatment with *ān shén wán* (Spirit-Quieting Pill) and *bā wèi wán* (Eight-Ingredient Pill)."

This quotation also discusses how kidney yáng exhaustion and inability to contain and absorb can cause panting.

🕮 *Yī Xué Xīn Wù* ("Medical Insights"), "Panting"

> "Beyond external contractions of cold evil, vacuity cold in the spleen and kidney can also cause panting, and is related to an interruption of fire… For cases when fire floats upward due to an insufficiency of true yáng in the kidney channel, conduct fire to return to its root. Use *guì fù bā wèi wán* (Cinnamon Bark and Aconite Eight-Ingredient Pill)."

Panting can arise from a vacuity of kidney yáng that is preventing kidney qì from absorbing, and causing vacuity fire to float upward. Therefore, treat this condition with *guì fù bā wèi wán* (Cinnamon Bark and Aconite Eight-Ingredient Pill) to downbear qì and calm panting.

文献评述

《医学入门•内伤类•喘》曰："肾冷元气不能纳：下元虚冷，肾气不得归元者，九味安肾九、八味丸; 甚者，黑锡丹以镇坠之。"指出肾阳虚冷，元气不纳而致气喘的治法。

《证治准绳•杂病•喘》曰："真元耗损，喘生于肾气之上奔。真阳虚惫，肾气不得归元，固有以金石镇坠，助阳接真而愈者，然亦不可峻骤，且先与安肾丸、八味丸。"也论述肾阳虚惫，不能摄纳可致气喘。

《医学心悟•喘》曰："然而外感寒邪，以及脾肾虚寒，皆能令喘，未便概以火断也。...肾经真阳不足而火上泛者，引火归根，桂附八味丸。"喘因肾阳虚，肾气不纳，虚火上浮而起，故用桂附八味丸以降气平喘进行治疗。

Summary of Impaired Absorption due to Yáng Vacuity

1. Yáng Vacuity and Impaired Absorption

   Hasty panting that is prolonged and recurrent, exhalation more than inhalation, which is exacerbated by movement, inability to maintain continuous breathing.

2. Deficient Warming

   Physical cold and cold limbs, green-blue facial complexion and purple lips.

3. Disturbed Qì Transformation

   Coughing with profuse clear white phlegm, possibly increased urination at night, or puffy face and swollen limbs.

3. Yáng Qì Failing to Nourish the Essence-Spirit

   Fatigued and feeble spirit.

4. Insecurity of External Defense

   Intermittent spontaneous sweating.

5. Lower Back and Knees Deprived of Nourishment

   Emaciation and lack of luster in the body, limp aching lower back and knees.

6. Exhaustion of Kidney Yáng

   Pale white or moist black tongue fur, fine faint or weak sunken pulse.

阳虚失纳
阳虚失纳—喘促日久，反复发作，呼多吸少，动则尤甚，气不得续
温煦不及—形寒肢冷，面青唇紫
气化失调—咳痰清稀量多色白，或夜尿多，或面浮肢肿
阳气不养精神—神疲乏力
卫外不固—时自汗出
形体腰膝失养—形瘦无华，腰膝酸软
肾阳衰惫—舌苔淡白或黑润，脉微细或沉弱

1.9 Yáng Floating Upward (Upcast Yáng)

The kidney is the root of earlier heaven. Yīn and yáng, and water and fire, reside together in a single abode. Nevertheless, the upper body belongs to yáng and the lower body belongs to yīn. If debilitation of kidney yáng reaches a critical extreme and yīn cold exuberates internally, since the kidney is located in the lower body, yīn cold then lives in the lower body alone. Because exuberant yīn repels yáng, vacuous yáng is unable to abide in the lower body and instead floats upward. This manifests in the pathomechanical changes of yīn exuberating in the lower body and yáng floating upward.

Long ago, the *Huáng Dì Nèi Jīng* ("The Yellow Emperor's Inner Canon") recognized the pathomechanical changes of "upcast yáng." As the chapter, "Five Colors" in the *Líng Shū* ("The Magic Pivot") points out: "In cases when red color appears on both cheeks, in a thumb-sized spot, the condition might be minor, but it invariably ends in sudden death." Bright red color in both cheeks is a sign of vacuous yáng floating astray. While this text does not mention by name the pathomechanism "yáng floating upward," it clearly describes vacuity yáng floating upward to cause what is termed "the last radiance of the setting sun."

When kidney yáng debilitation causes yīn to exuberate in the lower body and vacuous yáng to float upward, yáng harasses the heart spirit and becomes depressed in the head and face. This results in a red face as if painted, and in heart vexation and dry retching.

Debilitation of kidney yáng causes an internal exuberance of yīn cold and a breakdown of warming. The result is fear of cold and reversal cold of the limbs.

If the exuberance of yīn cold is extreme, fire fails to engender earth. This results in clear-food diarrhea and enduring and incessant diarrhea.

Due to yīn exuberating in the lower body, bladder qì transformation breaks down. Therefore we see white-colored urine.

When an internal exuberance of yīn cold and debilitation of yáng qì reaches an extreme, yáng qì lacks strength to agitate the blood in the vessels. The result is a fine sunken pulse, or reverse flow with no pulse.

The chapter, "Identifying Pulse Symptoms and Treatments of Lesser Yīn Disease" in the *Shāng Hán Lùn* ("On Cold Damage") states:

> "When lesser yīn disease presents with diarrhea and a faint pulse, give *bái tōng tāng* (Scallion Yáng-Freeing Decoction). When it presents with incessant diarrhea, reverse flow with no pulse, dry retching, and vexation, *bái tōng jiā zhū dǎn zhī tāng* (Scallion Yáng-Freeing Decoction plus Pig's Bile) governs it."

This quotation clearly points out the pulse signs in the pathomechanism of upcast yáng.

The "Treatise on Yīn and Yáng" in the *Yī Guàn* ("Thorough Knowledge of Medicine") also points out:

> When yīn exuberates in the lower body, it drives yáng into the upper body. This is known as a combination of cold well water with thunder and lighting. Since it causes the patient to have a red face, thirst, vexation and agitation, and panting and cough, who would not say that it is an extreme of fire exuberance? But who would know that it is a condition driven by yīn cold within the kidney? I do not know how many patients have died as a result of taking cold medicinals."

This quotation explains with absolute clarity how yīn exuberance in the lower body drives yáng into the upper body and causes upcast yáng.

Yáng floating upward is treated by warming the kidney and dispersing cold, and by breaking yīn and freeing yáng. Recommended formulas are *bái tōng tāng* (Scallion Yáng-Freeing Decoction) or *bái tōng jiā zhū dǎn zhī tāng* (Scallion Yáng-Freeing Decoction Plus Pig's Bile) from the *Shāng Hán Lùn* ("On Cold Damage").

Bái Tōng Tāng 白通汤 Scallion Yáng-Freeing Decoction
cōng bái (葱白 Allii Fistulosi Bulbus, scallion white)
gān jiāng (干姜 Zingiberis Rhizoma, dried ginger)
fù zǐ (附子 Aconiti Radix Lateralis Praeparata, aconite)

Bái Tōng Jiā Zhū Dǎn Zhī Tāng 白通加猪胆汁汤 Scallion Yáng-Freeing Decoction Plus Pig's Bile
cōng bái (葱白 Allii Fistulosi Bulbus, scallion white)
gān jiāng (干姜 Zingiberis Rhizoma, dried ginger)
fù zǐ (附子 Aconiti Radix Lateralis Praeparata, aconite)
rén niào (人尿 Hominis Urina, human urine)
zhū dǎn zhī (猪胆汁 Suis Bilis, pig's bile)

阳浮于上（戴阳）

肾为先天之本，阴阳水火同居一宅。然上属阳而下属阴，若肾阳虚衰至极，阴寒内盛，肾位在下，阴寒独居于下，阴盛格阳，令虚阳不能下留而上浮，出现阴盛于下，阳浮于上的病机变化。《黄帝内经》早已认识到了"戴阳"的病机变化。如《灵枢•五色篇》指出："赤色出两颧，大如拇指者，病虽小愈，必卒死。"两颧鲜红，则为虚阳浮越之兆，虽未提出"阳浮于上"的病机名称，但清楚描述了虚阳上浮，"回光反照"的病机变化。肾阳虚衰，阴盛于下，虚阳上浮，扰动心神，郁于头面，则面红如妆，心烦干呕; 肾阳虚衰，阴寒内盛，温煦失职，则畏寒，四肢厥冷; 阴寒盛极，火不生土，则下利清谷，久利不止; 阴盛于下，膀胱气化失职，故小便色白; 阴寒内盛，阳气虚衰至极，无力鼓动血脉，则脉沉微，或厥逆无脉。如《伤寒论•辨少阴病脉证并治》曰："少阴病，下利，脉微者，与白通汤。利不止，厥逆无脉，干呕，烦者，白通加猪胆汁汤主之。"明确提出戴阳病机的脉症。《医贯•阴阳论》也指出："阴盛于下，逼阳于上，井水寒，而雷电合也。今人病面红、口渴、烦躁、喘咳者，谁不曰火盛之极？抑孰知其为肾中阴寒所逼乎？以寒凉之药进而毙者，吾不知其几矣。"十分清晰地说明阴盛于下，逼阳于上而致戴阳的病机变化。 治法以温肾散寒，破阴通阳为原则。方药选用《伤寒论》白通汤（葱白、干姜、附子），或白通加猪胆汁汤（葱白、干姜、附子、人尿、猪胆汁）。

Literature Review of Yáng Floating Upward

📖 *Shāng Hán Lùn* ("On Cold Damage"), "Identifying Pulse Symptoms and Treatments of Lesser Yīn Disease"

> "When in lesser yīn disease diarrhea ceases, and the head is dizzy, and there is frequent spontaneous veiling [cloudiness and dizziness in the head and eyes, as if obstructed], [this bodes] death.."

Zhāng Lù-Yù explained in a commentary on this passage in the *Shāng Hán Xù Lùn* ("Clues On Cold Damage"):

> "Yīn and yáng in the human body are attached to each other. When yīn collapses in the lower body, all yáng rises and gathers in the head. Stirring chaotically, yáng causes dizziness in the head, frequent spontaneous veiling, and yáng desertion in the upper body, resulting in death."

This quotation describes in detail the pathomechanism by which kidney yáng vacuity causes yīn exuberance in the lower body and yáng floating upward.

📖 *Yī Guàn* ("Thorough Knowledge of Medicine"), "Treatise on Yīn and Yáng"

> "If patients manifest with great heat, dryness, thirst, and dry tongue, is this not a yáng pattern? Once I observed a red facial complexion, which I identified as upcast yáng. When I diagnosed the pulse, it was slow, weak, and forceless, with a large gap between the inch and the bar. I knew that this was related to a yīn exuberance in the lower body that was driving yáng into the upper body. It was thus a false yáng pattern. I used medicinals for false cold and thereby followed the nature of the disease to reverse its direction. The patient immediately recovered."

This quotation explicitly mentions the pathomechanism of "upcast yáng" by name and describes its pathomechanical changes and the special characteristics of facial complexion and pulse.

📖 *Xuè Zhèng Lùn* ("On Blood Patterns"), "Treatise on the Pathomechanisms of the Viscera and Bowels"

> "The pupil is ascribed to the kidney. When it is vacuous, it means that spirit water is dissipated, or that an internal obstruction has occurred. When vacuous yáng invades the upper body, it causes sore pharynx and red cheeks."

This quotation also describes the pathological changes of kidney yáng vacuity and vacuous yáng floating upward.

文献评述

《伤寒论•辨少阴病脉证并治》曰："少阴病，下利不止而头眩，时时欲冒者，死。"张路玉《伤寒绪论》对此条注释时说："人身阴阳，相为依附者也。阴亡于下，则诸阳之上聚于头者，纷然而动，所以头眩，时时自冒，阳脱于上而主死也。"对肾阳虚，阴盛于下，阳浮于上的病机作了详细的阐述。

《医贯•阴阳论》曰："如人大热发燥口渴舌燥，非阳证乎？余视其面色赤，此戴阳也。切其脉，迟弱而无力，寸关豁大而无伦，此系阴盛于下，逼阳于上，假阳之证。余以假寒之药，从其性而折之，顷刻平矣。"明确的提出了"戴阳"的病机名称，论述了戴阳的病机变化及色脉特征。

《血证论•脏腑病机论》曰："瞳人属肾，虚则神水散缩，或发内障。虚阳上犯，为咽痛颊赤。"也描述了肾阳亏虚，虚阳上浮的病机变化。

Summary of Yáng Floating to the Upper Body

1. Vacuous Yáng Floating Upward
   Red face, as if painted, heart vexation and dry retching.
2. Impaired Warming
   Fear of cold, reversal cold of the limbs.
3. Fire Failing to Engender Earth
   Clear-food diarrhea; in severe cases, incessant diarrhea.
4. Breakdown of Qì Transformation
   White-colored urine.
5. Forceless Activation
   Sunken faint pulse, or reverse flow with no pulse.

阳浮于上

虚阳上浮—面红如妆，心烦干呕

温煦失职—畏寒，四肢厥冷

火不生土—下利清谷，甚则下利不止

气化失司—小便色白

鼓动无力—脉沉微，或厥逆无脉

1.10 Yáng Repelled to the Outside (Repelled Yáng)

The kidney is the root of earlier heaven, and water and fire live reside together in a single abode. To maintain their normal physiological functions, yīn and yáng in the kidney must be balanced and harmonious, with yīn being calm and yáng being sound. If kidney yáng is debilitated to an extreme, yīn and yáng lose their balance. Yīn cold becomes extremely exuberant and occupies the inside of the body by itself. It repels weak yáng and makes it float and stretch to the outside. This can manifest in the pathomechanism of yīn exuberating within and repelling yáng to the outside.

When kidney yáng is debilitated, yīn exuberates internally while yáng floats to the outside. As a result, vacuous yáng floats astray into the exterior, and the location where floating yáng accumulates experiences a corresponding superabundance of yáng qì. This results in generalized heat effusion, no fear of cold, but fear of heat instead, and desire to cover up with clothes and blankets.

When yáng qì floats astray into the upper body, qì and blood gush upward and the blood vessels fill up. The result is red face and eyes.

If the internal exuberance of yīn cold has not yet damaged the fluids, there is bland taste in the mouth with absence of thirst. However, if the internal exuberance of yīn cold prevents qì from transforming liquid, and liquid fails to bear upward, yáng manifestations such as dry mouth and thirst with a liking for hot drinks result. When yáng qì strays to the outside, liquid can desert together with qì. The result is putting forth oily sweat.

Failure of yáng qì to reach the limbs results in reversal cold of the extremities and a faint pulse verging on expiry.

The chapter, "Identifying Pulse Symptoms and Treatments of Lesser Yīn Disease" in the *Shāng Hán Lùn* ("On Cold Damage") states:

> "Lesser yīn disease presents with clear-food diarrhea, interior cold and external heat, reversal of the extremities, a faint pulse verging on expiry, a paradoxical lack of aversion to cold in the body, and a red facial complexion. If these signs are accompanied by abdominal disease, dry retching, sore pharynx, or diarrhea that has ceased but the pulse fails to move outward, *tōng mài sì nì tāng* (Vessel-Freeing Counterflow Cold Decoction) governs it."

This quotation points out that the key aspects of the pathomechanism of yīn exuberating internally and repelling yáng to the outside are interior cold and external heat, generalized heat effusion, and no fear of cold, but fear of heat.

The "Record of Transmitting Loyalty; True and False Cold and Heat" in the *Jǐng Yuè Quán Shū* ("Jǐng-Yuè's Complete Compendium") states:

> "In false heat, water extreme resembles fire… All cases of true heat originally manifest with heat effusion, and yet false heat also manifests with heat effusion. Symptoms of both these patterns also include red face, vexation and agitation, constipation, inhibited voidings of reddish urine, and possibly hasty breathing, sore swollen throat, or heat effusion with a tight rapid pulse. An ignorant person who sees these symptoms will interpret them as heat and recklessly use cold and cooling medicinals.
>
> "When the patient swallows these, death is inevitable. Such a person is unaware that the condition, in spite of generalized heat effusion, is caused by interior cold repelling yáng, or possibly by vacuous yáng failing to constrain, which frequently presents with this symptom… For this reason, whenever a patient presents with generalized heat effusion and a rapid pulse that fails to beat when pressed, theses are all signs of exuberant yīn repelling yáng, and not of heat."

This is an extremely incisive discussion of the pathomechanical changes of yīn exuberance repelling yáng, based on the clinical manifestations of true cold and false heat.

Yáng repelled to the outside is treated by supplementing the kidney and invigorating yáng, and by returning yáng and stemming counterflow. The recommended formula is *tōng mài sì nì tāng* (Vessel-Freeing Counterflow Cold Decoction) from the *Shāng Hán Lùn* ("On Cold Damage").

Tōng Mài Sì Nì Tāng 通脉四逆汤 Vessel-Freeing Counterflow Cold Decoction
fù zǐ (附子 Aconiti Radix Lateralis Praeparata, aconite)
gān jiāng (干姜 Zingiberis Rhizoma, dried ginger)
gān cǎo (甘草 Glycyrrhizae Radix, licorice)

格阳于外（格阳）

肾为先天之本，水火同居一宅，肾中阴阳必须平衡协调，阴平阳秘，才能维持正常的生理功能。如肾阳虚衰至极，阴阳失调，阴寒极盛独居于内，排斥弱阳，向外浮张，则可出现阴盛于内，格阳于外的病机变化。肾阳虚衰，阴盛于内，阳浮于外，虚阳浮越在表，浮阳聚积之处，阳气相对有余，则全身发热，不怕冷，反怕热，欲盖衣被; 阳气浮越于上，气血上涌，血脉充盈，则面目红赤; 阴寒内盛，津液未伤，则口淡不渴; 若阴寒内盛，气不化津，津不上承，阳表现为口干、口渴喜热饮; 阳气外越，津随气脱，则汗出如油; 阳气不达四肢，则手足逆冷，脉微欲绝。如《伤寒论•辨少阴病脉证并治》曰：“少阴病，下利清谷，里寒外热，手足厥逆，脉微欲绝，身反不恶寒，其人面色赤。或腹病，或干呕，或咽痛，或利止脉不出者，通脉四逆汤主之。”指出了阴盛于内，格阳于外，“里寒外热”，全身发热，不怕冷，反怕热的病机要点。《景岳全书•传忠录•寒热真假篇》也说：“假热者，水极似火也。...凡真热本发热，而假热亦发热，其症则亦为面赤烦躁，亦为大便不通，小便赤涩，或为气促，咽喉肿痛，或为发热，脉见紧数等症。昧者见之，便认为热，妄投寒凉，下咽必毙。不知身虽有热而里寒格阳，或虚阳不敛者多有此证。...故凡身热脉数，按之不鼓击者，此皆阴盛格阳，即非热也。”非常精辟地从真寒假热的临床表现，论述了阴盛格阳的病机变化。治法宜补肾壮阳，回阳救逆。方药用《伤寒论》通脉四逆汤（大附子、干姜、甘草）。

Literature Review of Yáng Repelled to the Outside

📖 *Shāng Hán Lùn* (“On Cold Damage”), “Identifying Pulse Symptoms and Treatments of Greater Yáng Disease”

> “When a patient suffers great generalized heat effusion but desires clothes and blankets, the heat is in the skin, and the cold is in the bones and marrow.”

This quotation discusses the pathomechanical changes of true cold and false heat, caused by yīn exuberating internally and repelling yáng to the outside.

📖 *Yī Xué Zhèng Zhuàn* (“The Orthodox Tradition of Medicine”), “Identifying True and False in Disease”

> “In false heat, water extreme resembles fire, and yīn patterns resemble yáng. There is heat on the outside, but cold on the inside. The pulse is faint and weak, or rapid and vacuous, or large, floating, and without root, or stringlike, scallion-stalk, and interrupted. In spite of blazing heat in the body, the spirit appears tranquil; in spite of delirious raving, the sound of the speech is faint.

> Other possible signs are vacuity mania and tilting as if about to fall, which stops when you restrain the patient; false macules resembling mosquito bites that are red and broken up; a liking for cold drinks but not drinking a lot of water; a red tongue and face; not covering up completely at night; or profuse disinhibited urination and stool that is not bound. In patients with these signs, aversion to heat is not real heat. Properly understood, it is indicative of a cold pattern. This is called extreme cold paradoxically transforming into extreme heat, paradoxically concurrent with heat transformation, and is also referred to as exuberant yīn repelling yáng."

This quotation discusses how yīn exuberating internally and repelling yáng to the outside causes floating yáng on the outside, forming the numerous manifestations of false heat. It is of greatest significance for differentiating patterns of true cold and false heat.

🕮 *Yī Zōng Jīn Jiàn* ("The Golden Mirror of Medicine"), "Heart Approach to Cold Damage in Rhyme: Yīn Exuberating and Repelling Yáng"

> "When yīn qì is overly exuberant, yáng qì does not receive construction [qì]. Failing to obtain construction, it does not enter [yīn]. Failing to enter [yīn], repelled yáng moves to the outside. Therefore, this condition is called exuberant yīn repelling yáng. What is called shallow red color refers to the superficial red color of the facial complexion. Its external sign is a red face with heat effusion and vexation, very similar to yáng heat. Internal signs are absence of thirst, clear-food diarrhea, clear white urine, clear white nails, reversal cold of the limbs, and a faint floating pulse verging on expiry. These signs are attributed to yīn cold vacuity patterns."

This quotation describes incisively the pathomechanism and clinical manifestations of yīn exuberance repelling yáng.

文献评述

《伤寒论•太阳病脉证并治》曰："病人身大热，反欲得衣被，热在皮肤，寒在骨髓也。"论述阴盛于内，格阳于外，真寒假热的病机变化。

《医学正传•病有真假辨》曰："假热者，水极似火，阴证似阳也。外虽热而内则寒。脉微而弱，或数而虚，或浮大无根，或弦芤断绝，身虽炽热而神色自静，语虽谵妄而声音则微，或虚狂起倒，禁之则止，或蚊迹假斑而色红细碎，或喜冷饮而饮水不多，或舌面赤而夜被不彻，或小水多利而大便不结。此则恶热非热，明是寒证，所谓寒极反兼热化，亦曰阴盛格阳也。"论述阴盛于内，格阳于外，浮阳在外，形成多种假热的表现，对真寒假热证的鉴别有十分重要的意义。

《医宗金鉴•伤寒心法要诀•阴盛格阳》曰："阴气太盛，阳气不得相营也。不相营者，不相入也。既不相入，则格阳于外，故曰阴盛格阳也。色浅赤，谓面色见浮浅之红赤色也。其外证面赤发热而烦，颇类阳热，其内则不渴，下利清谷，小便清白，爪甲青白，四肢厥冷，脉浮微欲绝，一派阴寒虚证。"深刻阐述了阴盛格阳的病机和临床表现。

Summary of Yáng Repelled to the Outside

1. Yáng Floating into the Exterior
   Generalized heat effusion, no fear of cold, but fear of heat instead, desire to cover up with clothes and blankets.
2. Vacuous Yáng Floating Upward
   Red face and eyes.
3. Fluids not yet Damaged
   Bland taste in the mouth with absence of thirst.
4. Qì Failing to Transform Liquid
   Dry mouth, thirst with a liking for hot drinks.
5. Liquid Deserting Together with Qì
   Putting forth oily sweat.
6. Failure of Yáng Qì to Reach the Limbs
   Counterflow cold of the extremities, faint pulse on the verge of expiry.

格阳于外

阳浮在表—全身发热，不怕冷，反怕热，欲盖衣被

虚阳上浮—面目红赤

津液未伤—口淡不渴

气不化津—口干、口渴喜热饮

津随气脱—汗出如油

阳气不达四肢—手足逆冷，脉微欲绝

1.11 Surging Counterflow Qì Ascent (Running Piglet Qì)

The kidney is the water viscus and stores within it original yáng and original yīn. When yīn is calm and yáng is sound, visceral qì is balanced and harmonious. If kidney yáng is debilitated, however, kidney qì also cannot be quiet. Because it is the nature of qì to rise lightly, it has a tendency to stir internally and to surge up into the chest region like a running piglet. This forms the pathomechanism of surging counterflow qì ascent.

When cold-damp settles in the lower body, the kidney channel is affected by congealing cold qì stagnation. When there is stoppage, there is pain. Therefore, we observe conglomeration lumps and pain in the lesser abdomen.

In spite of the fact that qì is tied up by dampness and cold, there are times when it throws these off and the condition therefore transmutes and transforms. Consequently kidney qì stirs internally and surges upward, and the patient subjectively feels qì surging up from the lesser abdomen into the heart and chest. This manifests in appearance like a running piglet. Since it arises whenever qì stirs, upward or downward surges occur at any time and lessen gradually at times. When qì is normalized, the pain stops and the lumps disperse.

The upsurges of kidney qì harass the spirit-mind. The result is vexation and oppression verging on death.

Cold exuberance with surging counterflow qì ascent manifests in a pale white tongue, glossy white tongue fur, and faint sunken pulse.

This type of running piglet qì pathomechanism is different from the "kidney accumulation" running piglet mentioned above: The previously mentioned running piglet that is caused by static blood accumulating in the kidney is related to kidney cold blood stasis. The condition here, which is caused by an insufficiency of kidney yáng without there being any accumulation lumps, is related to kidney cold qì counterflow.

The chapter, "Pulse Symptoms and Treatments of Running Piglet Qì" in the *Jīn Guì Yào Lüe* ("Essential Prescriptions of the Golden Coffer") points out: "As stated by the master, running piglet disease begins in the lesser abdomen and surges up into the throat. During episodes, the patient verges on death, only to recover afterwards. It is always contracted from panic." The foot lesser yīn kidney channel pinches the umbilicus in its upward course and ascends into the throat. When a person experiences panic, kidney yáng qì is damaged and the qì of lower burner water-cold surges up in counterflow, forming running piglet.

The discussion, "Symptoms of Running Piglet Qì" in the *Zhū Bìng Yuán Hòu Lùn* ("Origin and Indicators of Disease") states:

> "Running piglet qì is accumulated qì in the kidney that arises from panic, anxiety, and thought. Panic damages the spirit, and the heart is where the spirit is stored. Anxiety and thought damage the mind, and the kidney is where the mind is stored. When the spirit and mind are stirred, qì accumulates in the kidney and then wanders up and down like the running of a piglet. Therefore, it is called 'running piglet.'"

This quotation describes how running piglet is caused by panic damaging the kidney, which results in kidney vacuity and in qì accumulating in the kidney.

Surging counterflow qì ascent is treated by warming the kidney and calming surging, and by warming the liver and supplementing the spleen. The recommended formula is *bēn tūn wán* (Running Piglet Pill) from the *Zá Bìng Yuán Liú Xī Zhú* ("Incisive Light on the Source of Miscellaneous Disease").

Bēn Tūn Wán 奔豚丸 Running Piglet Pill
fù zǐ (附子 Aconiti Radix Lateralis Praeparata, aconite)
chuān wū (川乌 Aconiti Radix, aconite main root)
ròu guì (肉桂 Cinnamomi Cortex, cinnamon bark)
bā dòu shuāng (巴豆霜 Crotonis Fructus Pulveratus, croton frost)
dīng xiāng (丁香 Caryophylli Flos, clove)
dú huó (独活 Angelicae Pubescentis Radix, pubescent angelica)
fú líng (茯苓 Poria, poria)
zé xiè (泽泻 Alismatis Rhizoma, alisma)
hòu pò (厚朴 Magnoliae Officinalis Cortex, officinal magnolia bark)
shí chāng pú (石菖蒲 Acori Tatarinowii Rhizoma, acorus)
chuān liàn zǐ (川楝子 Toosendan Fructus, toosendan)
huáng lián (黄连 Coptidis Rhizoma, coptis)
yán hú suǒ (延胡索 Corydalis Rhizoma, corydalis)
quán xiē (全蝎 Scorpio, scorpion)

冲气上逆（奔豚气）

肾为水脏，内藏元阳元阴，阴平阳秘，则脏气平和。如肾阳虚衰，肾气亦不得安宁，气性轻扬，故易内动，向上攻冲至胸部，如豚之奔跑，形成冲气上逆的病机变化。寒湿客于下，肾经寒凝气滞，不通则痛，则少腹有瘕块作痛。气虽被湿寒所缚，却有挣脱之时，故病情发生变化，肾气内动上冲，自觉有气从少腹上冲心胸，出现如豚奔走之状。气动则作，故上下无时，时或渐减，气顺则痛止块消;肾气上冲，扰乱神志，则烦闷欲死。寒盛冲气上逆，则舌淡白，苔白滑，脉沉微。此种奔豚气的病机与前所述“肾积”奔豚有所区别，前节所述为瘀血积肾所致奔豚，是肾寒血瘀;此因肾阳不足，无积结包块，是肾寒气逆。如《金匮要略•奔豚气病脉证治》指出：“师曰：奔豚病从少腹起，上冲咽喉，发作欲死，复还止，皆从惊恐得之。”足少阴肾经挟脐上行，上行于咽喉，惊恐得之，肾阳受伤，下焦水寒之气，向上冲逆，便成奔豚。《诸病源候论•奔豚气候》论曰：“夫奔豚气者，肾之积气，起于惊恐忧思所生。若惊恐则伤神，心藏神也。忧思则伤志，肾藏志也。神志伤动，气积于肾，而气上下游走，如豚之奔，故曰奔豚。”对因惊恐伤肾，引起肾虚，气积于肾，发为奔豚的病机变化进行了论述。治法宜温肾平冲，温肝补脾。方药选用《杂病源流犀烛》奔豚丸（附子、川乌、肉桂、巴豆霜、丁香、独活、茯苓、泽泻、厚朴、石菖蒲、川楝、黄连、延胡索、全蝎）。

Literature Review of Surging Counterflow Qì Ascent

📖 *Zá Bìng Yuán Liú Xī Zhú* (“Incisive Light on the Source of Miscellaneous Disease”), “Section on the Kidney: Running Piglet”

> “Kidney accumulation is called running piglet. It begins in the lesser abdomen, rises up to the heart, and resembles a running piglet in appearance, surging up or down at any time. When enduring, it results in panting counterflow, bone wilting, shortage of qì, and a sunken and slippery pulse. Suitable formulas are *bēn tūn wán* (Running Piglet Pill) and *zēng sǔn wǔ jī wán* (Modified Five Accumulations Pill). It is always caused by kidney vacuity and by the passing of dampness evil from the spleen down to the kidney.”

What this text calls "kidney accumulation" does not refer to tangible accumulation lumps formed from static blood, but to accumulated qì that is caused by a vacuity of kidney yáng and internal exuberance of yīn cold. In this sense, this passage does in fact discuss the pathomechanism of running piglet that is caused by kidney yáng debilitation and surging counterflow qì ascent.

📖 *Yī Zōng Jīn Jiàn* ("The Golden Mirror of Medicine"), "Corrective Notes on the *Jīn Guì Yào Lüe* ("Essential Prescriptions of the Golden Coffer"): Pulse Symptoms and Treatments of Running Piglet Qì"

> "Running piglet is a kidney disease. The name comes from the fact that the disease surges up from the lesser abdomen into the throat like a piglet scurrying and jostling. During attacks, kidney qì ascends and overwhelms the heart, bringing the patient to the verge of death. When the attack is over, qì is debilitated, [yet] returns to the kidney, and the condition stops. Therefore, this disease differs in its severity, but is always contracted from panic. Since fright damages the heart and fear damages the kidney, both viscera are jointly affected."

This quotation describes how the pathomechanism of running piglet is caused by panic damaging the kidney, debilitation of kidney yáng, and surging counterflow qì ascent.

文献评述

《杂病源流犀烛•肾部•奔豚》曰："肾之积，曰奔豚，发小腹，上至心，如豚奔走状，上下无时，久则喘逆，骨痿，少气，脉沉而滑，宜奔豚丸、增损五积丸。皆由肾虚，脾家湿邪下传客肾所致。"此处的"肾之积"，不是指瘀血形成的有形积块，而是由于肾阳虚，阴寒内盛形成的积气，所以此段条文实际上论述了肾阳虚衰，冲气上逆，形成奔豚的病机变化。

《医宗金鉴•订正金匮要略注•奔豚气病脉并治》曰："奔豚者，肾病也，以其病从少腹上冲咽喉，有如豚窜奔突之状，故名之也。发作则肾气上乘于心而欲死，作已则气衰复还于肾而止，故其病虽有微甚不同，然必皆从惊恐得之。盖惊伤心，恐伤肾，两脏交病也。"对惊恐伤肾，肾阳虚衰，冲气上逆，形成奔豚的病机进行了论述。

Summary of Surging Counterflow Qì Ascent
1. Upsurge of Kidney Qì Subjective feeling of qì surging from the lesser abdomen into the heart and chest, manifesting like a running piglet. 2. Erupting When Qì Stirs Surging up or down at any time, lessening gradually at times. 3. Harassing the Spirit-Mind Vexation and oppression verging on death. 4. Cold Exuberance with Surging Counterflow Qì Ascent Pale white tongue, glossy white tongue fur, faint sunken pulse.

冲气上逆
肾气上冲—自觉有气从少腹上冲心胸，出现如豚奔走之状 气动则作—上下无时，时或渐减 扰乱神志—烦闷欲死 寒盛冲气上逆—舌淡白，苔白滑，脉沉微

1.12 Thoroughfare-Controlling Disharmony

The kidney governs reproduction. Since the thoroughfare and controlling vessels and the uterus are all closely related to reproduction, they are indirectly subordinated to the kidney. The "Treatise of Heavenly Truth from Remote Antiquity" in the *Sù Wèn* ("Plain Questions") states: "The controlling vessel and thoroughfare vessel are both extraordinary vessels. When kidney qì is plentiful, the thoroughfare and controlling vessels flow freely and channel blood gradually develops a surplus, which descends at night."

If kidney yáng is debilitated, however, it is unable to warm and to fill and nourish the thoroughfare and controlling vessels. This can manifest in the pathomechanisms of thoroughfare-controlling disharmony and evil obstructing the uterus.

冲任不调

肾主生殖，冲任、胞宫皆与生殖有密切关系，间接隶属于肾。如《素问•上古天真论》曰"任脉、冲脉，皆奇经脉也，肾气充盛，冲任流通，经血渐盈，夜时而下。”如肾阳虚衰，不能温煦、充养冲任，即可出现冲任失调，邪阻胞宫之病机变化。

1.12.1 Thoroughfare-Controlling Disharmony

The kidney is the root of earlier heaven and commands and regulates the physiological functions of every single viscus and bowel in the entire body. The controlling vessel summarily controls all the yīn channels of the body. It constitutes the "sea of yīn vessels." The thoroughfare vessel is the key thoroughfare of qì and blood and is able to regulate the qì and blood in the twelve channels. It is therefore called the "sea of the twelve channels." The kidney and the thoroughfare and controlling vessels are very closely linked. If kidney yáng is debilitated and vacuous yáng floats upward, this can disturb the physiological functions of the thoroughfare and controlling vessels, manifesting in the pathomechanism of thoroughfare-controlling disharmony.

When kidney yáng is vacuous, the thoroughfare and controlling vessels are deprived of nourishment, the channels suffer from chaotic counterflow, and vacuous yáng floats and spreads out. This results in disordered menstruation, frequent baking heat with perspiration, and menopausal symptoms in women.

When kidney yáng is insufficient and warming breaks down, the result is physical cold, fear of cold, and a pale white facial complexion.

Due to a vacuity of kidney yáng, vacuity fire can ascend counterflow along the thoroughfare and controlling vessels and harass the clear orifices. The result is clouded and dizzy head and vision.

Vacuous yáng harassing the upper body can lead to non-interaction of the heart and kidney. The result is oppression in the chest, heart vexation, and reduced sleep and increased dreaming.

When yáng qì is unable to support and nourish the heart spirit, the heart spirit is inhibited. This manifests in listlessness of the essence-spirit, burning preoccupation, and depression.

The lower back is the house of the kidney, and vacuity of kidney yáng results in limp aching lower back and knees.

Debilitation of kidney yáng manifests in a slippery white tongue fur, fat pale tongue, and a weak and forceless vacuous cubit pulse.

The chapter, "Symptoms of Women's Miscellaneous Diseases" in the *Zhū Bìng Yuán Hòu Lùn* ("Origin and Indicators of Disease") states:

> "Women's menstrual irregularities are caused by taxation damage to qì and blood, resulting in vacuity of the body and contraction of wind. The qì of wind-cold settles in the uterus and damages the thoroughfare and controlling vessels... If wind and cold exploit this [vacuity], evil overpowers the blood... cold causes the blood to bind... and the menstrual fluid is therefore now profuse, now scant. This means irregularity."

This quotation describes the pathomechanism by which wind-cold evil settles in the lower burner and causes kidney yáng vacuity cold, chaotic counterflow in the controlling and thoroughfare vessels, and menstrual irregularities.

The chapter, "Origin and Development of Disease in the Thoroughfare Vessel" in the *Zá Bìng Yuán Liú Xī Zhú* ("Incisive Light on the Source of Miscellaneous Disease") also states:

> "When cold qì settles in the vessels and stops flow, qì stirs, rises to Pass Head (guān yuán, CV-4) and rises straight up along the abdomen. This manifests in mounting-conglomerations, enuresis, propping fullness and vexation in the rib-sides, infertility in women, and stirring qì above and below, to the right and to the left."

This quotation points out how debilitation of kidney yáng and cold qì settling in the thoroughfare vessel causes chaotic counterflow of channel qì and leads to numerous pathomechanical changes like infertility in women.

The chapter, "Origin and Development of Disease in the Controlling Vessel" in the same text also points out:

> "The controlling vessel indeed rises out of true yīn, and yīn is not engendered without yáng... The classic states that yīn qì is halved at the age of forty. Because it is said that yáng reaches an extreme and then becomes debilitated, at which point it is assailed by yīn, it is therefore called yīn half. Now this yīn is orifice yīn and not true yīn. Although this is a debilitation of true yīn, it is in reality a debilitation of true yáng. For this reason, disease of the controlling vessel is not a disease of yīn, but in reality one caused by an absence of yáng within yīn."

This quotation describes the pathomechanism of kidney yáng debilitation with vacuity cold in the controlling vessel.

Thoroughfare-controlling disharmony is treated by warming yáng and supplementing the kidney, and by regulating the thoroughfare and controlling vessels. The recommended formula is *yòu guī wán* (Right-Restoring [Life Gate] Pill) from the *Jǐng Yuè Quán Shū* ("Jǐng-Yuè's Complete Compendium") with modifications.

Yòu Guī Wán 右归丸 Right-Restoring [Life Gate] Pill
shú dì huáng (熟地黄 Rehmanniae Radix Praeparata, cooked rehmannia)
shān yào (山药 Dioscoreae Rhizoma, dioscorea)
gǒu qǐ zǐ (枸杞子 Lycii Fructus, lycium)
tù sī zǐ (菟丝子 Cuscutae Semen, cuscuta)
lù jiǎo jiāo (鹿角胶 Cervi Cornus Gelatinum, deerhorn glue)
xù duàn (续断 Dipsaci Radix, dipsacus)
dǎng shēn (党参 Codonopsis Radix, codonopsis)
bǔ gǔ zhī (补骨脂 Psoraleae Fructus, psoralea)
yín yáng huò (淫羊藿 Epimedii Herba, epimedium)
fù zǐ (附子 Aconiti Radix Lateralis Praeparata, aconite) [cooked]
xiān máo (仙茅 Curculiginis Rhizoma, curculigo)
ròu guì (肉桂 Cinnamomi Cortex, cinnamon bark)

冲任失调

肾为先天之本，对全身各个脏腑的生理功能都有统帅调节的作用。任脉总任一身之阴经，为"阴脉之海"; 冲脉为气血的要冲，能调节十二经之气血，又有"十二经脉之海"之称。肾与冲任二脉的关系非常密切，如肾阳虚衰，虚阳上浮，则可导致冲任二脉的生理功能受到干扰，出现冲任失调的病机变化。肾阳虚，冲任失养，经脉逆乱，虚阳浮张，则月经紊乱，时时烘热汗出，表现出妇女更年期的症状; 肾阳不足，温煦失职，则形冷畏寒，面色淡白; 肾阳虚，虚火沿冲任脉上逆，扰乱清窍，则头目昏眩; 虚阳上扰，导致心肾不交，则胸闷心烦，少寐多梦; 阳气不能奉养心神，心神不畅，则表现为精神萎靡，焦虑抑郁; 腰为肾之府，肾阳虚则腰酸膝软; 肾阳虚衰，则苔白滑，舌淡胖，尺脉虚弱无力。如《诸病源候论•妇人杂病诸候》曰："妇人月经不调，由劳伤气血，致体虚受风，风冷之气，客于胞内，伤冲脉、任脉，...有风冷乘之，邪搏于血，...寒则血结，...故月水乍多乍少，为不调也。"论述了风冷之邪客下焦，肾阳虚寒，冲任逆乱引起月经不调的病机。《杂病源流犀烛•冲脉病源流》也曰："寒气客脉不通，气因鸣动应手，起关元，随腹直上，疝瘕遗溺，胁支满烦，女子绝孕，动气在上下左右。"指出了肾阳虚衰，寒气客于冲脉，经气逆乱，可导致的女子绝孕等多种病机变化; 该书《任脉病源流》也指出："是任脉固起于真阴，而阴无阳不生，...经曰：年四十而阴气自半。言乎阳极而衰，为阴所袭，故曰阴半。盖此阴已为窍阴，非真阴也。此虽真阴衰，实真阳衰也。故任脉为病，非阴之自病，实由于阴中无阳。"对肾阳虚衰，任脉虚寒的病机变化作了阐述。治疗宜补肾温阳，调理冲任。方药选用《景岳全书》右归丸（熟地、山药、枸杞子、菟丝子、鹿角胶、续断、党参、补骨脂、淫羊藿、熟附子、仙茅、肉桂）加减。

Literature Review of Thoroughfare-Controlling Disharmony

📖 *Zá Bìng Yuán Liú Xī Zhú* ("Incisive Light on the Source of Miscellaneous Disease"), "The Origin and Development of Disease in the Thoroughfare Vessel"

> "How do you deal with an invasion of the kidney? If you promote sweating, you will invariably cause the rise of cold, absence of sweating, great vexation in the heart, bitter pain in the joints, dizzy vision and aversion to cold, vomiting after eating, and inability to eat grains. If you use precipitation, you will cause abdominal fullness and distention, suddenly arising dizziness in the head, non-transformation of grain and water after eating, and glomus below the heart. All these symptoms are caused by throughfare qì invading the kidney and harming it."

This quotation describes the pathomechanism by which an abnormal exuberance of yīn cold in the thoroughfare vessel causes chaotic counterflow invading the kidney. Because of the close relationship between the thoroughfare vessel and the kidney, a vacuity of kidney yáng and abnormal exuberance of yīn cold can also lead to the pathomechanism of chaotic counterflow in the thoroughfare vessel.

📖 *Yī Xué Yuán Liú Lùn* ("Medical Source Theory"), "Gynecology"

> "Whenever you treat women, you must first understand the thoroughfare and controlling vessels. Further: The thoroughfare and controlling vessels both begin within the uterus and rise up in the interior of the back. They constitute the sea of the channels. They are the place where all blood is engendered and where the fetus is tied. If you understand the state of the thoroughfare and controlling vessels, then you have a good grasp on the root, and afterwards can know where all the myriad diseases that they engender arise."

This quotation expounds that chaotic counterflow of the thoroughfare and controlling vessels is the basic pathomechanism leading to gynecological diseases. Debilitation of kidney yáng is one of the causes leading to chaotic counterflow of the thoroughfare and controlling vessels and can therefore lead to the many symptoms of women's interrupted menstrual cycle or early or late menstruation.

文献评述

《杂病源流犀烛•冲脉病源流》曰："犯肾则奈何?汗之必寒起，无汗，心中大烦，骨节苦疼，目晕恶寒，食则反吐，谷不能进。下之腹胀满，卒起头晕，食则清谷不化，心下痞。皆冲气犯肾，肾受其害。"论述冲脉阴寒偏盛，逆乱犯肾的病机。由于冲脉与肾关系密切，反之肾阳虚，阴寒偏盛，亦可引起冲脉逆乱的病机。

《医学源流论•妇人科》曰："凡治妇人，必先明冲任之脉。又云; 冲任脉皆起于胞中，上循背里，为经脉之海。此皆血之所从生，而胎之所由系。明于冲任之故，则本原洞悉，而后其所生之病，千条万绪，可以知其所从起。"论述冲任逆乱是引起妇科疾病的基本病机。肾阳虚衰，又是引起冲任逆乱的原因之一，故可引起妇人绝经期前后的多种症状。

Summary of Thoroughfare-Controlling Disharmony

1. Chaotic Counterflow in the Thoroughfare and Controlling Vessels
   Disordered menstruation, frequent baking heat with sweating.
2. Yáng Failing to Warm
   Physical cold and fear of cold, pale white facial complexion.
3. Vacuity Fire Harassing the Orifices
   Dizzy head and vision.
4. Vacuous Yáng Harassing the Heart
   Oppression in the chest, vexation in the heart, reduced sleep and increased dreaming.
5. Heart Spirit Deprived of Nourishment
   Listlessness of the essence-spirit, burning preoccupation, depression.
6. Lower Back Deprived of Nourishment
   Aching lower back and limp knees.
7. Debilitation of Kidney Yáng
   Glossy white tongue fur, fat pale tongue, vacuous, weak, and forceless cubit pulse.

冲任失调
冲任逆乱—月经紊乱，时时烘热汗出
阳失温煦—形冷畏寒，面色淡白
虚火扰窍—头目昏眩
虚阳扰心—胸闷心烦，少寐多梦
心神失养—精神萎靡，焦虑抑郁
腰府失养—腰酸膝软
肾阳虚衰—苔白滑，舌淡胖，尺脉虚弱无力

1.12.2 Uterine Vacuity Cold

The kidney governs reproduction and is closely related to the uterus. Furthermore, the thoroughfare and controlling vessels both begin in the uterus. For this reason, when kidney yáng is depleted and yáng vacuity engenders internal cold and an abnormal exuberance of yīn cold, this can often lead to the pathomechanism of uterine vacuity cold.

When kidney yáng is debilitated, the *tiān-guǐ* [the principle of reproductive viability] arrives only with difficulty. The result is menstrual irregularities, indifferent sexual desire, and infertility in spite of long-term conjugality.

Congealing cold qì stagnation in the uterus and stoppage in the channels results in delayed menstruation and abdominal pain during menstruation, which are exacerbated by exposure to cold.

If kidney yáng is vacuous and yīn cold exuberant, the girdling vessel loses its retention. Therefore, we see clear thin vaginal discharge, possibly like white ooze.

If kidney yáng is vacuous, its function of transforming qì by steaming is disordered and blood fails to luxuriate the upper body. This results in a withered yellow or dark facial complexion.

When yáng qì is unable to outthrust, congealing cold obstructs the network vessels. This causes aching lower back and limp legs, icy cold and pain in the limbs, and fatigue and lack of strength.

Uterine vacuity cold manifests in a pale white tongue, glossy white tongue fur, and a deep and fine or deep and slow pulse.

The chapter, "Symptoms of Women's Miscellaneous Diseases; Uterine Cold Infertility" in the *Zhū Bìng Yuán Hòu Lùn* ("Origin and Indicators of Disease") states:

> "Uterine cold infertility is caused by improper rest and recuperation or dietary irregularities, due to which the body is overwhelmed by wind and taken by cold. Alternatively, excessive taxation damage allows the qì of wind-cold to overwhelm the blood in its channels and bind it in the uterus. This results in coldness of the uterus leading to infertility."

This quotation describes the pathomechanism by which vacuity cold in the uterus and loss of warming causes inability to conceive.

The "Treatise on Prescriptions for Women's White Turbidity and White Ooze" in the *Fù Rén Dà Quán Liáng Fāng* ("Compendium of Good Remedies for Women") states:

> "*Suǒ jīng wán* (Lock Essence Pill) treats vacuity in the lower origin, white turbidity in the urine, or dribbling white discharge and urinary frequency… *gù jīng wán* (Menses-Securing Pill): Treats vacuity cold of uterine qì, white turbidity in the urine or immoderate urination, and similar symptoms."

This quotation specifically recognizes the pathomechanical change of white turbidity and white ooze resulting from kidney yáng insufficiency and cold congealing in the uterus.

Uterine vacuity cold is treated by warming the channels and the uterus, and by boosting qì and supplementing blood. Recommended formulas are *wēn bāo yǐn* (Warm the Uterus Beverage) from the *Fù Qīng Zhǔ Nǚ Kē* ("Fù Qīng-Zhǔ's Gynecology") or *ài fù nuǎn gōng wán* (Mugwort and Cyperus Palace-Warming Pill) from the *Rén Zhāi Zhí Zhǐ Fù Yí Fāng Lùn* "Supplement to 'Rén-Zhāi Clear Guidance Formulary."

Wēn Bāo Yǐn 温胞饮
Warm the Uterus Beverage

bā jǐ tiān (巴戟天 Morindae Officinalis Radix, morinda)
bǔ gǔ zhī (补骨脂 Psoraleae Fructus, psoralea)
tù sī zǐ (菟丝子 Cuscutae Semen, cuscuta)
ròu guì (肉桂 Cinnamomi Cortex, cinnamon bark)
fù zǐ (附子 Aconiti Radix Lateralis Praeparata, aconite)
dù zhòng (杜仲 Eucommiae Cortex, eucommia)
bái zhú (白术 Atractylodis Macrocephalae Rhizoma, white atractylodes)
qiàn shí (芡实 Euryales Semen, euryale)
rén shēn (人参 Ginseng Radix, ginseng)

Ài Fù Nuǎn Gōng Wán 艾附暖宫丸 Mugwort and Cyperus Palace-Warming Pill
xiāng fù (香附 Cyperi Rhizoma, cyperus)
ài yè (艾叶 Artemisiae Argyi Folium, mugwort)
dāng guī (当归 Angelicae Sinensis Radix, Chinese angelica)
huáng qí (黄其芪 Astragali Radix, astragalus)
wú zhū yú (吴茱萸 Evodiae Fructus, evodia)
chuān xiōng (川芎 Chuanxiong Rhizoma, chuanxiong)
sháo yào (芍药 Paeoniae Radix, peony)
shú dì huáng (熟地黄 Rehmanniae Radix Praeparata, cooked rehmannia)
ròu guì (肉桂 Cinnamomi Cortex, cinnamon bark)
xù duàn (续断 Dipsaci Radix, dipsacus)

胞宫虚寒

肾主生殖，与胞宫关系密切，冲任二脉又皆起于胞宫，故肾阳亏虚，阳虚而生内寒，阴寒偏盛，多可导致胞宫虚寒的病机变化。肾阳虚衰，“天癸”难至，则月经不调，性欲淡漠，婚久不孕；寒凝气滞于胞宫，经脉不通，则月经推迟，经行腹痛，遇寒加剧；肾阳虚，阴寒盛，带脉失束，故带下清稀，或如白淫；肾阳虚，蒸腾气化功能失常，血不上荣，则面色萎黄或晦暗；阳气不能外达，寒凝络阻，故腰酸腿软，四肢冰冷疼痛，倦怠无力。胞宫虚寒，则舌淡白，苔白滑，脉沉细或沉迟。如《诸病源候论•妇人杂病诸候•子脏冷无子候》曰：“子脏冷无子者，由将摄失宜，饮食不节，乘风取冷，或劳伤过度，致风冷之气，乘其经血，结于子脏。子脏则冷，故无子。”论述胞宫虚寒，失于温煦，不能受孕的病机。《妇人大全良方)= •妇人白浊白淫方论》曰：“锁精丸：治下元虚弱，小便白浊，或白带淋漓，小便频数。…固精丸：治胞气虚寒，小便白浊，或小便无度等症。”对肾阳不足，寒凝胞宫导致的白浊白淫的病机变化有一定的认识。治法宜温经暖宫，益气补血。方药选用《傅青主女科》温胞饮（巴戟天、补骨脂、菟丝子、肉桂、附子、杜仲、白术、芡实、人参），或选用《仁斋直指方论》艾附暖宫丸（香附、艾叶、当归、黄芪、吴茱萸、川芎、白芍药、地黄、肉桂、续断）。

Literature Review of Uterine Vacuity Cold

📖 *Jǐng Yuè Quán Shū* ("Jǐng-Yuè's Complete Compendium"), "Regular Patterns of Women: The Channels"

> "In all cases of coldness of the blood, the menses invariably arrive after their time. Why is this caused by cold? Owing to an insufficiency of yáng qì, cold arises from the center, and engendering and transformation are untimely. This is what is referred to as cold."

This quotation indicates how a vacuity of yáng qì, insufficient engendering and transformation, and uterine vacuity cold lead to menstrual irregularities.

📖 *Rén Zhāi Zhí Zhǐ Fù Yí Fāng Lùn* "Supplement to Rén-Zhāi Clear Guidance Formulary: Descendants"

> "*Ài fù nuǎn gōng wán* (Mugwort and Cyperus Palace-Warming Pill) treats women's uterine vacuity cold, white ooze vaginal discharge, withered yellow facial complexion, aching pain in the limbs, fatigue and lack of strength, decreased intake of food and drink, menstrual irregularities, colorless blood, intermittent abdominal pain, and enduring infertility."

This quotation describes in detail how uterine vacuity cold causes infertility in spite of long-term marriage, and menstrual irregularities.

📖 *Yī Fǎ Yuán Tōng* ("Medical Methods to Free the Garden"), "Section on Gynecology: Vaginal Discharge"

> "Possibly caused by excessive sexual intercourse, vanquished essence flows downward and reduces kidney yáng. In a patient with such a condition, you will certainly see dizzy head and fearful heart, decreased intake of food and drink, and lack of strength in the limbs. The pulse will invariably be extremely effulgent in the two inch positions and weak in the two cubit positions, floating above and not subdued below. Vaginal discharge will invariably be clear, pale, and cold, neither malodorous nor sticky. This condition is treated by greatly supplementing original yáng and by promoting absorption of kidney qì. Use formulas like *qián yáng dān* (Subdue Yáng Elixir) with *gù zhǐ* (Psoraleae Fructus) and *yì zhì* (Alpiniae Oxyphyllae Fructus) added, or *huí yáng yǐn* (Yáng-Returning Beverage) with *fú líng* (Poria) and *dāng guī* (Angelicae Sinensis Radix) added."

This quotation discusses the pathomechanism by which kidney yáng vacuity and uterine vacuity cold give rise to white vaginal discharge.

文献评述

《景岳全书•妇人规•经脉类》曰："凡血寒者，经必后期而至。然何以为寒？亦惟阳气不足，则寒从中生，而生化失期，是即所谓寒也。"指出阳气亏虚，生化不足，胞宫虚寒而致月经失调的病机变化。

《仁斋直指方论•子嗣》曰："艾附暖宫丸：治妇人子宫虚冷，带下白淫，面色痿黄，四肢酸痛，倦怠无力，饮食减少，经脉不调。血无颜色，肚腹时痛，久无子息。" 对胞宫虚寒所致的婚久不孕、经脉不调等病机改变作了详细的描述。

《医法园通•女科门•带下》曰："或房事过度而败精下流则损肾阳，如此之人，定见头眩心惕，饮食减少，四肢无力，脉必两寸旺而两尺弱甚，浮于上而不潜于下，其下之物，必清淡而冷，不臭不粘，法宜大补元阳，收纳肾气，如潜阳丹加故纸、益智，回阳饮加茯苓、安桂。"论述肾阳虚，胞宫虚寒，引起白带的病机。

Summary of Uterine Vacuity Cold

1. *Tiān-Guǐ* Failing to Arrive

   Menstrual irregularities, indifferent sexual desire, infertility in spite of long-term conjugality.

2. Stoppage in the Channels

   Delayed menstruation, abdominal pain during menstruation, exacerbated by exposure to cold.

3. Girdling Vessel Losing Retention

   Thin clear vaginal discharge, possibly like white ooze.

4. Abnormal Steaming

   Withered yellow or dark facial complexion.

5. Congealing Cold Obstructing the Network Vessels

   Aching lower back and limp legs, cold and pain in the limbs, fatigue and lack of strength.

6. Uterine Vacuity Cold

   Pale white tongue, glossy white tongue fur, deep and fine or deep and slow pulse.

胞宫虚寒
天癸不至—月经不调，性欲淡漠，婚久不孕
经脉不通—月经推迟，经行腹痛，遇寒加剧
带脉失束—带下清稀，或如白淫
蒸腾失常—面色萎黄或晦暗
寒凝络阻—腰酸腿软，四肢冷痛，倦怠乏力
胞宫虚寒—舌淡白，苔白滑，脉沉细或沉迟

1.12.3 Congealing Cold Blood Stasis

The kidney is the root of earlier heaven. It brews and houses original yīn and original yáng, encloses the life gate, and has the ability to promote the normal movement of qì and blood. When kidney yáng is insufficient, the thoroughfare and controlling vessels lack warming by original yáng and gradually incur vacuity cold. Since the thoroughfare and controlling vessels both begin in the uterus, this can lead to cold congealing in the uterus. As soon as cold evil arises, it tends to congeal and stagnate. Impeding the normal movement of qì and blood, it forms the pathomechanism of congealing cold blood stasis.

When kidney yáng is insufficient, vacuity cold in the thoroughfare and controlling vessels prevents it from promoting the normal movement of qì and blood. Congealing cold causes stasis obstruction, which inhibits the flow in the channels. This results in delayed menstruation, cold pain in the lesser abdomen that refuses pressure, and pain relieved by exposure to heat.

When cold congeals in the uterus, menstrual blood is depressed. This results in scant menses of dark pale color and with clots.

When yáng qì is damaged by cold, it becomes unable to outthrust, and the entire body and limbs are deprived of warmth. The result is fear of cold and liking for warmth, lack of warmth in the limbs, and cold pain in the joints.

Abnormally severe vacuity cold manifests in a dark pale tongue body and a slow sunken pulse. Abnormally severe stasis obstruction manifests in a dark tongue body with stasis macules and stasis speckles, and a fine rough pulse.

The chapter, "Symptoms of Women's Miscellaneous Diseases; Lesser Abdominal Pain" in the *Zhū Bìng Yuán Hòu Lùn* ("The Origin and Indicators of Disease") states:

> "Lesser abdominal pain is caused by the evil qì of wind-cold, which overwhelms the region of the uterine network vessels, contends with blood and qì, and collects and binds in the lesser abdomen. Because wind vacuity begins to stir and strikes the blood, there is pain."

This quotation discusses the pathomechanism by which congealing cold in the uterus and stasis obstruction of qì and blood lead to menstrual pain.

The chapter, "Regular Patterns of Women; Kidney Vacuity Chaotic Menstruation" in the *Jǐng Yuè Quán Shū* ("Jǐng-Yuè's Complete Compendium") also states:

> "When sexual passions in women have caused menstrual irregularities, the disease is always located in the kidney channel. This pattern is extremely frequent and must be identified and treated… If the condition is related to an insufficiency of true yīn in the right kidney (which corresponds to true yáng) causing menstrual irregularities, use formulas like *yòu guī yǐn* (Right-Restoring [Life Gate] Beverage), *yòu guī wán* (Right-Restoring [Life Gate] Pill), or *bā wèi dì huáng wán* (Eight-Ingredient Rehmannia Pill) to govern it."

This quotation reflects a thorough understanding of the pathomechanism of kidney yáng vacuity causing internally arising cold and congealing cold blood stasis, resulting in such changes as menstrual irregularities.

Congealing cold blood stasis is treated by warming the channels and dispersing cold, and by dispelling stasis and regulating menstruation. Recommended formulas are *jiāng fù sì wù tāng* (Ginger and Aconite Four Agents Decoction) from the *Yīn Lèi Yuán Róng* ("Supreme Commanders of the Fortress of Medicine") or *nǚ jīn dān* (Women's Immortality Elixir) from the *Hán Shì Yī Tōng* ("Han's Clear View of Medicine").

Jiāng Fù Sì Wù Tāng 姜附四物汤
Ginger and Aconite Four Agents Decoction

gān jiāng (干姜 Zingiberis Rhizoma, dried ginger)
fù zǐ (附子 Aconiti Radix Lateralis Praeparata, aconite)
dāng guī (当归 Angelicae Sinensis Radix, Chinese angelica)
chuān xiōng (川芎 Chuanxiong Rhizoma, chuanxiong)
shú dì huáng (熟地黄 Rehmanniae Radix Praeparata, cooked rehmannia)
bái sháo (白芍 Paeoniae Radix Alba, white peony)

Nǜ Jīn Dān 女金丹 Women's Immortality Elixir
gǎo běn (藁本 Ligustici Rhizoma, Chinese lovage)
dāng guī (当归 Angelicae Sinensis Radix, Chinese angelica)
bái sháo (白芍 Paeoniae Radix Alba, white peony)
rén shēn (人参 Ginseng Radix, ginseng)
bái wēi (白薇 Cynanchi Atrati Radix, black swallowwort)
chuān xiōng (川芎 Chuanxiong Rhizoma, chuanxiong)
mǔ dān pí (牡丹皮 Moutan Cortex, moutan)
ròu guì (肉桂 Cinnamomi Cortex, cinnamon bark)
bái zhǐ (白芷 Angelicae Dahuricae Radix, Dahurian angelica)
bái zhú (白朮 Atractylodis Macrocephalae Rhizoma, white atractylodes)
fú líng (茯苓 Poria, poria)
yán hú suǒ (延胡索 Corydalis Rhizoma, corydalis)
chì shí zhī (赤石脂 Halloysitum Rubrum, halloysite)
mò yào (没药 Myrrha, myrrh)
xiāng fù (香附 Cyperi Rhizoma, cyperus)
gān cǎo (甘草 Glycyrrhizae Radix, licorice)

寒凝血瘀

肾为先天之本，蕴藏元阴元阳，内附命门，能推动气血的正常运行。肾阳不足，冲任则无元阳温煦而亦渐致虚寒，冲任起于胞宫，则可导致寒凝胞宫。寒邪既生，易凝易滞，阻碍气血正常运行，形成寒凝血瘀的病机变化。肾阳不足，冲任虚寒，不能推动气血正常运行，寒凝瘀阻，经脉不畅，则月经后期，小腹冷痛拒按，得热痛减; 寒凝胞宫，经血郁滞，则经血量少，色淡暗有块; 寒伤阳气，不能外达，全身、四肢失于温煦，则畏寒喜暖，四肢不温，关节冷痛。若虚寒偏重，则舌质暗淡，脉沉迟。若瘀阻偏重，则舌质晦暗，有瘀斑、瘀点，脉细涩。如《诸病源候论•妇人杂病诸候•小腹痛候》曰："小腹痛者，此由胞络之间，风冷邪气乘之，搏于血气，停结小腹，因风虚发动，与血相击故痛。"论述了寒凝胞宫，气血瘀阻，引起痛经的病机。《景岳全书•妇人规•肾虚经乱》也曰："妇人因情欲房室，以致经脉不调者，其病皆在肾经，此证最多，所当辨而治之。…若右肾真阴（应为真阳）不足，而经有不调者，宜右归饮、右归丸、八味地黄丸之类主之。"对肾阳虚则寒内生，寒凝血瘀而引起月经不调等病机变化深有认识。治法宜温经散寒，祛瘀调经。方药选用《医垒元戎》姜附四物汤（干姜、附子、当归、川芎、熟地、白芍），或选用《韩氏医通》女金丹（藁本、当归、白芍、人参、白薇、川芎、丹皮、桂心、白芷、白术、茯苓、延胡索、赤石脂、没药、香附、甘草）。

Literature Review of Congealing Cold Blood Stasis

📖 *Zhū Bìng Yuán Hòu Lùn* ("The Origin and Indicators of Disease"), "Symptoms of Women's Miscellaneous Diseases: Menstrual Stoppage"

> "Regarding wind-cold damage to channel blood, since it is the nature of blood to perfuse when exposed to warmth and to be blocked when exposed to cold, blood binds internally when it is overpowered by cold. This results in menstrual stoppage."

This is an incisive discussion of the pathomechanism by which congealing cold in the uterus and stasis obstruction of qì and blood lead to menstrual obstruction.

📖 *Shèng Jì Zǒng Lù* ("Sages' Salvation Records"), "Entry on Women's Qì and Blood"

> "In cases of abdominal pain at the onset of menstruation in maidens, when *tiān-guǐ* first arrives, construction and defense are not yet harmonized and the heart spirit is disquieted, which allows cold qì to intrude. Their blood and qì do not flow freely, which causes menstrual fluid to bind in the umbilical and abdominal region. This results in acute stabbing pain in the abdomen."

This quotation discusses how congealing cold and stagnant qì stop the flow of menses, qì, and blood, which leads to abdominal pain.

文献评述

《诸病源候论•妇人杂病诸候•月水不通候》曰："风冷伤其经血，血性得温则宣通，得寒则闭塞，既为冷所搏结，血结在内，则令月水不通。"对寒凝胞宫，气血瘀阻引起月经闭阻的病机作了深刻论述。

《圣济总录•妇人血气门》曰："室女月水来腹痛者，以天癸乍至，荣卫未和，心神不宁，间为寒气所客，其血与气两不流利，致令月水结搏于脐腹间，㽲（指腹中急痛）刺疼痛。"对寒气凝滞，经水气血不通，引起腹痛的病机变化作了论述。

Summary of Congealing Cold Blood Stasis

1. Cold Congealing in the Channels
   Delayed menstruation, cold pain in the lesser abdomen that refuses pressure, pain relieved by exposure to heat.
2. Depression of Menstrual Blood
   Scant menstrual bood of dark palc color and with clots.
3. Yáng Failing to Outthrust
   Fear of cold and liking for warmth, lack of warmth in the limbs, cold pain in the joints.
4. Congealing Cold Blood Stasis
   Dark pale tongue body with slow sunken pulse or a dark tongue body with stasis macules and stasis speckles, fine rough pulse.

寒凝血瘀

寒凝经脉—月经后期，小腹冷痛拒按，得热痛减

经血郁滞—经血量少，色淡暗有块

阳不外达—畏寒喜暖，四肢不温，关节冷痛

寒凝血瘀—舌质暗淡，脉沉迟或舌质晦暗，有瘀斑、瘀点，脉细涩

Chapter Two

Debilitation of Kidney Qì

Kidney qì refers to original qì in the kidney and constitutes the origin of the body. It is able to promote the growth and development of the body and stimulate the physiological activities of the bowels and viscera, the channels and network vessels, and the tissues and organs. Thus, it is the motivating force for maintaining the body's vital activities. Kidney qì also governs hibernation and is the root of receiving and storing, having the function of sealing, storing, securing, and containing. Constitutional insufficiency, immaturity of kidney qì in young age, weakening of the body in old age, excessive vexation and taxation damage from sexual activity, enduring or severe illness, and lack of or inappropriate treatment can all lead to the pathomechanism of debilitation of kidney qì.

Already at the time of the *Nèi Jīng* ("The Inner Canon"), kidney qì vacuity was mentioned explicitly by name and its manifestations discussed. The chapter, "The Spirit" in the *Líng Shū* ("The Magic Pivot"), for example, states that "kidney qì vacuity results in reversal."

"Treatise on Vital Qì Connecting with Heaven" in the *Sù Wèn* ("Plain Questions") also states: "Owing to an excessive exertion of strength, kidney qì is damaged and the lumbar vertebrae are damaged."

In addition, the "Treatise of Heavenly Truth from Remote Antiquity" in the *Sù Wèn* ("Plain Questions") states: "In men… at the age of fifty-eight, kidney qì is debilitated. The hair falls out and the teeth are desiccated." This quotation indicates the close relationship between kidney qì vacuity and age-related debilitation.

In the chapter, "Discussing Kidney Foot Lesser Yīn Disease Patterns" in the *Mài Jīng* ("The Pulse Canon") the Jìn period author Wáng Shū-Hé stated: "Vacuity of kidney qì leads to reverse flow… Vacuity of kidney qì causes a person to dream of seeing boats and drowning people, of being submerged in water, and of that which they fear." The understanding of kidney qì vacuity in this text for the most part resembled that of the *Nèi Jīng* ("The Inner Canon").

In the chapter, "Various Symptoms of Diseases of the Five Viscera and Six Bowels; Symptoms of Kidney Disease" in the *Zhū Bìng Yuán Hòu Lùn* ("Origin and Indicators of Disease"), the Suí dynasty author Cháo Yuán-Fāng pointed out: "Vacuity of kidney qì leads to reversal, coldness in the back and lower back, pain in the chest, and tinnitus and deafness. These signs indicate kidney qì vacuity." This quotation described in depth the pathomechanism and clinical manifestations of kidney qì vacuity.

Subsequently, the various medical texts like the *Dān Xī Xīn Fǎ* ("Dān Xī's Heart-Approach"), *Jǐng Yuè Quán Shū* ("Jǐng-Yuè's Complete Compendium"), *Shí Shì Mì Lù* ("Secret Records from the Stone Chamber"), and *Zhèng Zhì Huì Bǔ* ("Combined Supplements to Patterns and Treatment") further elaborated on the pathomechanism of kidney qì vacuity. According to differences in the special traits of the pathomechanism, we can further divide kidney qì depletion into six types: functional decline, loss of acuity in the ears and eyes, kidney qì failing to absorb, insecurity of the essence gate, enuresis, and stirring fetus.

肾气虚衰

肾气是指肾中元气，是构成人体的本元，能推动人体的生长发育，激发脏腑、经络等组织器官的生理活动，是维持人体生命活动的原动力。肾气主蛰伏，为收藏之本，具有封藏固摄的功能。凡禀赋不足，年幼肾气未充，年老体弱，烦劳过度，房事损伤，久病重病，失治误治，均可导致肾气虚衰的病机变化。早在《内经》时代，就已正式提出肾气虚的名称，论述了肾气虚的表现。如《灵枢•本神》曰："肾气虚则厥。"《素问•生气通天论》又曰："因而强力，肾气乃伤，高骨乃坏。"此外《素问•上古天真论》云："丈夫...五八肾气衰，发堕齿槁。"指出肾气虚与衰老有密切关系。晋代王叔和《脉经•论肾足少阴经病证》曰："肾气虚则厥逆。...肾气虚则梦见舟船溺人，得其梦伏水中，若有畏怖。"对肾气虚的认识与《内经》大体相似。隋代巢元方《诸病源候论•五脏六腑病诸候•肾病候》则指出："肾气不足则厥，腰背冷，胸内痛，耳鸣苦聋，是为肾气之虚也。"对肾气虚的病机和临床症状有了深入的阐述。其后《丹溪心法》、《景岳全书》、《石室秘录》、《证治汇补》等诸多医著对肾气虚病机更有所发挥。肾气亏虚，根据其病机特点不同，可进一步分为功能减退、耳目失聪、肾气不纳、精关不固、小便遗失、胎动不安等六类病机变化。

2.1 Functional Decline

Original qì in the kidney has the function of promoting and stimulating the vital activities in the human body. Therefore, the "Treatise of the Arcane Book of the Orchid Chamber of the Spirit Tower" in the *Sù Wèn* ("Plain Questions") states: "The kidney holds the office of labor, whence agility emanates." When kidney qì is depleted, the physiological functions in the entire body are impacted. This can lead to a reduction in organ functions and activities.

The kidney lives in the lower back, and when kidney qì is insufficient, the lower back is deprived of nourishment and its functional activities are reduced. This results in limp aching lower back and knees, which persists continuously, and a liking for [the area] being rubbed and pressed.

Movement exacerbates the consumption of qì further, and rest allows qì to be stored instead of dissipated. Therefore, symptoms are aggravated by fatigue and relieved by rest.

When kidney qì is plentiful, the essence-spirit is prosperous. However, when kidney qì is insufficient, qì fails to nourish the spirit, and spirit qì is debilitated. This manifests in listlessness of the essence-spirit and fatigued spirit and thinking of sleeping.

When kidney qì is debilitated, original qì is reduced and fails to manage breathing. The result is shortness of breath and shortage of qì, and fatigue and lack of strength.

The kidney governs the bones. When kidney qì is depleted, it is unable to nourish the bones. This results in limp aching sinews and bones, and in lack of strength in walking.

Owing to poor qì transformation, the waterways are stopped. This manifests in hypertonicity in the lesser abdomen and inhibited urination.

When kidney qì is debilitated, its function of securing and containing the bladder is reduced and the bladder's opening and closing is immoderate. As a result of this, we can see increased urination.

Vacuity of kidney qì manifests in a pale tongue, white tongue fur, and a forceless cubit pulse.

As the "Treatise on the Essential Subtleties of the Pulse" in the *Sù Wèn* ("Plain Questions") states, "The lower back is the house of the kidney. If the patient is unable to turn or rock it, it means that the kidney is exhausted." This quotation describes how kidney vacuity and lower back deprived of nourishment manifests in aching lower back and limp knees.

The chapter, "Lumbar Pain" in the *Yī Biǎn* ("Lancing Stones of Medicine") also states:

> "When the classic states, 'The lower back is the house of the kidney, and if the patient is unable to turn or rock it, it means that the kidney is exhausted,' this means that lumbar pain is in fact a disease of the kidney and bladder. If the greater yáng channel is vacuous, the various guest evils of wind, cold, and dampness can all do harm. This is especially common in those with kidney vacuity. Its symptoms are wilting and weakness in the lower back and limbs, generalized fatigue, limp aching legs and knees, a pulse that is forceless but surging and fine, and pain that is long, drawn-out, indistinct, and not severe."

This quotation not only suggests that kidney qì vacuity is an important pathomechanism leading to lumbar pain, but it also describes with great precision its clinical manifestations.

Reduced functionality is treated by supplementing the kidney and boosting qì. Recommended formulas are *shèn qì wán* (Kidney Qì Pill) from the *Jīn Guì Yào Lüe* ("Essential Prescriptions of the Golden Coffer") or the secret formula *zhuàng běn dān mì fāng* (Secret Elixir Formula to Invigorate the Root) from the *Lán Shì Mì Cáng* ("Secret Treasure of the Orchid Chamber").

Shèn Qì Wán 肾气丸
Kidney Qì Pill

shú dì huáng (熟地黄 Rehmanniae Radix Praeparata, cooked rehmannia)
shān zhū yú (山茱萸 Corni Fructus, cornus)
shān yào (山药 Dioscoreae Rhizoma, dioscorea)
zé xiè (泽泻 Alismatis Rhizoma, alisma)
fú líng (茯苓 Poria, poria)
mǔ dān pí (牡丹皮 Moutan Cortex, moutan)
guì zhī (桂枝 Cinnamomi Ramulus, cinnamon twig)
fù zǐ (附子 Aconiti Radix Lateralis Praeparata, aconite)

Zhuàng Běn Dān Mì Fāng 壮本丹秘方 Secret Elixir Formula to Invigorate the Root
dù zhòng (杜仲 Eucommiae Cortex, eucommia)
ròu cōng róng (肉苁蓉 Cistanches Herba, cistanche)
bā jǐ tiān (巴戟天 Morindae Officinalis Radix, morinda)
bǔ gǔ zhī (补骨脂 Psoraleae Fructus, psoralea)
xiǎo huí xiāng (小茴香 Foeniculi Fructus, fennel)
qīng yán (青盐 Halitum, halite)

功能减退

肾中元气，有推动、激发人体生命活动的作用，故《素问•灵兰秘典》云："肾者作强之官，伎巧出焉。"肾气虚衰，人身整体生理功能活动受到影响，则会导致脏腑功能活动衰减。肾居腰府，肾气不足，腰府失养，功能活动减弱，则腰膝酸软，绵绵不绝，喜揉喜按；动则耗气更甚，卧则气藏不散，故劳累加重，卧则减退；肾气充足，则精神昌盛，肾气不足，气不养神，神气衰微，则出现精神萎靡，神疲思睡；肾气虚衰，元气衰减，不司呼吸，则气短少气，困倦乏力；肾主骨，肾气亏虚，不能养骨，则筋骨酸软，行走乏力；气化不行，水道不通，故表现为少腹拘急，小便不利；肾气虚衰，对膀胱固摄作用减弱，膀胱开合失度，则反见小便增多。肾气虚弱，则舌淡，苔白，尺脉无力。如《素问•脉要精微论》曰："腰者肾之府，转摇不能，肾将惫矣。"描述了肾虚腰府失养，出现腰酸膝软的病机变化。《医碥•腰痛》也云："经曰：腰者肾之府也，转摇不能，肾将惫矣，是腰痛乃肾与膀胱病也。太阳经虚，则风寒湿诸客邪皆得为患，而肾虚之所患尤多。腰肢痿弱，小体（应当指身体）=疲倦，脚膝酸软，脉或洪细，细皆无力，痛亦悠悠隐隐不甚，是其候也。"不仅认为肾气虚是引起腰痛的重要病机，而且对其临床症状描述十分准确。治法宜补肾益气。方药选用《金匮要略》肾气丸（熟地黄、山萸肉、怀山药、泽泻、茯苓、丹皮、桂枝、附子），或选《兰室秘藏》壮本丹秘方（杜仲、肉苁蓉、巴戟天、补骨脂、茴香、青盐）。

Literature Review of Reduced Functionality

📖 *Zhū Bìng Yuán Hòu Lùn* ("Origin and Indicators of Disease"), "The Various Symptoms of Disease in the Back and Lower Back: Pain in the Lower Back and Leg"

> "Insufficiency of kidney qì is caused by contracting wind evil. Taxation damage results in kidney vacuity, and vacuity results in contraction of wind-cold. Wind-cold struggles with right qì, and this causes pain in the lower back and leg."

This quotation discusses how wind evil or excessive taxation damaging the kidney and insufficiency of kidney qì lead to lumbar pain.

📖 *Jǐng Yuè Quán Shū* ("Jǐng-Yuè's Complete Compendium"), "Schema of Miscellaneous Patterns: Lumbar Pain"

> "In patterns of lumbar pain, whenever it is long and drawn-out, deeply distressing, and occurs repeatedly and incessantly, it means vacuity of the kidney… When anxiety, thought, and preoccupation are followed by pain, it means vacuity of qì. When taxation and activity are followed by pain, it means debilitation of the liver and kidney."

It also states:

> "The lower back is the house of the kidney, and the kidney stands in exterior-interior relationship with the bladder. Therefore it is ascribed to greater yáng among the channels, and in terms of the viscera, it is ascribed to kidney qì. Furthermore, it is the key meeting point between the thoroughfare, controlling, governing, and girdling vessels. Thus all conditions with lumbar pain are caused by insufficiency of true yīn (which here should be understood to refer to insufficiency of kidney qì), and are best governed by banking up and supplementing kidney qì."

This quotation describes in detail how insufficiency of kidney qì leads to lumbar pain.

📖 *Shòu Shì Bǎo Yuán* ("Prolonging Life and Preserving the Origin"), "Examples of Vacuity and Repletion in the Vessels of the Five Viscera and Six Bowels: Vacuity and Repletion in the Vessel of the Kidney"

> "Insufficiency of kidney qì results in reversal, coldness in the back and lower back, pain in the chest, and tinnitus and deafness. These signs indicate a vacuity of kidney qì."

This quotation precisely discusses the pathomechanism of kidney qì vacuity causing cold pain in the back and lower back.

文献评述

《诸病源候论•腰背病诸候•腰脚疼痛候》曰："肾气不足，受风邪之所为也。劳伤则肾虚，虚则受于风冷，风冷与真气交争，故腰脚疼痛。"论述了风邪或过劳伤肾，肾气不足，引起腰痛的病机变化。

《景岳全书•杂证谟•腰痛》曰："腰痛证，凡悠悠戚戚，屡发不已者，肾之虚也。...忧愁思虑而痛者，气之虚也。劳动即痛者，肝肾之衰也。"又曰："腰为肾之府，肾与膀胱为表里，故在经则属太阳，在脏则属肾气，而又为冲任督带之要会。所以凡病腰痛者，多由真阴之不足（此处应理解为肾气不足），最宜以培补肾气为主。"对肾气不足导致的腰痛之病机改变进行了详细的描述。

《寿世保元•五脏六腑脉病虚实例•肾脏脉病虚实》曰："肾气不足则厥，腰背冷，胸内痛，耳鸣苦聋，是为肾气之虚也。"明确论述了肾气亏虚，腰背冷痛的病机改变。

Summary of Reduced Functionality

1. Lower Back Deprived of Nourishment

   Limp aching lower back and knees, which persists continuously, liking for being rubbed and pressed.

2. Consumption of Qì Upon Movement

   Symptoms aggravated by fatigue, relieved by rest.

3. Debilitation of Spirit Qì

   Listlessness of the essence-spirit, fatigued spirit and thinking of sleeping.

4. Debilitation of Original Qì

   Shortness of breath and shortage of qì, fatigue and lack of strength.

5. Inability to Nourish the Bones

   Limp aching sinews and bones, lack of strength in walking.

6. Poor Qì Transformation

   Hypertonicity in the lesser abdomen, inhibited urination, or paradoxically increased urination.

7. Kidney Qì Vacuity

   Pale tongue, white tongue fur, forceless cubit pulse.

功能减退
腰府失养—腰膝酸软，绵绵不绝，喜揉喜按
动则耗气—劳累加重，卧则减轻
神气衰微—精神萎靡，神疲思睡
元气衰减—气短少气，困倦乏力
不能养骨—筋骨酸软，行走乏力
气化不行—少腹拘急，小便不利，或小便反多
肾气虚弱—舌淡，苔白，尺脉无力

2.2 Loss of Acuity in the Ears and Eyes

The kidney opens at the ears and governs listening and identifying sounds. As the chapter, "Outward Manifestations and Diseases Caused by the Five Viscera" in the *Líng Shū* ("The Magic Pivot") states, "The ears are the office of the kidney." The chapter, "Vessel Measurement" in the *Líng Shū* ("The Magic Pivot") also states: "Kidney qì flows to the ears. When the kidney is harmonious, the ears are able to hear the five notes." Exposure to the five taxations and seven damages or excessive fatigue can damage kidney qì and lead to loss of acuity in the ears and eyes.

When kidney qì is debilitated, it is unable to promote the upward movement of qì and blood to fill the ears, and the ear orifices lose their acuity. The result is poor hearing, tinnitus, and deafness.

When kidney qì is vacuous, it is unable to promote the upward movement of qì and blood to nourish the head, eyes, and orifices of the heart, and the clear orifices are deprived of nourishment. This results in dizzy head and vision, dim vision, heart palpitations, shortness of breath, insomnia, and forgetfulness.

The lower back is the house of the kidney. When kidney qì is vacuous, the lower back is deprived of nourishment, which results in aching and pain in the lower back.

When kidney qì is insufficient, it is unable to promote the upward movement of qì and blood to luxuriate the face, or its promoting function lacks strength. The result is qì vacuity with blood stasis, and stasis obstruction in the blood vessels of the face, which manifests in a somber white or soot-black facial complexion.

When kidney qì is vacuous, defensive yáng is consequently also debilitated, and the external defense is not secure. This results in intermittent spontaneous sweating.

Debilitation of kidney qì manifests in a pale tongue, white tongue fur, and a fine weak pulse.

The "Entry on the Ears; Ear Vacuity" in the *Shèng Jì Zǒng Lù* ("Sages' Salvation Records") states:

> "As soon as kidney qì is vacuous, wind evil interferes with it. When this is further complicated by thought and preoccupation taxing the heart, qì binds in the vessels and is unable to flow freely. As a result, there is muddled and dim hearing, and tinnitus when qì attacks."

This quotation describes the pathomechanism by which kidney qì vacuity and obstruction of the qì dynamic lead to tinnitus.

The "Schema of Miscellaneous Patterns: Eyes" in the *Jǐng Yuè Quán Shū* ("Jǐng-Yuè's Complete Compendium") states:

> "In cases of what is called internal obstruction [any of a number of diseases of the eye manifesting in poor vision], inspection of the pupils may show that the root has no cover, only the eyeballs are colored blue, or perhaps slightly green, or the pupils are scattered and enlarged. These and other patterns lacking in heat and congestion, as well as symptoms such as dim vision, or frequent black flowery vision are all caused by an insufficiency of kidney qì, which leads to an absence of light in the pupils."

This passage describes how an insufficiency of kidney qì leads to dim vision, internal obstruction, and absence of light.

The chapter, "If there is no phlegm, dizziness does not arise" in the *Zhī Yí Lù* ("Records of Inquiry") explains:

> "In kidney vacuity, sexual desires have been immoderate, which has prevented kidney qì from returning to the origin and caused it to run in counterflow upward instead. The classic states, 'Sudden dizzy vision and unstable shaking of the head are due to repletion above and vacuity below; located in the foot lesser yīn and greater yáng channels.' It further states, 'Insufficiency in the sea of marrow causes dizzy vision'."

This quotation discusses the pathomechanism by which kidney qì vacuity and counterflow ascent leads to dizzy head and vision.

Loss of acuity in the ears and eyes is treated by supplementing the kidney and nourishing qì, and by sharpening hearing and brightening the eyes. The recommended formula is *bǔ shèn wán* (Kidney-Supplementing Pill) from the *Qiān Jīn Yào Fāng* ("A Thousand Gold Pieces Prescriptions").

Bǔ Shèn Wán 补肾丸
Kidney-Supplementing Pill

bā jǐ tiān (巴戟天 Morindae Officinalis Radix, morinda)
tù sī zǐ (菟丝子 Cuscutae Semen, cuscuta)
shé chuáng zǐ (蛇床子 Cnidii Fructus, cnidium seed)
ròu cōng róng (肉苁蓉 Cistanches Herba, cistanche)
yáng shèn (羊肾 Caprae seu Ovis Renes, goat's kidney)
ròu guì (肉桂 Cinnamomi Cortex, cinnamon bark)
fù zǐ (附子 Aconiti Radix Lateralis Praeparata, aconite)
shān zhū yú (山茱萸 Corni Fructus, cornus)
shēng dì huáng (生地黄 Rehmanniae Radix, rehmannia)
mǔ dān pí (牡丹皮 Moutan Cortex, moutan)
fú líng (茯苓 Poria, poria)
zé xiè (泽泻 Alismatis Rhizoma, alisma)
shí hú (石斛 Dendrobii Herba, dendrobium)
dāng guī (当归 Angelicae Sinensis Radix, Chinese angelica)
rén shēn (人参 Ginseng Radix, ginseng)
yuǎn zhì (远志 Polygalae Radix, polygala)
shí chāng pú (石菖蒲 Acori Tatarinowii Rhizoma, acorus)
fáng fēng (防风 Saposhnikoviae Radix, saposhnikovia)
huáng qí (黄其芪 Astragali Radix, astragalus)
wū yào (乌药 Linderae Radix, lindera)
gān jiāng (干姜 Zingiberis Rhizoma, dried ginger)
xì xīn (细辛 Asari Radix, asarum)
gān cǎo (甘草 Glycyrrhizae Radix, licorice)

耳目失聪

肾开窍于耳，主听声辨音。如《灵枢•五阅五使》曰："耳者，肾之官也"。《灵枢•脉度》亦曰："肾气通于耳，肾和则耳能闻五音矣。"如逢五劳七伤，劳累过度，则可导致肾气损伤，耳目失聪的病机变化。肾气虚衰，不能推动气血上充于耳，耳窍失聪，则为听力减退，耳鸣耳聋；肾气虚，不能推动气血上养头目心窍，清窍失养，则头目眩晕，视物不明，心悸气短，失眠健忘；腰为肾之府，肾气虚，腰府失养，则腰酸疼痛；肾气不足，不能推动气血上荣于面，或推动乏力，气虚血瘀，面部血脉瘀阻，则出现面色苍白，或面色黧黑；肾气虚，卫阳亦随之虚衰，卫外不固，则时有自汗。肾气虚衰，则舌淡，苔白，脉细弱。如《圣济总录•耳门•耳虚门》云："肾气既虚，风邪干之，复以思虑劳心，气脉内结，不得疏通，则耳内浑焞（音吞，听觉不清之意），与气相击耳鸣。"阐述了肾气虚，气机阻塞，引起耳鸣的病机。《景岳全书•杂证谟•眼目》曰："有所谓内障者，察其瞳子则本无遮隔，唯其珠色青蓝，或微兼绿色，或瞳人散大，别无热壅等证，而病目视不明，或多见黑花等证，此悉由肾气不足，故致瞳子无光。"对肾气不足引起眼目不明，内障无光的病机变化进行了描述。《质疑录•无痰不作眩》说："肾虚者，房欲过度，则肾气不归元而逆奔于上，经云：徇蒙招尤目眩，上实下虚，过在足少阴、巨阳。又曰：髓海不足，目为之眩是也。"论述肾气虚上逆致头晕目眩的病机。治法为补肾养气，聪明耳目。方药选用《千金方》补肾丸（巴戟、菟丝子、蛇床子、肉苁蓉、羊肾、桂心、附子、山茱萸、干地黄、丹皮、茯苓、泽泻、石斛、当归、人参、远志、菖蒲、防风、黄芪、乌药、干姜、细辛、甘草）。

Literature Review of Loss of Acuity in the Ears and Eyes

📖 *Líng Shū* ("The Magic Pivot"), "Inquiry About Statements"

> "When ascending qì is insufficient, the brain is not full. Consequently, the ears suffer from tinnitus, the head suffers from leaning over, and the eyes suffer from dizzy vision."

Insufficiency of ascending qì refers to the pathocondition of depleted kidney qì that is unable to ascend and fill the head, eyes, and five offices. This leads to tinnitus and dizzy vision.

📖 *Jǐng Yuè Quán Shū* ("Jǐng-Yuè's Complete Compendium"), "Schema of Miscellaneous Patterns: Ear Patterns"

> "Deafness is always caused by qì being blocked and not flowing to the ears… Vacuity results in qì not being full. Lack of fullness results in block."

This quotation sets forth the pathomechanism by which qì vacuity and qì block result in deafness and tinnitus. Since the kidney opens at the ears, it of course also includes the pathomechanism of kidney qì depletion.

📖 *Yī Lín Shéng Mò* ("Level Line Ink of the Forest of Medicine"), "Ears"

> "The ears are ascribed to the foot lesser yīn channel... Vanquishing of kidney qì results in deafness; insufficiency of kidney qì results in tinnitus."

This quotation succinctly poses that debilitation of kidney qì can induce the pathomechanical changes of tinnitus and deafness.

文献评述

《灵枢•口问》曰："上气不足，脑为之不满，耳为之苦鸣，头为之苦倾，目为之眩"。上气不足，即指肾气亏虚，不能上充头目五官，所以引起耳鸣目眩。

《景岳全书•杂证谟•耳证》曰："耳聋证，总因气闭不通耳。...虚则气不充，不充则闭也。"对气虚气闭则耳聋耳鸣的病机变化进行了深刻的分析，肾开窍于耳，当然也包括肾气亏虚的病机变化。

《医林绳墨•耳》曰："耳属足少阴肾经，...肾气虚败则耳聋，肾气不足则耳鸣。"明确提出肾气虚衰，可致耳鸣耳聋的病机变化。

Summary of Loss of Acuity in the Ears and Eyes

1. Loss of Acuity in the Ears
   Poor hearing, tinnitus, deafness.
2. Eyes Deprived of Nourishment
   Dizzy head and vision, dim vision.
3. Heart Orifices Deprived of Nourishment
   Heart palpitations, shortness of breath, insomnia, forgetfulness.
4. Lower Back Deprived of Nourishment
   Aching and pain in the lower back.
5. Qì Vacuity and Failure to Luxuriate
   Somber white or soot-black facial complexion.
6. Insecurity of External Defense
   Intermittent spontaneous sweating.
7. Insufficiency of Kidney Qì
   Pale tongue, white tongue fur, fine weak pulse.

耳目失聪
耳窍失聪—听力减退，耳鸣耳聋
目窍失养—头目眩晕，视物不明
心窍失养—心悸气短，失眠健忘
腰府失养—腰酸疼痛
气虚失荣—面色苍白，或面色黧黑
卫阳不固—时有自汗
肾气不足—舌淡，苔白，脉细弱

2.3 Kidney Qì Failing to Absorb

The lung governs the exhalation of qì; the kidney governs the absorption of qì. The lung is the governor of qì; the kidney is the root of qì. Kidney qì is in charge of absorption and thereby ensures that inhalation and exhalation are even and have a fixed depth to prevent shallow breathing. The lung and the kidney are mutually engendering as mother and child. The kidney's governance of containment and absorption works in concert with the lung's perfusion and depuration. Together, they maintain the normal inhalation and exhalation functions in the body.

Enduring disease spreading to the kidney or physical weakness in old age can manifest in the pathomechanism of kidney qì insufficiency and qì failing to contain and absorb. When kidney qì is debilitated, containment and absorption break down. The result is chronic hasty panting that is further exacerbated by movement, long exhalations and short inhalations, and inability to maintain continuous breathing.

The kidney is linked to the lung above. When kidney qì is vacuous, lung qì is also vacuous, and the external defense is not secure. This results in frequent spontaneous sweating.

When kidney qì is debilitated, it lacks strength to promote movement. The movement of qì and blood is inhibited, the limbs and body are deprived of nourishment, and blood stagnates in the face. As a result, the limbs are cold and the face is green-blue.

When kidney qì is vacuous, the lower back is deprived of nourishment. This results in limp aching lower back and knees.

When kidney qì is debilitated, qì fails to transform water, and water-damp gathers internally and spills out into the skin. The result is puffy swelling in the limbs and body.

When kidney qì is insufficient, qì transformation in the bladder is inhibited. This results in inhibited urination.

Vacuity of kidney qì results in a pale tongue body, white tongue fur, and fine sunken pulse.

The "Treatise on Disharmony" in the *Sù Wèn* ("Plain Questions") states:

> "The kidney is the water viscus. It governs fluids and it governs panting while lying down. The kidney vessel follows the mouth of the stomach upward to pour into the lung. If kidney qì is insufficient, qì is not contained and absorbed, and water qì ascends counterflow, intruding into the stomach and distressing the lung. Therefore, the person is unable to lie down and suffers panting."

This quotation is an early description of the pathomechanism by which kidney disease leads to panting.

It was not until the Southern Sòng period that Yáng Rén-Zhāi first proposed the notion of a pathomechanism related to kidney governing qì absorption. In the chapter, "Cough" in *Rén Zhāi Zhí Zhǐ Fù Yí Fāng Lùn* ("Supplement to 'Rén-Zhāi Clear Guidance Formulary'"), he stated:

> "Whenever coughing is violent and severe, moving and stretching the hundred bones, and is accompanied by the subjective sensation that qì is running counterflow from below the umbilicus to the upper body, this means that the kidney is vacuous and unable to receive qì and return it to the origin. It is best treated with *bǔ gǔ zhī* (Psoraleae Fructus) or *ān shén wán* (Spirit-Quieting Pill) to govern it. Do not limit treatment to quieting the lung."

This quotation discusses explicitly how kidney qì failing to absorb causes qì counterflow and panting.

Kidney qì failing to absorb is treated by supplementing and boosting kidney qì, and by promoting qì absorption and returning it to the source. The recommended formula is *gù shèn shè qì tāng* (Secure the Kidney and Contain Qì Decoction) from the *Lín Zhèng Zhǐ Nán Yī Àn* ("A Clinical Guide with Case Histories").

Gù Shèn Shè Qì Tāng 固肾摄气汤
Secure the Kidney and Contain Qì Decoction

shú dì huáng (熟地黄 Rehmanniae Radix Praeparata, cooked rehmannia)
shān zhū yú (山茱萸 Corni Fructus, cornus)
wǔ wèi zǐ (五味子 Schisandrae Fructus, schisandra)
fú líng (茯苓 Poria, poria)
chē qián zǐ (车前子 Plantaginis Semen, plantago seed)
niú xī (牛膝 Achyranthis Bidentatae Radix, achyranthes)
bǔ gǔ zhī (补骨脂 Psoraleae Fructus, psoralea)
hé táo rén (核桃仁 Juglandis Semen, walnut)

肾气不纳

肺主呼气，肾主纳气。肺为气之主，肾为气之根。肾气主司摄纳，能使呼吸调匀，具有一定的深度，防止呼吸表浅。肺肾母子相生，肾主摄纳，与肺之宣肃两相呼应，共同维持人体正常的呼吸功能。如久病及肾，或年老体弱，则可出现肾气不足，气不摄纳的病机改变。肾气虚衰，摄纳无权，则久病喘促，动则更甚，呼长吸短，气不得续; 肾上连肺，肾气虚，肺气亦虚，卫外不固，则汗常自出; 肾气虚衰，无力推动，气血运行不畅，肢体失养，面部血滞，则肢冷面青; 肾气虚，腰府失养，则腰膝酸软; 肾气虚衰，气不化水，水湿内停，外溢肌肤，则肢体浮肿; 肾气不足，膀胱气化不利，则小便不利。肾气虚弱，则舌质淡，苔白，脉沉细。如《素问•逆调论》曰：“肾者，水脏，主津液，主卧与喘也。”肾脉循胃口上注肺，如肾气不足，气不摄纳，水气上逆，客胃迫肺，故不得卧而喘，早期论述了肾病致喘的病机变化。直至南宋，杨仁斋首次提出了“肾主纳气”的病机概念，如《仁斋直指附遗方论•咳嗽》云：“凡咳嗽暴重，动引百骸，自觉气从脐下逆奔而上者，此肾虚不能收气归元也，当以补骨脂、安肾丸主之，毋徒从事于宁肺。”明确论述了肾气不纳，气逆而喘的病机变化。治法宜补益肾气，纳气归原。方药选用《临证指南医案•喘》固肾摄气汤（熟地、山萸肉、五味子、茯苓、车前子、怀牛膝、补骨脂、胡桃肉）。

Literature Review of Kidney Qì Failing to Absorb

🕮 *Zhèng Zhì Zhǔn Shéng* ("The Level-Line of Pattern Identification and Treatment"), "Panting"

"Lung vacuity results in shortage of qì and panting. If the condition endures without cure, it spreads from the lung to the kidney, resulting in a dual vacuity of the lung and kidney. Alternatively, taxation and desire can damage the kidney, so that essential qì is despoliated internally and the root is not secure. Both of these cause qì absorption to be marked by profuse emission and scant intake, which results in counterflow qì running into the upper body and panting."

This quotation elaborates on the pathomechanism by which kidney qì failing to absorb causes qì counterflow and panting.

🕮 *Jǐng Yuè Quán Shū* ("Jǐng-Yuè's Complete Compendium"), "Schema of Miscellaneous Patterns: Hasty Panting"

"Vacuity panting is not related to the presence of evil, but to a vacuity of original qì... Vacuity panting [manifests in] shortness and discontinuity of breath, ... flusteredness and qì timidity, low voice and shortness breath, anxiety as if qì were about to expire, difficulty in inhalation and exhalation. The symptoms are exacerbated by physical movement and there is panting with rapid movement, but relief when a deep breath can be drawn... All patterns of vacuity panting are invariably caused by qì vacuity. Qì vacuity panting accounts for 7 or 8 out of 10 cases. If inspection reveals no wind evil on the outside and no repletion heat on the inside, this always indicates a pattern of vacuity panting.

"Vacuity of spleen and lung qì does not go beyond the middle and upper burner and a branch depletion of the source of transformation. Its disease is therefore still superficial. However, in a vacuity of liver and kidney qì, the disease issues from the lower burner, and the root and branch are both diseased. This disease is therefore deep and you must quickly rescue the root to join and assist true qì and hope for a return to life."

This quotation sets forth in detail the pathomechanism and clinical manifestations of vacuity panting that results from kidney qì debilitation and qì failing to contain and absorb.

🕮 *Lín Zhèng Zhǐ Nán Yī Àn* ("A Clinical Guide with Case Histories"), "Panting"

"An old man presented with a fine pulse that was weak at the cubit, emaciated body and reduced eating, and hasty breathing and rapid

> panting upon physical movement. Most commonly, ungratifying exhalation and panting is a lung disease, and most cases relate to guest contraction [contraction of external evil]. In the present case, movement resulted in yáng transforming. Yīn was weak and unable to absorb, so inhalation of qì caused panting.
>
> "How can you dismiss kidney disease? The treatment method is to promote containment and absorption and to secure the true. For disease in the upper body, you must make the lower burner full. This is the significance of the method of gathering kidney qì."

The fact that movement resulted in qì panting meant that kidney qì failed to absorb. The treatment method of gathering kidney qì is precisely that of supplementing the kidney to promote qì absorption. This explains a typical case of enduring cough with panting that is related to kidney qì failing to absorb.

文献评述

《证治准绳•喘》曰："肺虚则少气而喘，若病仍迁延不愈，由肺及肾，则肺肾俱虚，或劳欲伤肾，精气内夺，根本不固，皆使气摄纳出多入少，逆气上奔而发喘。"明确阐述了肾虚不纳，气逆而喘的病机变化。

《景岳全书•杂证谟•喘促》曰："虚喘者无邪，元气虚也。...虚喘者气短而不续。...虚喘者慌张气怯，声低息短，皇皇然若气欲断，提之若不能升，吞之若不相及，劳动则甚，而唯急促似喘，但得引长一息为快也。...凡虚喘之证，无非由气虚耳。气虚之喘，十居七八，但察其外无风邪，内无实热而喘者，即皆虚喘之证。若脾肺气虚者，不过在中上二焦，化源未亏，其病犹浅。若肝肾气虚，则病出下焦而本末俱病，其病则深，此当速救其根以接助真气，庶可回生也。"详细描述了肾气虚衰，气不摄纳而致虚喘的病机变化及临床表现。

《临证指南医案•喘》曰："翁，脉细尺弱，形瘦食少，身动即气促喘急。大凡出气不爽而喘为肺病，客感居多。今动则阳化，由乎阴弱失纳，乃吸气入而为喘，肾病何辞，治法惟以收摄固真，上病当实下焦，宗肾气方法意。"动则气喘，为肾气失纳，治法宗肾气，即补肾纳气，说明此为久病咳喘，肾气不纳的典型病案。

Summary of Kidney Qì Failing to Absorb
1. Containment and Absorption Failure Chronic hasty panting, further exacerbated by movement, long exhalations and short inhalations, inability to maintain continuous breathing.
2. Insecurity of External Defense Sweating.
3. Inhibited Flow of Qì and Blood Cold limbs and green-blue face.
4. Lower Back Deprived of Nourishment Limp aching lower back and knees.
5. Qì Failing to Transform Water Puffy swelling of the limbs and body, inhibited urination.
6. Kidney Qì Vacuity Pale tongue, white tongue fur, fine sunken pulse.

肾气不纳
摄纳无权—久病喘促，动则更甚，呼长吸短，气不得续
卫外不固—汗出
气血不畅—肢冷面青
腰府失养—腰膝酸软
气不化水—肢体浮肿，小便不利
肾气虚弱—舌质淡，苔白，脉沉细

2.4 Insecurity of the Essence Gate

The kidney stores the essence of earlier heaven and governs birth, growth, development, and reproduction. Kidney qì has the function of regulating both the stockpiling and diffusion of kidney essence, which reflects one aspect of the kidney's function of governing securing and containing. Physical weakness in old age can gradually debilitate kidney qì. Taxation from immoderate sexual intercourse can damage kidney qì. Either of these can lead to a breakdown in securing and containing, causing qì to fail to contain essence due to insecurity of the essence gate.

The chapter, "Beginnings of the Hundred Diseases" in the *Líng Shū* ("The Magic Pivot") states: "Excessive physical exertion, as during sexual intercourse, and sweating in the bath damage the kidney." When kidney qì is debilitated and unable to secure and contain, the essence gate loses its ability to restrain, and semen flows spontaneously. The result is seminal emission and incessant seminal efflux.

Frequent seminal emission easily leads to depletion of semen. In addition, kidney qì is already vacuous, which further prevents it from promoting the upward movement of the subtle essences to nourish the head and eyes. This results in clouded head and flowery vision.

When kidney qì is debilitated, the lower back is deprived of nourishment and the essence-spirit does not receive assistance. This results in limp aching lower back and knees, and lassitude of the spirit.

Insufficiency of kidney qì manifests in a pale tongue with white fur and a fine weak sunken pulse.

The chapter, "Seminal Emission" in the *Jǐng Yuè Quán Shū* ("Jǐng-Yuè's Complete Compendium") states:

> "Seminal emission due to dreaming is called dream emission. Spontaneous seminal discharge that is not due to dreaming is called seminal efflux. ... Seminal efflux is always related to kidney qì failing to keep composure."

This passage points out that insecurity of kidney qì can lead to seminal emission and seminal efflux.

The chapter, "Internal Damage and External Contraction; The Origin and Development of Damage from Sexual Desire" in the *Zá Bìng Yuán Liú Xī Zhú* ("Incisive Light on the Source of Miscellaneous Disease") also explains:

> "The kidney storing essence is related to the kidney's ability to foster life. Both gathering and dispersing are controlled by the kidney. If kidney qì is debilitated, essential qì of the entire body is lacking. Therefore essence moves frenetically and is discharged at any time. The formula for *zhū líng wán* (Polyporus Pill) is constructed exactly for this condition."

This quotation sets forth the pathomechanical changes of insufficiency of kidney qì and inability to contain essence.

Insecurity of the essence gate is treated by supplementing and boosting kidney qì, and by securing the kidney and astringing essence. The recommended formula is *jīn suǒ gù jīng wán* (Golden Lock Essence-Securing Pill) from the *Yī Fāng Jí Jiě* ("Medical Formulas Gathered and

Explained") in combination with *wǔ zǐ yǎn zōng wán* (Five-Seed Progeny Pill) from the *Zhèng Zhì Zhǔn Shéng* ("The Level-Line of Pattern Identification and Treatment").

Jīn Suǒ Gù Jīng Wán 金锁固精丸 Golden Lock Essence-Securing Pill
shā yuàn zǐ (沙苑子 Astragali Complanati Semen, complanate astragalus seed)
qiàn shí (芡实 Euryales Semen, euryale)
lián xū (莲须 Nelumbinis Stamen, lotus stamen)
lóng gǔ (龙骨 Mastodi Ossis Fossilia, dragon bone)
mǔ lì (牡蛎 Ostreae Concha, oyster shell)

Wǔ Zǐ Yǎn Zōng Wán 五子衍宗丸 Five-Seed Progeny Pill
tù sī zǐ (菟丝子 Cuscutae Semen, cuscuta)
wǔ wèi zǐ (五味子 Schisandrae Fructus, schisandra)
gǒu qǐ zǐ (枸杞子 Lycii Fructus, lycium)
fù pén zǐ (覆盆子 Rubi Fructus, rubus)
chē qián zǐ (车前子 Plantaginis Semen, plantago seed)

精关不固

肾藏先天之精，主生长发育生殖，肾气具有调节控制肾精存储和宣泄的功能，此是肾主固摄功能的一种体现。如年高体弱，肾气日渐虚衰，或房事不节，劳伤肾气，即可引起固摄无权，气不摄精，精关不固的病机变化。如《灵枢•百病始生》曰："用力过度，若入房，汗出浴，则伤肾。"肾气虚衰，不能固摄，精关失制，精液自流，则遗精、滑精不止; 经常遗精，精液易亏，加之肾气已虚，更不能推动精微物质上养头目，则头昏眼花; 肾气虚衰，腰府失养，精神不济，则腰膝酸软，倦怠神疲; 肾气不足，则舌淡苔白，脉沉细弱。如《景岳全书•遗精》指出："因梦而出精者，谓之梦遗; 不因梦而精自出者，谓之精滑。...滑精者无非肾气不守而然。"明确指出了肾气不固可致遗精滑精的病机改变。《杂病源流犀烛•内伤外感门•色欲伤源流》也说："肾藏精，盖肾能摄精气以育人伦者也。或育或散，皆主于肾，今肾气衰，则—身之精气，无所管摄，故妄行而出不时，猪苓丸一方，正为此设。"明确指出了肾气不足，不能摄精的病机变化。治法宜补益肾气，固肾涩精。方药选用《医方集解》金锁固精丸（沙苑蒺藜、芡实、莲须、龙骨、牡蛎），合《证治准绳》五子衍宗丸（菟丝子、五味子、枸杞子、覆盆子、车前子）。

Literature Review of Insecurity of the Essence Gate

📖 *Zhū Bìng Yuán Hòu Lùn* ("Origin and Indicators of Disease"), "Symptoms of Vacuity-Taxation Scant Semen"

> "The kidney governs the bones and marrow, and stores essence. Vacuity taxation weakens kidney qì and therefore causes scant semen. When examining the pulse, if the cubit pulse on the left hand indicates yīn expiry, it means an absence of kidney pulse. If there is heat on the underside of the feet and tension on the inside of both thighs, the governance of essence and qì is exhausted, which is caused by taxation damage."

The chapter, "Symptoms of Vacuity-Taxation Seminuria" states:

> "[Vacuity-taxation seminuria] is caused by debilitation of kidney qì. The kidney stores essence, and its qì flows to the genitals. When taxation damage makes the kidney vacuous so that it is unable to store essence, this causes semen to be discharged with urine."

The chapter, "Symptoms of Vacuity-Taxation Spillage of Essence and Noticeable Seminal Loss" also explains:

> "Vacuity of kidney qì is the reason for spillage of essence. When one can see, smell, and feel it, there is stirring of kidney qì. The kidney stores essence, and when it is vacuous and therefore unable to control essence, this causes symptoms that one can see via the outward spillage of essence."

The chapter, "Symptoms of Vacuity-Taxation Seminal Loss" further points out:

> "When kidney qì is reduced so that it is unable to store essence, this is the reason for leaking of essence. This condition manifests with bowstring tension in the lesser abdomen, yīn head cold, pain in the eye socket, and hair loss. When the pulse is rapid and scattered, this is the pulse of seminal loss. Whenever the pulse is scallion-stalk, stirred, faint, and tight, it indicates seminal loss in men."

The passages above analyze in considerable detail how vacuity of kidney qì and inability to receive essence leads to scant essence, seminuria, spillage of essence, and seminal loss. At the same time, they identify vacuity and insecurity of the kidney as the basic pathomechanism for seminal emission.

📖 *Míng Yī Zhǐ Zhǎng* ("Illuminating Medicine in the Palm of Your Hand"), "Red and White Turbidity, Seminal Efflux, and Dream Emission Patterns"

> "Dream emission means dreaming of [sexual] intercourse and emitting semen. Seminal efflux refers to spontaneous spilling of semen that is not due to dreaming of sexual intercourse. Both conditions are caused by vacuity of the true origin and by vacuity fire raging, which leads to desertion in the sea of essence."

Vacuity of the true origin refers to a vacuity of kidney qì. This passage thus describes how vacuity of kidney qì and insecurity of the essence gate can lead to dream emission and seminal efflux.

文献评述

《诸病源候论•虚劳少精候》曰："肾主骨髓，而藏于精。虚劳肾气虚弱，故精液少也。诊其脉，左手尺中阴绝者，无肾脉也。苦足下热，两髀里急，主精气竭少，为劳伤所致也。"《虚劳尿精候》曰："肾气衰弱故也。肾藏精，其气通于阴。劳伤肾虚，不能藏于精，故因小便而精液出也。"《虚劳溢精见闻精出候》又说："肾气虚弱，故精溢也。见闻感触，则动肾气。肾藏精，今虚弱不能制于精，故因见闻而精溢出也。"《虚劳失精候》还指出："肾气虚损，不能藏精，故精漏失。其病小腹弦急，阴头寒，目眶痛，发落。诊其脉数而散者，失精脉也。凡脉芤动微紧，男子失精也。"上述文字对肾气虚弱，摄精不能而导致的少精、尿精、溢精、失精等病机变化进行了较深刻的分析，并把肾虚不固作为遗精的基础病机。

《明医指掌•赤白浊精滑梦遗证》曰："梦遗者，梦与人交而遗其精也。精滑者，不因梦交而精自泄也。皆因真元虚，虚火流行，以致精海脱滑。"真元虚，即指肾气虚，指出肾气虚，精关失固，可致梦遗滑精。

Summary of Insecurity of the Essence Gate
1. Qì Failing to Receive Essence Seminal emission, incessant seminal efflux. 2. Head and Eyes Deprived of Nourishment Clouded head and flowery vision. 3. Kidney Vacuity and Loss of Nourishment Limp aching lower back and knees, fatigued body and spirit. 4. Insufficiency of Kidney Qì Pale tongue, white tongue fur, fine weak sunken pulse.

精关不固
气不摄精—遗精、滑精不止 头目失养—头昏眼花 肾虚失养—腰膝酸软，倦怠神疲 肾气不足—舌淡苔白，脉沉细弱

2.5 Enuresis

The kidney governs water and containment and absorption. It stands in exterior-interior relationship with the bladder. Thus it has an important regulating effect on both the engenderment and elimination of urine. Kidney qì has a securing and containing effect on the bladder. It is able to restrain the bladder, manage its opening and closing, and prevent the loss of urine. Damage to the kidney from debility in old age or enduring disease can lead to insufficiency of kidney qì, retention failure in the bladder, and subsequently enuresis.

When kidney qì is insufficient, the bladder is unable to secure and contain. This results in frequent urination, urinary incontinence, or frequent profuse nocturia, and clear white urine.

When kidney qì is unable to secure and contain, subtle essences flow downward. The result is white turbidity in the urine and emaciation.

When kidney qì is vacuous, the essence-spirit and the lower back are deprived of nourishment. This results in limp aching lower back and knees and exhaustion of the essence-spirit.

Vacuity of kidney qì manifests in a pale tongue, thin white tongue fur, and a fine weak sunken pulse.

In ancient texts, enuresis is referred to by such names as "emission of urine" or "urinary incontinence." The "Treatise Explaining the Five Qì" in the *Sù Wèn* ("Plain Questions"), for example, states: "Inhibition of the bladder means dribbling block. Failure to retain means emission of urine." This passage describes the pathomechanism of insufficiency of kidney qì and failure of the bladder's retentive power leading to enuresis.

The chapter, "Enuresis" in the "Schema of Miscellaneous Patterns" in the *Jǐng Yuè Quán Shū* ("Jǐng-Yuè's Complete Compendium") also states:

> "Enuresis patterns include spontaneous emission, which means loss of urine during sleep, as well as incontinence, which means that the qì gate is insecure, causing frequent urination and inability to retain urine. Furthermore, there is qì desertion in the upper body, which causes loss of retention in the lower burner and subsequent unconscious loss of urine. These are symptoms of extreme vacuity. To summarize, these three are all related to vacuity patterns and are merely differentiated by the degree of severity.
>
> "Spontaneous emission of urine during dreams is mostly found in young patients. If you wait until their qì is strong and secure, you might be able to treat it with just a little recuperation and have nothing to worry about. However, if it is a case of incessant urination and of the bladder failing to store, this must be related to qì vacuity. Qì is the mother of water and if water is unable to amass, it is because qì is unable to secure. This is a sign of loss of composure, which is highly irregular and in severe cases leads to qì desertion and loss. If it is unnoticed, it is particularly serious. This disease not only afflicts patients with wind patterns and weak qì from age-related debilitation, but is also common after serious illness. This is what Zhāng Zhòng-Jǐng referred to when he stated that 'lower burner exhaustion results in enuresis and incontinence.'"

When kidney qì is insufficient, water is able to amass, and opening and closing are regular. When kidney qì is insufficient, qì is not secure or contained. Therefore, the symptom of enuresis occurs frequently. Thus, this quotation incisively discusses the pathomechanism by which insufficiency of kidney qì leads to enuresis.

Enuresis is treated by supplementing and boosting kidney qì, and by securing the bladder and checking enuresis. The recommended formula is *sāng piāo xiāo sǎn* (Mantis Egg-Case Powder) from the *Běn Cǎo Yǎn Yì* ("Expanded Herbal Foundation"), with the addition of *fù pén zǐ* (Rubi Fructus), *bǔ gǔ zhī* (Psoraleae Fructus), and *yì zhì rén* (Alpiniae Oxyphyllae Fructus).

Sāng Piāo Xiāo Sǎn 桑螵蛸散 Mantis Egg-Case Powder
sāng piāo xiāo (桑螵蛸 Mantidis Ootheca, mantis egg-case) *yuǎn zhì* (远志 Polygalae Radix, polygala) *shí chāng pú* (石菖蒲 Acori Tatarinowii Rhizoma, acorus) *lóng gǔ* (龙骨 Mastodi Ossis Fossilia, dragon bone) *rén shēn* (人参 Ginseng Radix, ginseng) *fú shén* (茯神 Poria cum Pini Radice, root poria) *dāng guī* (当归 Angelicae Sinensis Radix, Chinese angelica) *guī bǎn* (龟版 Testudinis Plastrum, tortoise plastron) Plus: *fù pén zǐ* (覆盆子 Rubi Fructus, rubus) *bǔ gǔ zhī* (补骨脂 Psoraleae Fructus, psoralea) *yì zhì rén* (益智仁 Alpiniae Oxyphyllae Fructus, alpinia)

小便遗失

肾主水，主摄纳，与膀胱互为表里，对小便的生成和排泄具有重要调节的作用。肾气对膀胱有固摄作用，能约束膀胱，启司开合，防止尿液遗失。如年老体衰，或久病伤肾，则可导致肾气不足，膀胱失约，小便遗失的病机变化。肾气不足，膀胱不能固摄，则小便频数，或小便失禁，或夜尿频多，小便清白; 肾气不能固摄，精微物质下流，则小便白浊，形体消瘦; 肾气虚弱，精神、腰府失养，则腰膝酸软，精神疲惫; 肾气虚弱，则舌淡，苔薄白，脉沉细弱。小便遗失，古谓之“遗溺”、“小便不禁”等病证名称。如《素问•宣明五气》曰：“膀胱不利为癃，不约为遗溺。”论述了肾气不足，膀胱不约，小便遗失的病机改变。《景岳全书•杂证谟•遗溺》也云：“遗溺一证，有自遗者，以睡中而遗失也; 有不禁者，以气门不固，而频数不能禁也。又有气脱于上，则下焦不约，而遗失不觉者，此虚极之候也。总之，三者皆属虚证，但有轻重之辨耳。若梦中自遗者，唯幼稚多有之，俟其气壮而固，或少加调理可愈，无足疑也。唯是水泉不止，膀胱不藏者，必以气虚而然。盖气为水母，水不能蓄，以气不能固也，此失守之兆，大非所宜，甚至气脱而遗，无所知觉，则尤其甚者也。此唯非风证及年衰气弱之人，或大病之后多有之。仲景曰：下焦竭则遗溺失禁，此之谓也。”肾气足则水能存蓄，开阖有度，肾气不足，气不固摄，故遗溺之症频作，明确论述了肾气不足，小便遗失的病机改变。治法宜补益肾气，固脬止遗。方药选用《本草衍义》桑螵蛸散（桑螵蛸、远志、菖蒲、龙骨、人参、茯神、当归、龟板）加覆盆子、补骨脂、益智仁。

Literature Review of Enuresis

📖 *Zhū Bìng Yuán Hòu Lùn* ("Origin and Indicators of Disease"), "Symptoms of Vacuity-Taxation: Vacuity-Taxation Dribble after Voiding"

> "The kidney governs water. In patients with taxation damage, kidney qì is vacuous and unable to store water, and there is vacuity cold in the uterus. Therefore, they suffer from water not stopping but continuing to dribble after voiding. A slow pulse that is moderate and fine means dribble after voiding."

This quotation is a description of the pathomechanism by which kidney qì vacuity and failure of the bladder's retentive power results in urinary incontinence.

📖 *Lèi Zhèng Zhì Cái* ("Systematized Patterns with Clear-Cut Treatments"), "Discussing the Treatment of Dribbling Urinary Block and Enuresis"

> "Enuresis patterns include spontaneous emission during sleep, frequent incontinence due to qì failing to contain, and loss of retention in the lower burner as a result of upward desertion of qì, which causes unnoticed loss of urine. Spontaneous emission during sleep is found mostly in young patients. If you wait until their qì is strong and secure, possibly regulating and supplementing the heart and kidney, patients will recover on their own. However, incessant flow of urine and storage failure of the bladder is mostly related to debilitation in old age and weakness of qì. Since qì is the mother of water, a failure of water to amass is caused by qì being unable to secure and contain."

This quotation describes the pathomechanism by which insecurity of kidney qì and retention failure in the bladder cause enuresis.

文献评述

《诸病源候论•虚劳候•虚劳小便余沥候》曰："肾主水，劳伤之人，肾气虚弱，不能藏水，胞内虚冷，故小便后水液不止而有余沥。迟脉缓细者，小便余沥也。"对肾气虚弱，膀胱不约而小便不禁的病机进行了论述。

《类证治裁•闭癃遗溺论治》曰：“若遗溺一症，有睡中自遗者，有气不摄而频数不禁者，有气脱于上则下焦不约，而遗失不知者。睡中自遗，幼稚多有，俟其气壮乃固，或调补心肾自愈。惟水泉不止，膀胱不藏，多是年衰气弱，以气为水母，水不能蓄，由气不固摄也。”论述肾气不固，膀胱失约，小便遗失的病机变化。

Summary of Enuresis
1. Loss of Retention in the Bladder Urinary frequency, possibly urinary incontinence, or frequent profuse nocturia, clear white urine. 2. Subtle Essences Flowing Downward White turbidity in the urine, emaciation. 3. Kidney Vacuity and Loss of Nourishment Limp aching lower back and knees, exhaustion of the essence-spirit. 4. Kidney Qì Vacuity Pale tongue, thin white tongue fur, fine weak sunken pulse.

小便遗失
膀胱不约—小便频数，或小便失禁，或夜尿频多，小便清白 精微下流—小便白浊，形体消瘦 肾虚失养—腰膝酸软，精神疲惫 肾气虚弱—舌淡，苔薄白，脉沉细弱

2.6 Stirring Fetus

The kidney stores essential qì and governs birth, growth, development, and reproduction. The thoroughfare vessel is the sea of blood, and the controlling vessel governs the uterus. Both these vessels are subordinated to the kidney and depend on the movement-promoting function of qì in the kidney. This causes essence and blood to pour into the thoroughfare and controlling vessels and to nourish the fetus in the uterus.

Only when kidney qì is plentiful and has the strength to secure and contain, is it able to protect the healthy growth of the fetus, stabilize and secure its development, and prevent it from stirring in disorder. Therefore, the “Treatise of Heavenly Truth from Remote Antiquity” in the *Sù Wèn*

("Plain Questions") states: "When women reach the age of two sevens, *tiān-guǐ* [the principle of reproductive viability] arrives; the controlling vessel flows, the great thoroughfare vessel exuberates, and the menses descend in a timely manner. Therefore, she is able to bear children." When kidney qì is debilitated, the pathomechanical changes of insecurity of the fetal origin and stirring fetus can appear.

When kidney qì is insufficient, the containing and absorbing functions are reduced, the thoroughfare and controlling vessels are insecure, and the fetus loses its ties. This can result in stirring fetus, premature delivery, and miscarriage, and lead to habitual miscarriage.

When kidney qì is insufficient and its promotion of movement lacks strength, essence-blood is unable to nourish the embryo, and the formation, growth, and development of the fetus are disturbed. The result is atrophied fetus, a fetus that fails to grow, fetal feebleness, and poor fetal development.

When kidney qì is vacuous, it is unable to contain and control blood. The result is fetal spotting and the appearance of red vaginal discharge.

When kidney qì is insufficient, the lower back is deprived of nourishment. The result is aching lower back and sagging of the abdomen.

Kidney qì debilitation manifests in a pale tongue, white tongue fur, and insufficient cubit pulse.

The chapter, "Vomiting, Diarrhea, and Abdominal Pain" in the *Fù Qīng Zhǔ Nǚ Kē* ("Fù Qīng-Zhǔ's Gynecology") states:

> "What is the reason for pain in the uterus and ultimately miscarriage? This is absolutely related to securing by kidney qì. The uterus is tied to the kidney and linked to the heart. When kidney qì is secure, it interacts with the heart whose qì flows to the uterus. This is the reason why the fetus cannot abort in spite of its tendency to do so. Moreover, when kidney qì is able to secure, yīn fire invariably arrives to engender the spleen, and heart qì is able to reach. As a result, heart fire invariably arrives to rescue the stomach. Thus, if the spleen and stomach are vacuous but not yet expired, the fetus might stir but will not abort."

This quotation points out that when kidney qì is plentiful, the fetus is secure and does not stir. By contrast, it explains that when kidney qì is vacuous, fetal qì is insecure, which can result in stirring fetus.

The chapter, "Habitual Miscarriage" in the *Zhōng Yī Fù Kē Xué* ("Chinese Gynecology") also states:

> "Constitutional insufficiency of earlier heaven can prevent kidney qì from being full. Alternatively, immoderate sexual intercourse after

> conception and damage from indulging in desires can also cause kidney qì depletion. In either case, the thoroughfare and controlling vessels are insecure, and the fetus loses its ties. This leads to frequent pregnancies but frequent loss of the fetus, or in other words, habitual miscarriage."

This quotation succinctly points to the pathomechanism by which debilitation of kidney qì can lead to stirring fetus.

Stirring fetus is treated by securing the kidney and quieting the fetus. Recommended formulas are *shòu tāi wán* (Fetal Longevity Pill) from the *Yī Xué Zhōng Zhōng Cān Xī Lù* ("Records of Chinese Medicine with Reference to Western Medicine") or *bǔ shèn gù chōng wán* (Kidney-Supplementing Thoroughfare-Securing Pill) from the *Zhōng Yī Fù Kē Xué* ("Chinese Gynecology").

Shòu Tāi Wán 寿胎丸 Fetal Longevity Pill
tù sī zǐ (菟丝子 Cuscutae Semen, cuscuta)
sāng jì shēng (桑寄生 Taxilli Herba, mistletoe)
xù duàn (续断 Dipsaci Radix, dipsacus)
ē jiāo (阿胶 Asini Corii Colla, ass hide glue)

Bǔ Shèn Gù Chōng Wán 补肾固冲丸 Kidney-Supplementing Thoroughfare-Securing Pill
tù sī zǐ (菟丝子 Cuscutae Semen, cuscuta)
xù duàn (续断 Dipsaci Radix, dipsacus)
bā jǐ tiān (巴戟天 Morindae Officinalis Radix, morinda)
dù zhòng (杜仲 Eucommiae Cortex, eucommia)
dāng guī (当归 Angelicae Sinensis Radix, Chinese angelica)
shú dì huáng (熟地黄 Rehmanniae Radix Praeparata, cooked rehmannia)
lù jiǎo shuāng (鹿角霜 Cervi Cornu Degelatinatum, degelatinated deer antler)
gǒu qǐ zǐ (枸杞子 Lycii Fructus, lycium)
ē jiāo (阿胶 Asini Corii Colla, ass hide glue)
dǎng shēn (党参 Codonopsis Radix, codonopsis)
bái zhú (白术 Atractylodis Macrocephalae Rhizoma, white atractylodes)
dà zǎo (大枣 Jujubae Fructus, jujube)
shā rén (砂仁 Amomi Fructus, amomum)

胎动不安

肾藏精气，主生长发育与生殖。冲为血海、任主胞宫，冲任二脉隶属于肾，依靠肾中之气的推动作用，使精血灌注冲、任，濡养胞胎。肾气充足，固摄有力，才能保证胎儿的健康成长，稳固发育，不得乱动。故《素问•上古天真论》曰："女子二七，天癸至，任脉通，太冲脉盛，月事以时下，故有子。"肾气虚衰，则会出现胎元不固，胎动不安的病机变化。若肾气不足，摄纳功能衰减，冲任不固，胎失所系，则会引起胎动不安，早产堕胎，或屡有滑胎，引起习惯性流产; 肾气不足，推动乏力，精血不能充养胚胎，胎儿生长发育障碍，则胎萎不长，胎音微弱，发育不良; 肾气虚弱，不能统摄血液，则胎漏下血见红; 肾气不足，腰府失养，则腰酸腹坠。肾气虚衰，则舌淡，苔白，尺脉不足。如《傅青主女科•妊娠吐泻腹痛》曰："然胞胎疼痛而究不至下坠者，何也?全赖肾气之固也。胞胎系于肾而连于心，肾气固则交于心，其气通于胞胎，此胞胎之所以欲坠而不得也。且肾气能固，则阴火必来生脾，心气能通，则心火必来援胃; 脾胃虽虚而未绝，则胞胎虽动而不堕。"指出肾气充足，则胎固而不动，从而反证了肾气虚弱，胎气不固，可引起胎动不安。《中医妇科学•滑胎》也云："先天禀赋不足，肾气未充; 或因孕后房事不节，纵欲所伤，以致肾气亏虚，冲任不固，胎失所系，而致屡孕屡堕为滑胎。"明确指出肾气虚衰，可致胎动不安的病机。治法宜固肾安胎。方药选用《医学衷中参西录》寿胎丸（菟丝子、桑寄生、川续断、阿胶），或选《中医妇科学》补肾固冲丸（菟丝子、续断、巴戟天、杜仲、当归、熟地、鹿角霜、枸杞子、阿胶、党参、白术、大枣、砂仁）。

Literature Review of Stirring Fetus

📖 *Jǐng Yuè Quán Shū* ("Jǐng-Yuè's Complete Compendium"), "Regular Patterns of Women: Repeated Abortion"

> "Whenever you see repeated miscarriage in pregnancy, this must be related to a depletion of qì in the vessels. The reason for this depletion can lie in being endowed with constitutional weakness, in age-related debilitation of strength… or in lack of caution in sexual desires and resulting detriment of vital qì… All these can damage the qì vessels."

The kidney is the root of earlier heaven. The completion and securing of earlier heaven refers to an abundance of kidney qì, and insufficiency of earlier heaven thus means depletion of kidney qì. This quotation therefore indicates the pathomechanism by which kidney qì depletion and damage to qì in its channels can lead to recurrent miscarriage.

📖 *Fù Qīng Zhǔ Nǚ Kē* ("Fù Qīng-Zhǔ's Gynecology"), "Precipitation of Blood in Urine during Pregnancy, Termed Fetal Spotting"

> "When a pregnant woman presents with no stirring fetus or abdominal pain, but with frequent blood running out during urination, people assume that this is blood vacuity fetal spotting. Who is aware that this indicates that qì is vacuous and unable to contain blood! Blood is only able to protect and nurture the fetus, and the protecting and nurturing blood within the fetus must rely on qì to balance it. When qì is vacuous and falls downward, the blood nurturing the fetus will follow qì and also fall. When qì is vacuous and falls downward, but blood is not vacuous, it seems that it should not fall together with qì.
>
> "People are not aware that qì is the defense of blood and that blood depends on qì to be secure. When qì is vacuous, blood lacks its base, and without a base, there is restlessness… As a result of stirring, it is discharged and cannot be held back by anything. How could it not flow downward! If, on the other hand, qì is not vacuous, but blood is hot, this must result in great flooding, which is not limited to just slight spotting. The appropriate method of treatment is to supplement the insufficiency of qì and discharge the superabundance of fire. As a result, the bleeding does not have to be checked, but will invariably stop on its own."

This is a penetrating and thorough analysis of the pathomechanism by which qì vacuity (most importantly kidney qì vacuity), inability to contain blood, and blood falling with qì results in fetal spotting and bleeding.

文献评述

《景岳全书•妇人规•数堕胎》曰："凡妊娠之数见堕胎者，必以气脉亏损而然。而亏损之由，有禀质之素弱者，有年力之衰残者，…有色欲不慎而盗损其生气者，…皆能伤其气脉，气脉有伤而胎可无恙者，非先天之最完固者不能，而常人未之有也。"肾为先天之本，先天完固，说明肾气充足，先天不足，即肾气亏损。指出肾气亏损，伤其气脉，可致反复堕胎的病机。

《傅青主女科•妊娠小便下血病名胎漏》曰："妊妇有胎不动腹不疼，而小便中时常有血流出者，人以为血虚胎漏也，谁知气虚不能摄血乎！夫血只能荫胎，而胎中之荫血，必赖气以衡之，气虚下陷，则荫胎之血亦随气而陷矣。然则气虚下陷，而血未尝虚，似不应与气同陷也。不知气乃血之卫，血赖气以固，气虚则血无凭依，无凭依必躁急。...动则外出而莫能遏，又安得不下流乎！倘气不虚而血热，则必大崩，而不止些微之漏矣。治法宜补其气之不足，而泄其火之有余，则血不必止而自无不止。"对气虚（主要为肾气虚）不能摄血，血随气陷，导致胎漏出血的病机变化进行了深入详尽的分析.

Summary of Stirring Fetus

1. Insecurity of Kidney Qì

   Stirring fetus, premature delivery and miscarriage, possibly habitual miscarriage.

2. Kidney Qì Deprived of Nourishment

   Atrophied fetus, shaded fetus, fetal feebleness, poor fetal development.

3. Kidney Qì Failing to Contain

   Fetal spotting and the appearance of red vaginal discharge.

4. Lower Back Deprived of Nourishment

   Aching lower back and sagging abdomen.

5. Kidney Qì Debilitation

   Pale tongue, white tongue fur, insufficient cubit pulse.

胎动不安

肾气不固—胎动不安，早产堕胎，或屡有滑胎，引起习惯性流产

肾气失养—胎萎不长，胎音微弱，发育不良。

肾气失收—胎漏下血见红

腰府失养—腰酸腹坠

肾气虚衰—舌淡，苔白，尺脉不足

Chapter Three

Kidney Yīn Depletion

Kidney yīn is the root of the entire body's yīn humor and has the function of nourishing and moistening the viscera, bowels, and organs throughout the body. Kidney yīn and kidney yáng depend on each other for their existence, growth, and decline. By adopting and preserving the state of calm yīn and sound yáng, they maintain the normal physiological functions of the body. Weakening of the body in old age, damage to yīn from enduring disease, excessive sexual taxation, damage to yīn from heat disease, taking acrid or dry yīn-despoiling substances for a long time, or damage to yīn humor in any of the viscera that over time affects kidney yīn can all lead to the pathomechanism of kidney yīn debilitation.

The *Nèi Jīng* ("The Inner Canon") contains quite a few references to kidney yīn vacuity, such as in the "Treatise on Reversal" in the *Sù Wèn* ("Plain Questions"): "Debilitation of yīn qì in the lower body results in heat vexation." The "Treatise on Wilting" in the same text states: "The kidney is the water viscus. Water failing to overcome fire results in desiccation of the bone and vacuity of the marrow. Therefore, the legs fail to support the body and bone wilting occurs." The "Great Treatise on the Correspondences and Manifestations of Yīn and Yáng" in the same text further states: "At the age of forty, yīn qì is halved and general debilitation sets in." These quotations describe the pathomechanism of natural debilitation of kidney yīn in old age.

In the Yuán period, Zhū Dān-Xī pointed out in the *Gé Zhì Yú Lùn* ("Further Treatises on the Properties of Things") that "yáng is often in superabundance, and yīn is often insufficient." This alerted people that they should clear the heart and have few desires during ordinary times to safeguard yīn essence, and that it is even more important during times of illness to protect yīn qì and focus on enriching yīn and downbearing fire.

During the Míng dynasty, kidney yīn vacuity was further elucidated in terms of its disease causes, pathomechanisms, symptoms, and manifestations. For example, the "Schema of Miscellaneous Patterns; Fire Patterns" in the *Jǐng Yuè Quán Shū* ("Jǐng-Yuè's Complete Compendium") explained: "Yīn vacuity can cause heat effusion. This is because true yīn depletion means that water fails to restrain fire." The chapter, "Sleeplessness" in the same text further explained: "When true yīn and essence-blood are insufficient, yīn and yáng fail to intermingle, and the spirit is disquieted in its chamber." These quotations describe the pathomechanisms of yīn vacuity heat effusion and yīn vacuity sleeplessness.

The "Treatise on True Yīn" in the "Record on Seeking Rightness" in the *Lèi Jīng Fù Yì* ("Wings to the Classified Canon") states:

> "*Yòu guī wán* (Right-Restoring [Life Gate] Pill) treats insufficiency of true yīn kidney water, [which causes] failure to enrich and moisten construction and defense. This gradually leads to debilitating emaciation, intermittent vacuity heat and spontaneous and night sweating, failure of the spirit to keep to its abode and of blood to return to its origin, taxation detriment damaging yīn, urinary incontinence, qì vacuity clouding and dizziness, flowery vision and deafness, dry mouth and tongue, or aching lower back and limp legs. All patterns of internal exhaustion of essence and marrow and of desiccated fluids must quickly be treated by strengthening water to bank up original yīn of the left kidney. This formula governs it."

This quotation describes in detail the pathomechanical changes and treatment principles of kidney yīn vacuity.

The Qīng period witnessed a further development in knowledge about the disease causes and pathomechanisms of kidney yīn vacuity patterns, bringing it more nearly to completion. For example, in the "Kidney Section" of the *Bǐ Huā Yī Jìng* ("Bǐ-Huā's Medical Mirror"), Jiāng Hán-Tūn stated:

> "Heat in the kidney means that water is desiccated. This is included in the entry on cold damage and is rarely seen among discussions of miscellaneous pathoconditions. The pulse at the left and right cubit positions is invariably sunken and rapid, or floating and vacuous, and the tongue is black and without fluid. Its symptoms include dry mouth and throat, dim vision, inhibited urination, turbid urine, discharge of blood in the urine, and constipation."

In the chapter, "Vacuity Detriment Consumption" in the *Yī Biǎn* ("Lancing Stones of Medicine"), Hé Mèng-Yáo stated:

> "Regarding damage to any of the five viscera, damage to the kidney is the most severe. Kidney vacuity results in steaming bone tidal heat,

> tidal heat after noon or midnight, spontaneous and night sweating, emaciation, dry mouth and throat, hoarse voice, dispersion thirst and strangury-turbidity, seminal emission and blood loss, irascibility, dry cough with phlegm, sleeplessness with vexation and agitation, and abstraction and fearful throbbing. All these are caused by water vacuity and fire flaming."

Insufficiency of kidney yīn can thus manifest in a range of pathomechanical changes related to loss of nourishment in the viscera, bowels, and organs, which are caused by insufficiency of yīn humor. It is also possible that yīn-yáng disharmony manifests in yīn vacuity and yáng hyperactivity and internal engenderment of vacuity heat.

For this reason, kidney yīn depletion can manifest concretely in eight types of pathomechanisms: yīn liquid deprived of enrichment; sea of marrow deprived of nourishment; loss of acuity in the ears; insecurity of yīn essence; vacuity-related sexual hyperactivity; internal engenderment of vacuity heat; vacuity fire floating upward; and yīn vacuity heat vexation.

肾阴亏损

肾阴为全身阴液之根本，有滋养、濡润全身脏腑器官的作用，和肾阳相互依存，相互消长，通过保持阴平阳秘的功能状态，从而维持人体的正常生命活动。如因年老体弱，或久病伤阴，或房劳过度，或热病伤阴，或久服辛燥劫阴之品，或各脏阴液耗伤，久及肾阴等，均可导致肾阴虚衰的病机变化。《内经》有不少关于肾阴虚的描述，如《素问•厥论》曰："阴气衰于下，则为热烦。"《素问•痿论》曰："肾者，水脏也。今水不胜火，则骨枯而髓虚，故足不任身，发为骨痿。"《素问•阴阳应象大论》又曰："年四十而阴气自半也，起居衰矣。"对年老而肾阴自然虚衰的病机变化进行了描述。元代朱丹溪《格致余论》提出"阳常有余，阴常不足"论，提醒人们平时要清心寡欲，以保阴精，病时更要维护阴气，重视滋阴降火。明代对肾阴虚的病因病机、症状表现等方面有进一步阐发，如《景岳全书•杂证谟•火证》说："阴虚者能发热，此以真阴亏损，水不制火也。"《景岳全书•杂证谟•不寐》又说："真阴精血之不足，阴阳不交，而神有不安其室耳。"描述了阴虚发热，阴虚不寐的病机。《类经附翼•求正录•真阴论》曰："左归丸治真阴肾水不足，不能滋溉营卫，渐至衰羸，或虚热往来，自汗盗汗，或神不守舍，血不归原，或劳损伤阴，或遗淋不禁，或气虚昏晕，或眼花耳聋，或口燥舌干，或腰酸腿软。凡精髓内竭，津液枯涸等证，俱速宜壮水之主，以培左肾之元阴，此方主之。”详细论述了肾阴虚的各种病机变化及治疗原则。清代对肾阴虚证的病因病机的认识有了进一步的发展，使之趋于完善。如江涵暾《笔花医镜•肾部》曰：“肾之热，水将涸也。伤寒门有之，而杂症罕见，左尺右尺必沉数，或浮而空，舌黑无液，其症为口燥咽干，为目不明，为小便不利，为小便浊，为小便出血，为大便秘。”何梦瑶《医碥•虚损痨瘵》曰：“五脏之伤，肾为最重，肾虚则骨蒸潮热，或午后或子后潮热，自汗盗汗，形体消瘦，口干咽燥，声嘶音哑，消渴淋浊，遗精失血，易生嗔怒，干咳痰嗽，不眠烦躁，恍惚怔忡，皆水虚火炎所致。”肾阴不足，既可表现为因阴液不足而导致脏腑器官失去滋养的一系列病机变化；也可因阴阳失调而出现阴虚阳亢、虚热内生等病机改变。因此，肾阴亏损可具体表现为阴津失滋、髓海失养、耳窍失聪、阴精不固、生殖虚亢、虚热内生、虚火上浮、阴虚烦热等八种病机类型。

3.1 Yīn Liquid Deprived of Enrichment

Kidney yīn, which is also called original yīn or true yīn, is the root of yīn humor in the body and has the function of nourishing and moistening the viscera, bowels, tissues, and organs. In addition, kidney yīn is able to restrict yáng qì within the kidney and prevent kidney yáng from stirring too frenetically. Insufficiency of kidney yīn can lead to fluid depletion in the organism and to inability to nourish the four limbs and hundred bones. This can manifest in the pathomechanism of yīn liquid deprived of enrichment.

When kidney yīn is insufficient, the lower back and knees are deprived of nourishment and their functions are weakened. This causes limp and feeble aching lower back and knees.

Depletion of kidney yīn causes insufficiency of the fluids, preventing them from ascending and enriching the head and eyes and from moistening the orifices. The result is dizzy head and vision, dry mouth and throat, tinnitus, and deafness.

When kidney yīn is so depleted that yīn fails to restrain yáng, vacuity heat arises internally. This causes low-grade fever and vacuity taxation, reddening of the cheeks and night sweating, and possibly steaming bone tidal heat or heat in the palms and soles.

When yīn humor is depleted it is unable to descend and enrich stool and urine. The result is short voidings of scant urine and dry bound stool.

Kidney yīn vacuity results in a red tongue with scant fur and a fine rapid pulse.

The chapter, "Supplementing Arrays" in the *Jǐng Yuè Quán Shū* ("Jǐng-Yuè's Complete Compendium"), "Eight Tactical Arrays in the New Formularies" succinctly points out:

> "*Yòu guī wán* (Right-Restoring [Life Gate] Pill) treats insufficiency of true yīn kidney water, [which causes] failure to enrich and moisten construction and defense. This [condition] gradually leads to debilitation, possibly intermittent vacuity heat with spontaneous and night sweating, or failure of the spirit to keep to its abode and of blood to return to its origin, taxation detriment damaging yīn, urinary incontinence, qì vacuity clouding and dizziness, flowery vision and deafness, dry mouth and tongue, or aching lower back and limp legs. All patterns of internal depletion of essence and marrow and of desiccated fluids must quickly be treated by strengthening water to bank up original yīn of the left kidney. As a result, essence-blood will naturally become abundant. This formula is suitable for governing it."

This quotation includes a detailed discussion of the pathomechanical changes of yīn liquid deprived of enrichment and loss of luxuriance in construction, defense, and the viscera, all of which result from kidney yīn depletion.

The *Yīn Xū Zhèng Zhì* ("Yīn Vacuity Patterns and Treatment), "Treatment of Kidney-Related Yīn Vacuity Patters; Lumbar Pain" states:

> "Constitutional insufficiency and habitual depletion of kidney essence, failure to nourish later heaven and enrich earlier heaven, general vacuity after enduring illness that reduces kidney yīn, collapse of liquid and loss of blood that consumes kidney yīn, indulging in affects and desires that exhaust yīn essence, and depletion of essence-blood in the elderly can all lead to insufficiency of yīn essence in the kidney, impaired nourishment in the lumbar spine, and erupting pain."

This quotation directly discusses the pathomechanism by which kidney yīn depletion can lead to limp aching lower back and knees.

Yīn liquid deprived of enrichment is treated by enriching and nourishing kidney yīn. Recommended formulas are *liù wèi dì huáng wán* (Six-Ingredient Rehmannia Pill) from the *Xiǎo Ér Yào Zhèng Zhí Jué* ("Key to Diagnosis and Treatment of Children's Diseases") or *zuǒ guī yǐn* (Left-Restoring [Kidney Yīn] Beverage) from the *Jǐng Yuè Quán Shū* ("Jǐng-Yuè's Complete Compendium").

Liù Wèi Dì Huáng Wán 六味地黄丸 Six-Ingredient Rehmannia Pill
dà huáng (大黄 Rhei Radix et Rhizoma, rhubarb)
shān zhū yú (山茱萸 Corni Fructus, cornus)
shān yào (山药 Dioscoreae Rhizoma, dioscorea)
zé xiè (泽泻 Alismatis Rhizoma, alisma)
mǔ dān pí (牡丹皮 Moutan Cortex, moutan)
fú líng (茯苓 Poria, poria)

Zuǒ Guī Yǐn 左归饮 Left-Restoring [Kidney Yīn] Beverage
shú dì huáng (熟地黄 Rehmanniae Radix Praeparata, cooked rehmannia)
shān yào (山药 Dioscoreae Rhizoma, dioscorea)
gǒu qǐ zǐ (枸杞子 Lycii Fructus, lycium)
fú líng (茯苓 Poria, poria)
shān zhū yú (山茱萸 Corni Fructus, cornus)
zhì gān cǎo (炙甘草 Glycyrrhizae Radix cum Liquido Fricta, mix-fried licorice)

阴津失滋

肾阴，又称元阴，真阴，为人体阴液之根本，对脏腑组织器官起着滋养、滋润的作用。此外肾阴能够制约肾中阳气，防止肾阳过亢妄动。肾阴不足，引起机体津液亏虚，不能滋养四肢百骸，则会出现阴津失滋的病机变化。肾阴不足，腰膝失养，功能减弱，故腰膝酸软无力; 肾阴亏虚，津液不足，不能上滋头目，官窍失濡，则头晕目眩，口燥咽干，耳鸣耳聋; 肾阴亏虚，阴不制阳，虚热内生，故低热虚烦，颧红盗汗，或骨蒸潮热，或手足心热; 阴液亏损，不能下滋二便，则小便短少，大便干结。肾阴虚亏，则舌红苔少，脉细数。如《景岳全书•新方八阵•补阵》明确指出："左归丸，治真阴肾水不足，不能滋养营卫，渐至衰弱，或虚热往来，自汗盗汗，或神不守舍，血不归原，或虚损伤阴，或遗淋不禁，或气虚昏运，或眼花耳聋，或口燥舌干，或腰酸腿软，凡精髓内亏，津液枯涸等证，俱速宜壮水之主，以培左肾之元阴，而精血自充矣，宜此方主之。"虽明言方药，实际却对肾阴亏损导致阴津失滋，营卫脏器不荣的多种病机变化进行了详细地论述。《阴虚证治•肾系阴虚证治•腰痛》云："禀赋不足，肾精素亏，或后天失于调养，先天失于充滋，或久病体虚，损及肾阴，或亡津失血，耗损肾阴，或恣情纵欲，耗竭阴精，或年老之人，精血亏虚，皆可以导致肾的阴精不足，腰脊失养，发生疼痛。"直接论述肾阴亏损可致腰膝酸软的病机。治法宜滋养肾阴。方药选用《小儿药证直诀》六味地黄丸（地黄、山茱萸、怀山药、泽泻、丹皮、茯苓），或选《景岳全书》左归饮（熟地黄、怀山药、枸杞子、茯苓，山茱萸、炙甘草）。

Literature Review of Yīn Liquid Deprived of Enrichment

🕮 *Jǐng Yuè Quán Shū* ("Jǐng-Yuè's Complete Compendium"), "Schema of Miscellaneous Patterns: Lumbar Pain"

> "Eight or nine out of ten cases of lumbar pain are vacuity patterns. If inspection reveals no exterior evil and furthermore no damp-heat, and the condition is caused by age-related debilitation, taxation and hardship, loss due to sensual pursuits, or a depressed state of mind, then you know that it is a pattern of vacuity of true yīn."

Since true yīn is the same as kidney yīn, this quotation explains how vacuity of kidney yīn and loss of enrichment in the lower back can lead to lumbar pain.

🕮 *Shòu Shì Bǎo Yuán* ("Prolonging Life and Preserving the Origin"), "Vacuity Vexation"

> "Vacuity vexation is in most people caused by yīn vacuity engendering internal heat. In patients with vacuity taxation, kidney water is depleted and heart fire steams internally. Thus they invariably suffer from vexation and agitation."

This quotation clarifies how kidney yīn vacuity, failure of yīn to restrain yáng, and internal engenderment of vacuity heat can lead to vacuity vexation.

文献评述

《景岳全书•杂证谟•腰痛》曰："腰痛之虚证十居八九，但察其既无表邪，又无湿热，而年事以衰，或以劳苦，或以酒色斩丧，或心情忧郁所致者，则悉属真阴虚证。"真阴即肾阴，说明肾阴虚，腰府失滋，可致腰痛。

《寿世保元•虚烦》曰："令人虚烦，多是阴虚生内热所致。虚劳之人，肾水有亏，心火内蒸，其烦必躁。"阐明了肾阴虚，阴不制阳，虚热内生，可致虚烦的病机变化。

Summary of Yīn Liquid Deprived of Enrichment
1. Loss of Enrichment in the Lower Back and Knees Limp and feeble aching lower back and knees. 2. Loss of Enrichment in the Head and Eyes Dizzy head and vision, dry mouth and throat, tinnitus and deafness. 3. Yīn Vacuity Internal Heat Low-grade fever and vacuity vexation, reddening of the cheeks and night sweating, possibly steaming bone tidal heat or heat in the palms and soles. 4. Loss of Enrichment to Urine and Stool Short voidings of scant urine, dry bound stool. 5. Kidney Yīn Depletion Red tongue with scant fur, fine rapid pulse.
阴津失滋
腰膝失滋—腰膝酸软无力 头目失滋—头晕目眩，口燥咽干，耳鸣耳聋 阴虚内热—低热虚烦，颧红盗汗，或骨蒸潮热，或手足心热 二便失滋—小便短少，大便干结 肾阴虚亏—舌红苔少，脉细数

3.2 Sea of Marrow Deprived of Nourishment

The kidney stores true yīn and essence-blood. It governs the bones, engenders marrow, and penetrates to the brain. Lack of kidney yīn results in a reduction of essence-blood, which in turn deprives the bones, marrow, and brain of nourishment. This forms the pathomechanism of kidney yīn insufficiency and sea of marrow deprived of nourishment.

Already in the Spring and Autumn period (770-476 BCE), physicians were acutely aware of the physiological and pathological relationship of kidney yīn with essence and marrow. For example, the chapter, "The

Five Dribbling Urinary Stoppages and the Differences Between Liquid and Humor" in the *Líng Shū* ("The Magic Pivot"), states:

> "The essence of the five grains combines with humor and forms a paste. This internally percolates into the empty spaces of the bones, supplements and boosts brain marrow, and flows down into the inguinal region. When yīn and yáng are not harmonious, humor spills and flows downward into the genitals, and marrow and humor are both reduced and descend. If they descend beyond their normal limit, this results in vacuity, which in turn causes lumbar and back pain and lower leg ache."

This quotation expounds clearly how the subtle essences of the five grains that are engendered by the spleen and stomach transform into yīn essence in the kidney, percolate into the bones, and nourish the marrow and brain.

When yīn humor is insufficient and the sea of marrow is deprived of nourishment, this can lead to limp aching lower back and knees.

Numerous pathogenic factors like debility in old age, warm-heat scorching liquid, lack of or inappropriate treatment, or damage to yīn from enduring illness all cause insufficiency of kidney yīn true water. As a result, the fluids dry up, yīn vacuity affects essence, essence fails to engender marrow, and essence and marrow are internally exhausted. This manifests in the pathomechanical changes of essence and marrow deprived of nourishment.

When kidney yīn is depleted, yīn fails to transform essence, essence fails to engender marrow, and marrow fails to nourish the brain. The result is forgetfulness and reduced sleep, dizzy head, flowery vision, and deafness.

Insufficiency of kidney yīn causes lack of yīn essence and failure to enrich the marrow of the bones and the lower back and knees. The result is weak wilting useless lower limbs, limp and feeble aching lower back and knees, and marked emaciation of the body.

When kidney yīn is insufficient, it is unable to ascend and nourish heart yīn. The heart and kidney fail to interact, heart fire becomes abnormally hyperactive and harasses the heart spirit, and the spirit fails to keep to its abode. As a result, the heart spirit is without governance.

Insufficiency of kidney yīn prevents liquid from bearing upward. This results in a dry mouth and tongue.

When vacuity heat arises internally, the result is coming and going vacuity heat, night sweating and reddening of the cheeks, and vexing heat in the five hearts.

Insufficiency of kidney yīn results in a red tongue with scant fur and a fine rapid pulse.

The chapter, "Vacuity Detriment" in the *Jǐng Yuè Quán Shū* ("Jǐng-Yuè's Complete Compendium") states: "Vacuity of essence is identical with yīn vacuity. All cases of fire exuberance and water depletion, when construction, defense, and fluids are dessicated, are yīn vacuity patterns." This quotation discusses precisely the pathomechanical transformation and progression from yīn vacuity to essence vacuity.

The treatise, "On Wilting" in the *Sù Wèn* ("Plain Questions") further states: "The kidney is the water viscus. Water failing to overcome fire results in desiccation of the bone and vacuity of marrow. Therefore, the legs fail to support the body, and bone wilting occurs." This is an early description of the pathomechanism by which kidney yīn vacuity leads to emptiness of bone marrow.

Sea of marrow deprived of nourishment is treated by strengthening water and enriching yīn, and by supplementing essence and replenishing marrow. Recommended formulas are *yòu guī wán* (Right-Restoring [Life Gate] Pill) from the *Jǐng Yuè Quán Shū* ("Jǐng-Yuè's Complete Compendium") or *zī yīn bǔ suǐ tāng* (Enrich Yin and Supplement Marrow Decoction) from the *Yī Chún Shèng Yì* ("Enriching the Meaning of the Wine of Medicine") without *zhī mǔ* (Anemarrhenae Rhizoma) and *huáng bǎi* (Phellodendri Cortex), but with *mò hàn lián* (Ecliptae Herba) and *nǚ zhēn zǐ* (Ligustri Lucidi Fructus).

Yòu Guī Wán 左归丸
Right-Restoring [Life Gate] Pill

shú dì huáng (熟地黄 Rehmanniae Radix Praeparata, cooked rehmannia)
shān yào (山药 Dioscoreae Rhizoma, dioscorea)
shān zhū yú (山茱萸 Corni Fructus, cornus)
guī bǎn (龟版 Testudinis Plastrum, tortoise plastron)
niú xī (牛膝 Achyranthis Bidentatae Radix, achyranthes)
tù sī zǐ (菟丝子 Cuscutae Semen, cuscuta)
gǒu qǐ zǐ (枸杞子 Lycii Fructus, lycium)
lù jiǎo jiāo (鹿角胶 Cervi Cornus Gelatinum, deerhorn glue)

Zī Yīn Bǔ Suǐ Tāng 滋阴补髓汤
Enrich Yin and Supplement Marrow Decoction

shēng dì huáng (生地黄 Rehmanniae Radix, rehmannia)
guī bǎn (龟版 Testudinis Plastrum, tortoise plastron)
huáng bǎi (黄柏 Phellodendri Cortex, phellodendron)
zhī mǔ (知母 Anemarrhenae Rhizoma, anemarrhena)
hǔ jìng gǔ (虎胫骨 Tigris Patella, tiger's kneecap)
gǒu qǐ zǐ (枸杞子 Lycii Fructus, lycium)
dāng guī (当归 Angelicae Sinensis Radix, Chinese angelica)
dǎng shēn (党参 Codonopsis Radix, codonopsis)
fú líng (茯苓 Poria, poria)
jīn máo gǒu jǐ (金毛狗脊 Cibotii Rhizoma, cibotium)
bái zhú (白术 Atractylodis Macrocephalae Rhizoma, white atractylodes)
xù duàn (续断 Dipsaci Radix, dipsacus)
niú xī (牛膝 Achyranthis Bidentatae Radix, achyranthes)
zhū jǐ suǐ (猪脊髓 Suis Spinae Medulla, pig's spine marrow)
huáng bǎi (黄柏 Phellodendri Cortex, phellodendron)

Plus:
mò hàn lián (墨旱莲 Ecliptae Herba, eclipta)
nǚ zhēn zǐ (女贞子 Ligustri Lucidi Fructus, ligustrum)

髓海失养

肾藏真阴，蕴藏精血，肾主骨生髓通于脑，肾阴缺乏，精血随之减少，对骨髓脑府的滋养就会减弱，形成肾阴不足，髓海失养的病机。早在春秋时期，医家就对肾阴与精髓的生理病理关系有了较深刻的认识。如《灵枢•五癃津液》曰："五谷之精液和合而为膏者，内渗入于骨空，补益脑髓，而下流于阴股。阴阳不和，则使液溢而下流于阴，髓液皆减而下，下过度则虚，虚故腰背痛而胫酸。"明确阐述，脾胃化生的五谷之精微，可转化为肾中阴精，渗入骨中，滋养髓脑。阴液不足，髓海失养，可致腰膝酸软。若年老虚衰，温热灼津，失治误治，久病伤阴等多种因素均导致肾阴真水不足，津液枯槁，阴虚及精，精不生髓，精髓内竭，出现精髓失养的病机变化。肾阴亏虚，阴不化精，精不生髓，髓不养脑，则健忘少寐，头晕、眼花、耳聋；肾阴不足，阴精缺乏，不能滋养骨髓、腰膝，则下肢痿弱不用，腰脊酸软无力，身体羸瘦；肾阴不足，不能上养心阴，心肾不交，心火偏亢，扰乱心神，神不守舍，则心神无主；肾阴不足，津不上承，则口燥舌干；虚热内生，则虚热往来，盗汗颧红，五心烦热。肾阴不足，则舌红少苔，脉细数。如《景岳全书•虚损》曰："精虚者，即阴虚也。凡病有火盛水亏，而见营卫燥津液枯者，即阴虚之证也。"明确论述了阴虚与精虚之间的病机转化过程。又如《素问•痿论》曰："肾者，水脏也。今水不胜火，则骨枯而髓虚，故足不任身，发为骨痿。"较早地论述了肾阴虚而致骨髓空虚的病机变化。治法宜壮水滋阴，益精填髓。方药用《景岳全书》之左归丸（大怀熟地，怀山药、山萸肉、龟板胶、川牛膝、菟丝子、枸杞子、鹿角胶），或选《医醇剩义》滋阴补髓汤（生地、龟板、黄柏、知母、虎胫骨、枸杞子、当归、党参、茯苓、金毛狗脊、白术、川断、牛膝、猪脊髓）去知母、黄柏加旱莲草、女贞子。

Literature Review of Sea of Marrow Deprived of Nourishment

📖 *Jǐng Yuè Quán Shū* ("Jǐng-Yuè's Complete Compendium"), "Schema of Miscellaneous Patterns: Vacuity Detriment"

> "Bone pain as if breaking means vanquishing of true yīn, since the kidney governs the bones."

The kidney governs the bones and stores true yīn. When kidney yīn is insufficient, essence-marrow is depleted and unable to nourish the bones. Therefore, it manifests in such pathological changes as skeletal pain as if breaking and aching lower back and limp legs.

📖 *Zhèng Yīn Mài Zhì* ("Pathoconditions: Causes, Pulses, and Treatments"), "Internal Damage Lumbar Pain"

> "When true water is insufficient, and furthermore yīn essence reduced, kidney vacuity and effulgent fire results in lumbar pain."

This quotation explains that insufficiency of true water, which is identical with kidney yīn depletion, can lead to insufficiency of yīn essence, sea of marrow deprived of nourishment, and aching lower back and knees.

文献评述

《景岳全书•杂证谟•虚损》曰："骨痛如折者，肾主骨，真阴败竭也。"肾主骨，藏真阴，肾阴不足，精髓亏虚，不能养骨，故出现骨骼疼痛如折、腰酸腿软等病机变化。

《症因脉治•内伤腰痛》曰："真水不足，复损阴精，则肾虚火旺而腰痛。" 说明真水不足，即肾阴亏虚，可致阴精不足，髓海失养，引起腰膝酸痛。

Summary of Sea of Marrow Deprived of Nourishment

1. Brain Deprived of Nourishment

   Forgetfulness and reduced sleep, dizzy head, flowery vision, deafness.

2. Bone Marrow Deprived of Nourishment

   Weak wilting, useless lower limbs, limp feeble aching lumbar spine, marked emaciation of the body.

3. Essence Spirit Deprived of Nourishment

   Failure of the spirit to keep to its abode, heart spirit lacking governance.

4. Liquid Failing to Bear Upward

   Dry mouth and tongue.

5. Internally Arising Vacuity Heat

   Coming and going vacuity heat, night sweating and reddening of the cheeks, vexing heat in the five hearts.

6. Insufficiency of Kidney Yīn

   Red tongue with scant fur, fine rapid pulse.

髓海失养

脑府失养—健忘少寐，头晕，眼花，耳聋

骨髓失养—下肢痿弱不用，腰脊酸软无力，身体羸瘦

精神失养—神不守舍，心神无主

津不上承—口燥舌干

虚热内生—虚热往来，盗汗颧红，五心烦热

肾阴不足—舌红少苔，脉细数

3.3 Loss of Acuity in the Ears

The ears are the upper orifice of the kidney, and are governed by the foot lesser yīn kidney channel. The kidney stores essence, which engenders marrow. The brain is the sea of marrow, and the ears penetrate to the brain. As long as kidney yīn engenders essence and this ascends to nourish the ears, both ears are acute and sharp and therefore able to identify sounds.

The "Great Treatise on the Correspondences and Manifestations of Yīn and Yáng" in the *Sù Wèn* ("Plain Questions") states: "The northern direction engenders cold, and is associated with the kidney among the viscera, and with the ears among the orifices." The chapter, "Outward Manifestations and Diseases Caused by the Five Viscera" in the *Líng Shū* ("The Magic Pivot") also states: "The ears are the office of the kidney."

Kidney essence is yīn and depends on being converted, enriched, and engendered from kidney yīn. If kidney yīn is insufficient, essence fails to bear upward, and the ears lose their acuity and become unable to hear and identify sounds. As a result, loss of hearing acuity can occur.

When kidney yīn is insufficient, yīn essence is deprived of enrichment, the sea of marrow loses its fullness, and the head, eyes, and ears are deprived of nourishment. Alternatively, insufficiency of kidney yīn can cause ministerial fire to ascend and harass the ears. Either situation results in ringing in the ears as if from cicadas or from tidal waves, or deafness and complete lack of hearing, as well as in dizzy head and vision.

The lower back is the house of the kidney. When kidney yīn is depleted, the lower back is deprived of enrichment. This results in limp aching lower back and knees.

Yīn vacuity engenders internal heat, and when vacuity heat harasses internally, the result is vacuity vexation and insomnia, vexing heat in the five hearts, and tidal heat and night sweating.

When vacuity heat flames upward and deprives yīn liquid of enrichment, the result is dry mouth and throat, dizzy head, and dim vision.

Yīn vacuity and loss of enrichment results in a red tongue with scant fur, and a fine and weak or rapid pulse.

The chapter, "Diseases of the Ear" in the *Jǐng Yuè Quán Shū* ("Jǐng-Yuè's Complete Compendium"), "Schema of Miscellaneous Patterns" points out:

> "When a person past middle age experiences increased ringing in the ears as if from wind or rain or from singing cicadas or from the sound of tidal waves, this always indicates yīn debilitation and kidney depletion. The classics say that yīn qì is halved at the age of forty. Halved precisely refers to debilitated."

This quotation describes how incessant tinnitus in elderly patients is caused by kidney yīn depletion.

Furthermore, the chapter, "Tinnitus and Deafness" in the *Yīn Xū Zhèng Zhì* ("Yīn Vacuity Patterns and Treatment) states:

> "In most cases [of tinnitus and deafness], essence has been depleted for a long time and kidney yīn is invariably vacuous. Consequently, wood is deprived of moistening and nourishment, and ministerial fire becomes abnormally exuberant and follows the channels to harass the upper body.
>
> "Alternatively, these conditions can arise because water is depleted and unable to assist fire, and vacuity fire harasses the inner body. Either of these can lead to tinnitus and deafness. Depletion of yīn essence manifests in ringing in the ears as if from cicadas, with a faint low sound that worsens gradually, and in severe cases in deafness. This is accompanied by dizzy head and vision, heart vexation and insomnia, seminal emission, dry mouth and throat, vexing heat in the five hearts, limp aching lower back and knees, a red tongue with scant fur, and a fine rapid pulse."

This quotation is a comprehensive summary and discussion of the pathomechanism and manifestations of tinnitus and deafness that result from kidney yīn depletion and loss of enrichment in the ears.

Loss of acuity in the ears is treated by enriching yīn and supplementing the kidney and by subduing yáng and sharpening the hearing. The recommended formula is *ěr lóng zuǒ cí wán* (Deafness Left-Benefiting Loadstone Pill) from the *Chòng Dìng Guǎng Wēn Rè Lùn* ("On Warm Heat: Revised and Expanded") with modifications.

Ěr Lóng Zuǒ Cí Wán 耳聋左慈丸
Deafness Left-Benefiting Loadstone Pill

shú dì huáng (熟地黄 Rehmanniae Radix Praeparata, cooked rehmannia)
shān zhū yú (山茱萸 Corni Fructus, cornus)
shān yào (山药 Dioscoreae Rhizoma, dioscorea)
mǔ dān pí (牡丹皮 Moutan Cortex, moutan)
zé xiè (泽泻 Alismatis Rhizoma, alisma)
fú líng (茯苓 Poria, poria)
cí shí (磁石 Magnetitum, loadstone)
shí chāng pú (石菖蒲 Acori Tatarinowii Rhizoma, acorus)
wǔ wèi zǐ (五味子 Schisandrae Fructus, schisandra)

耳窍失聪

耳为肾之上窍，由足少阴肾所主。肾藏精，精生髓，脑为髓海，两耳通脑，若肾阴生精上养耳窍，则两耳聪灵，能辨音识声。如《素问•阴阳应象大论》曰："北方生寒，在脏为肾，在窍为耳。"《灵枢•五阅五使》亦曰："耳者，肾之官也。"肾精属阴，有赖于肾阴之转化和滋生。如肾阴不足，精不上承，耳窍失养，不能听声辨音，则可出现耳窍失聪的病机变化。肾阴不足，阴精失滋，髓海失充，头目、耳窍失养，或肾阴不足，相火上扰耳窍，则为耳鸣如蝉如潮，或耳聋无所闻，头晕目眩; 腰为肾之府，肾阴亏虚，腰府失滋，则腰膝酸软; 阴虚生内热，虚热内扰，则虚烦不眠，五心烦热，潮热盗汗; 虚热炎上，阴津失滋，则口燥咽干，头晕目暗。阴虚失滋，则舌红少苔，脉细弱或细数。如《景岳全书•杂证谟•耳病》指出："人于中年之后，每多耳鸣，如风雨，如蝉鸣，如潮声者，是皆阴衰肾亏而然。经曰：人年四十而阴气自半。半，即衰之谓也。"对年老肾阴亏虚所致耳鸣不已的病机变化进行了阐述。又如《阴虚证治•耳鸣耳聋》曰："大凡精亏日久肾阴必虚，木失涵养，相火偏盛，循经上扰，或因水亏不得济火，虚火内扰，均可导致耳鸣、耳聋。阴精亏虚者，耳鸣如蝉，音低而微，逐渐加重，甚则耳聋，伴头晕目眩，心烦失眠，遗精，口咽发干，五心烦热，腰膝酸软，舌红少苔，脉细数。"对肾阴亏虚，耳窍失滋，引起耳鸣耳聋的病机及表现进行了全面的总结和论述。治法宜滋阴补肾，潜阳聪耳。方药选用《重订广温热论》耳聋左慈丸（熟地黄、山茱萸、怀山药、丹皮、泽泻、茯苓、磁石、石菖蒲、五味子）加减。

Literature Review of Loss of Acuity in the Ears

📖 *Dān Xī Xīn Fǎ* ("Dān Xī's Heart-Approach"), "Deafness"

> "In cases of deafness with yīn vacuity and fire surging, also use *sì wù tāng* (Four Agents Decoction)."

This quotation discusses the pathomechanical changes of deafness that results from the fact that yīn is vacuous and unable to engender essence-blood to nourish the ears, which leads to yīn vacuity fire becoming effulgent and harassing the ears.

📖 *Zá Bìng Yuán Liú Xī Zhú* ("Incisive Light on the Source of Miscellaneous Disease"), "The Origin and Development of Ear Disease"

> "The ears are ascribed to the foot lesser yīn channel and are the orifices entrusted to the kidney. What enables the ears to hear is essence, and when essential qì is harmonized and kidney qì is plentiful, the hearing is acute. But if taxation damages qì and blood, and wind evil exploits vacuity, this causes desertion of essence and exhaustion of the kidney. The result is deafness. This is the source of deafness…
>
> "*Liù wèi wán* (Six-Ingredient Pill) is suitable, with the addition of *zhī mǔ* (Anemarrhenae Rhizoma), *huáng bǎi* (Phellodendri Cortex), *yuǎn zhì* (Polygalae Radix), *shí chāng pú* (Acori Tatarinowii Rhizoma), all stir-fried with brine…
>
> "In cases of tinnitus from insufficiency of kidney essence and from yīn vacuity stirring fire, you must warm the kidney and boost essence. *Bǔ shèn wán* (Kidney-Supplementing Pill) or *zī shèn tōng ěr wán* (Kidney-Enriching Ear-Freeing Decoction) are suitable."

This quotation provides a clear review of the pathomechanism by which insufficiency of kidney yīn depletes kidney essence and prevents it from ascending to nourish the ears.

📖 *Zhōng Yī Lín Zhèng Bèi Yào* ("Essentials Clinical Patterns in Chinese Medicine"), "Ear Symptoms: Tinnitus"

> "Ringing in the ears as if from cicadas, from dashing water, or from bells and drums, are all subjective symptoms… This vacuity pattern is caused by yīn depletion and fire flaming, or from excessive use of the brain. This is what the *Nèi Jīng* ("The Inner Canon") refers to as 'insufficiency of the sea of marrow that results in spinning brain and ringing ears.' In most cases, it is accompanied by dizzy head and vision, heart palpitations, aching lower back, and a fine weak pulse."

This is a straightforward discussion of the manifestation of tinnitus and of the pathomechanism of yīn vacuity with loss of enrichment and ministerial fire harassing the orifices.

文献评述

《丹溪心法•耳聋》曰："阴虚火冲耳聋者，亦用四物汤"。对阴虚不能化生精血滋养耳窍，阴虚火旺，扰乱耳窍，引发耳聋的病机变化进行了论述。

《杂病源流犀烛•耳病源流》曰："耳属足少阴，肾之寄窍也。耳所致者精，精气调和，肾气充足，则耳聪。若劳伤气血，风邪乘虚，使精脱肾惫，则耳聋。是肾为耳聋之原也。…其由阴虚火动者别治，宜六味丸加知母、黄柏、远志、菖蒲，并盐水炒。…肾精不足，阴虚火动而鸣，须温肾益精，宜补肾丸、滋肾通耳丸。"清楚地分析了肾阴不足，肾精亏虚，不能上养耳窍的病机变化。

《中医临证备要•耳症状•耳鸣》曰："耳鸣如蝉噪，或如水激，或如钟鼓之声，均系自觉症状。…虚证由于阴亏火炎，或用脑过度，<内经>所谓'髓海不足则脑转耳鸣。'多伴有头晕目眩，心悸腰酸，脉象细弱。"清楚地论述了耳鸣的表现和阴虚失滋，相火扰窍的病机。

Summary of Loss of Acuity in the Ears

1. Orifices of the Head Deprived of Nourishment
   Ringing in the ears as if from cicadas or from tidal waves, or deafness and complete lack of hearing; dizzy head and vision.
2. Lower Back Deprived of Nourishment
   Limp aching lower back and knees.
3. Vacuity Heat Harassing Internally
   Vacuity vexation and insomnia, vexing heat in the five hearts, tidal heat and night sweating.
4. Vacuity Heat Flaming Upward
   Dry mouth and throat.
5. Yīn Vacuity and Loss of Enrichment
   Red tongue with scant fur, fine weak or rapid pulse.

耳窍失聪
头窍失养—耳鸣如蝉如潮，或耳聋无所闻，头晕目眩
腰府失养—腰膝酸软
虚热内扰—虚烦不眠，五心烦热，潮热盗汗
虚热炎上—口燥咽干
阴虚失滋—舌红少苔，脉细弱或细数

3.4 Insecurity of Yīn Essence

The kidney stores essential qì. It is only when yīn essence is sealed and yáng qì tightly secured that the kidney is able to supply the body's needs for growth and development. The kidney is the storehouse for fire and water, which implies kidney yīn and kidney yáng. Kidney yīn and kidney yáng convert into each other by growing and dispersing, and thereby maintain the balance of yīn and yáng in the body. If for any number of reasons kidney yīn is harmed, this is the onset of kidney yīn depletion and of yīn failing to transform essence. This can manifest in insufficiency of kidney essence. If kidney yīn depletion endures, the disease of yīn can affect yáng, progressing to the point of damaging kidney qì. When kidney qì is insufficient, securing and containing are without strength. As a result, the pathomechanism of insecurity of yīn essence arises.

The chapter, "The Spirit" in the *Líng Shū* ("The Magic Pivot") states: "The five viscera govern the storage of essence. Therefore, they may not be damaged. If they are damaged, they lose the ability to guard, and yīn becomes vacuous. Yīn vacuity results in lack of qì, and lack of qì results in death." This quotation offers an succinct summation of the pathomechanism by which yīn vacuity can lead to qì vacuity.

When kidney yīn depletion damages kidney qì, qì becomes vacuous, the essence gate is insecure, and yīn essence runs off. Alternatively, kidney yīn depletion can cause vacuity fire to stir frenetically and harass the essence chamber. This causes seminal efflux and premature ejaculation.

When kidney yīn is vacuous and unable to engender kidney qì, or when vacuity fire harasses and stirs, menstruation is insecure. This results in dribbling menstruation and clear thin menses as well as vaginal discharge.

When kidney yīn is depleted and kidney qì is vacuous, the bladder can become insecure. The result is incessant dribbling of urine.

When yīn essence is depleted, it is unable to ascend and nourish the head and eyes. The result is dizzy head and tinnitus.

Yīn vacuity and loss of nourishment can cause a reduction in organ functions. This results in fatigued and feeble spirit.

Depletion of kidney yīn results in a red tongue with scant fur, and a fine rapid pulse.

The chapter, "Vacuity Detriment" in the *Jǐng Yuè Quán Shū* ("Jǐng-Yuè's Complete Compendium"), "Schema of Miscellaneous Patterns" states:

> "If [vacuity detriment] is severe, it leads to symptoms such as cough with ejection of phlegm, seminal emission and night sweating, panting and loss of voice, sinew and bone pain, abstraction of the heart spirit, whittling of the flesh, dreaming of intercourse with ghosts, and menstrual block in women. Regardless of whether it is a yīn or a yáng pattern, when any disease reaches this extreme, the reason why it reaches this extreme is invariably found in vanquishing of true yīn."

Since true yīn is the same as kidney yīn, this quotation explains that insufficiency of kidney yīn can manifest in seminal emission.

The chapter, "Yīn Vacuity Vaginal Discharge" in the *Yīn Xū Zhèng Zhì* ("Yīn Vacuity Patterns and Treatment) states:

> "[Yīn vacuity vaginal discharge] is mostly caused by constitutional yīn vacuity, by the six excesses and seven affects transforming into fire and damaging yīn, by sexual intercourse, childbirth, and nursing consuming yīn essence, or by excessive consumption of warm and dry medicinals, which have dried out and damaged yīn liquid. Any of these may lead to depletion of kidney qì, frenetic stirring of the ministerial fire, yīn vacuity and failure to guard, and loss of security in the girdling vessel."

This quotation discusses the pathomechanism by which kidney yīn depletion and loss of security in the girdling vessel leads to vaginal discharge.

Insecurity of yīn essence is treated by enriching and supplementing qì and yīn, and by stemming desertion and checking emission. Recommended formulas are *gù yīn jiān* (Yīn-Securing Brew) from the *Jǐng Yuè Quán Shū* ("Jǐng-Yuè's Complete Compendium") or *jiā wèi liù wèi dì huáng tāng* (Supplemented Six-Ingredient Rehmannia Decoction) from the *Fù Kē Yù Chǐ* ("Jade Ruler of Gynecology").

Gù Yīn Jiān 固阴煎 Yīn-Securing Brew
rén shēn (人参 Ginseng Radix, ginseng)
shú dì huáng (熟地黄 Rehmanniae Radix Praeparata, cooked rehmannia)
shān yào (山药 Dioscoreae Rhizoma, dioscorea)
shān zhū yú (山茱萸 Corni Fructus, cornus)
yuǎn zhì (远志 Polygalae Radix, polygala)
zhì gān cǎo (炙甘草 Glycyrrhizae Radix cum Liquido Fricta, mix-fried licorice)
wǔ wèi zǐ (五味子 Schisandrae Fructus, schisandra)
tù sī zǐ (菟丝子 Cuscutae Semen, cuscuta)

Jiā Wèi Liù Wèi Dì Huáng Tāng 加味六味地黄汤 Supplemented Six-Ingredient Rehmannia Decoction
shēng dì huáng (生地黄 Rehmanniae Radix, rehmannia)
shān yào (山药 Dioscoreae Rhizoma, dioscorea)
shān zhū yú (山茱萸 Corni Fructus, cornus)
chē qián zǐ (车前子 Plantaginis Semen, plantago seed)
fú líng (茯苓 Poria, poria)
zé xiè (泽泻 Alismatis Rhizoma, alisma)
mǔ dān pí (牡丹皮 Moutan Cortex, moutan)
tù sī zǐ (菟丝子 Cuscutae Semen, cuscuta)
gǒu qǐ zǐ (枸杞子 Lycii Fructus, lycium)
huáng bǎi (黄柏 Phellodendri Cortex, phellodendron)
zhī mǔ (知母 Anemarrhenae Rhizoma, anemarrhena)

阴精不固

肾藏精气，阴精封藏，阳气固秘，才能保证人体生长发育的需要。肾为水火之藏，寓有肾阴肾阳，肾阴肾阳互相转化消长，以维持人体阴阳平衡。若各种原因导致肾阴损害，肾阴亏虚之初，阴不化精，可见肾精不足之病机变化，若肾阴久亏，阴病及阳，进而损伤肾气，肾气不足，固摄乏力，则出现阴精不固的病机变化。《灵枢•本神》曰："五脏主藏精者也，不可伤，伤则失守而阴虚，阴虚则无气，无气则死矣。"对阴虚可致气虚的病机变化进行了清晰的论述。

肾阴虚亏，损伤肾气，气虚精关不固，阴精流失，或肾阴亏虚，虚火妄动，扰乱精室，故见滑精早泄; 肾阴虚，不能化生肾气，或虚火扰动，经带不固，则月经淋漓，经带清稀; 肾阴亏，肾气虚，膀胱不固，则小便淋漓不尽; 阴精亏损，不能上养头目，则头晕耳鸣; 阴虚失养，脏腑功能减弱，则神疲乏力; 肾阴亏虚，则舌红少苔，脉细数。如《景岳全书•杂证谟•虚损》曰：“甚至咳嗽吐痰，遗精盗汗，气喘声喑，筋骨疼痛，心神恍惚，肌肉尽削，梦与鬼交，妇人月闭等证，则无论阴阳，凡病至极，皆所必至，总由真阴之败耳。”真阴即肾阴，说明肾阴不足，可出现遗精的病机改变。《阴虚证治•阴虚带下》曰：“多由素体阴虚，或六淫七情，化火伤阴，或房室产育，耗伤阴精，或过服温燥，燥伤阴津，以致肾阴亏虚，相火妄动，阴虚失守，带脉失固所致。”论述肾阴亏虚，带脉失固，引起带下的病机。治法宜滋补气阴，固脱止遗。方药选用《景岳全书》固阴煎（人参、熟地、山药、山萸肉、远志，炙甘草、五味子、菟丝子），或选《妇科玉尺》加味六味地黄汤（生地、山药、山茱萸、车前子、茯苓、泽泻、丹皮、菟丝子、枸杞子、黄柏、知母。）

Literature Review of Insecurity of Yīn Essence

📖 *Huà Tuó Shén Yī Mì Chuán* (“Secret Transmission of Hua Tuo”) : “Huà Tuó’s Divine Formula for Treating Seminal Emission”

> “The cause of this pathocondition is found in exhaustion of kidney water. In the upper body, it is unable to reach the heart; in the center, it is unable to moisten the liver; and in the lower body, it is unable to engender spleen-earth. For this reason, the jade gate fails to close, resulting in spontaneous emission without dreaming.”

This quotation describes how insufficiency of kidney yīn, lack of strength in securing and containing, and yīn essence running off manifests in seminal efflux and premature ejaculation.

📖 *Yīn Xū Zhèng Zhì* (“Yīn Vacuity Patterns and Treatment), “Menstrual Irregularities”

> “The monthly water depends completely on transformation from kidney water. As soon as there is a lack of kidney water, the menstrual fluid dries up or comes early or late, or dribbles at any time.”

This quotation discusses the pathomechanism by which insufficiency of kidney yīn and insecurity of the thoroughfare and controlling vessels can lead to menstrual irregularities.

📖 *Yīn Xū Zhèng Zhì* ("Yīn Vacuity Patterns and Treatment), "Strangury Patterns"

> "Owing to an insufficiency of kidney yīn, essence fails to transform qì, and the lower origin is insecure. Therefore we see turbid urine like water that rice has been washed in, strangury with urine that resembles fat, and roughness and pain in the urethra."

This quotation indicates the pathomechanism by which kidney yīn depletion, failure to transform qì, and insecurity of kidney qì results in dribbling and rough urination.

文献评述

《华佗神医秘传•华佗治遗精神方》曰："本症之原因，为肾水耗竭，上不能通心，中不能润于肝，下不能生于脾土，以致玉关不闭，无梦自遗。"论述肾阴不足，固摄乏力，阴精流失，出现滑精早泄的病机变化。

《阴虚证治•月经失调》曰："月水全赖肾水施化，肾水既乏，则经水日以干涸，或先或后，淋漓无时。"论述肾阴不足，冲任不固，可致月经失调的病机。

《阴虚证治•淋证》曰："因肾阴不足，精不化气，下元不固，故见小便浑浊如米泔，成淋出如脂，尿道涩痛不著。"指出肾阴亏虚，不能化气，肾气不固，引起淋涩的病机。

Summary of Insecurity of Yīn Essence

1. Yīn Vacuity-Related Insecurity of the Essence Gate
   Seminal efflux and premature ejaculation.
2. Yīn Vacuity-Related Insecurity of the Channels and Vessels
   Dribbling menstruation, clear thin menses and vaginal discharge.
3. Yīn Vacuity-Related Insecurity of the Bladder
   Incessant dribbling of urine.
4. Head and Eyes Deprived of Nourishment
   Dizzy head and tinnitus.
5. Viscera and Bowels Deprived of Nourishment
   Fatigued and feeble spirit.
6. Kidney Yīn Depletion
   Red tongue with scant fur, fine rapid pulse.

阴精不固
阴虚精关不固—滑精早泄
阴虚经带不固—月经淋漓，经带清稀
阴虚膀胱不固—小便淋漓不尽
头目失养—头晕耳鸣
脏腑失养—神疲乏力
肾阴亏虚—舌红少苔，脉细数

3.5 Vacuity-Related Reproductive Hyperactivity

The kidney stores essence and governs birth, growth, and reproduction. For the normal performance of reproductive functions, a balance of kidney yáng and kidney yīn is necessary. As the "Treatise on Vital Qì Connecting with Heaven" in the *Sù Wèn* ("Plain Questions") states, "Yīn stores essence and gives rise to qì. Yáng defends against the outside and provides security." If kidney yīn is insufficient, yīn fails to restrain yáng, kidney yáng becomes abnormally hyperactive, and the ministerial fire stirs frenetically and harasses the essence gate. This can lead to accentuated sexual functions. Because it is caused by yīn vacuity and yáng hyperactivity, this type of sexual hyperfunction is a false vacuity and manifests in the pathological changes of vacuity-type accentuation of reproductive functions.

When kidney yīn is depleted, yīn fails to restrain yáng, and the ministerial fire stirs frenetically. Distressed by vacuity fire, sexual functions are accentuated. In men, this manifests in increased persistent and frequent erection, priapism, and in severe cases, spontaneous discharge of semen at any time. In women, it manifests in increased sexual desire.

As a result of yīn vacuity internal heat, vacuity fire can harass the spirit so that the spirit fails to keep to its abode, [the patient] dreams of intercourse with ghosts. Vacuity fire harasses the essence chamber and prevents yīn essence from keeping its place. The result is frenetic dreaming with seminal emission.

When kidney yīn is insufficient, the formal body and the lower back are deprived of enrichment. This results in limp aching lower back and knees, and emaciation.

Owing to yīn vacuity and yáng hyperactivity, vacuity fire stirs and harasses. The result is night sweating during sleep and steaming bone tidal heat.

Yīn vacuity internal heat results in a red tongue with scant fur and lack of liquid, and a fine rapid pulse at the left cubit position.

The chapter, "On Dream Emission and Seminal Efflux" in the *Yī Guàn* ("Thorough Knowledge of Medicine") states:

> "There are people with constitutional source vacuity of earlier heaven. If this concurs with excessive sexual desire, it brings about vanquishing of kidney yīn. Yīn vacuity results in the stirring of ministerial fire. This is tied to the heart's sovereign fire above. When sovereign fire stirs, ministerial fire follows. As a result, essence leaves its place even without any sexual intercourse and lodges in the genital area. During sleep at night, as soon as it encounters ministerial fire, which has deposited there, and joins with it internally, it combines with yīn qì. Therefore, such patients dream as soon as they fall asleep and have emissions as soon as they dream."

This quotation discusses the pathomechanism by which kidney yīn depletion and frenetic stirring of the ministerial fire harasses the essence chamber and thereby brings about dream emission and seminal efflux.

The chapter, "Origin and Development of Disease in the Anterior and Posterior Yīn" in the *Zá Bìng Yuán Liú Xī Zhú* ("Incisive Light on the Source of Miscellaneous Disease") further states:

> "What some call yīn protraction is also called yīn erection. Because the anterior yīn contracts heat, the penis is persistently erect without retraction, or swollen and wilting, or rubbing against the thigh, making it difficult to walk. In severe cases, both rib-sides suffer from counterflow ascent of qì, and the extremities are fatigued and weak."

What this quotation calls "anterior yīn contracting heat" can refer to fire heat that is caused by kidney yīn insufficiency and yáng hyperactivity. This passage therefore explains that the pathomechanism of persistent and frequent erection is related to yīn vacuity and yáng hyperactivity.

Vacuity-related reproductive hyperactivity is treated by enriching yīn and supplementing the kidney, and by draining fire and checking seminal emission. The recommended formula is *sān cái tāng* (Heaven, Human, and Earth Decoction) in combination with *fēng suǐ dān* (Marrow-Sealing Elixir) from the *Yī Zōng Jīn Jiàn* ("The Golden Mirror of Medicine").

Sān Cái Tāng 三才汤 with *Fēng Suǐ Dān* 封髓丹 Heaven, Human, and Earth Decoction with Marrow Sealing Elixir
rén shēn (人参 Ginseng Radix, ginseng)
tiān dōng (天冬 Asparagi Radix, asparagus)
shú dì huáng (熟地黄 Rehmanniae Radix Praeparata, cooked rehmannia)
shā rén (砂仁 Amomi Fructus, amomum)
huáng bǎi (黄柏 Phellodendri Cortex, phellodendron)
zhì gān cǎo (炙甘草 Glycyrrhizae Radix cum Liquido Fricta, mix-fried licorice)

生殖虚亢

肾藏精，主生长发育与生殖，生殖功能的正常完成需要肾阳肾阴相对平衡。如《素问•生气通天论》曰："阴者，藏精而起亟也；阳者，卫外而为固也。"如肾阴不足，阴不制阳，肾阳偏亢，相火妄动，扰动精关，可导致性功能亢进。由于是因阴虚阳亢所致，此种性功能的增强具有虚假性，表现为生殖功能虚性亢进的病机变化。肾阴亏虚，阴不制阳，相火妄动，虚火逼迫，性功能亢进，则表现为男子阳强易举，举而不衰，甚者不时精液自出，女子性欲增强；阴虚内热，虚火扰神，神不守舍，梦与鬼交，扰动精室，阴精不守其位，则妄梦遗精；肾阴不足，形体、腰府失滋，则腰膝酸软，形体消瘦；阴虚阳亢，虚火扰动，则夜寐盗汗，骨蒸潮热。阴虚内热，则舌红少苔乏津，左尺脉细数。如《医贯•梦遗并滑精论》："今人先天禀赋原虚，兼之色欲过度，以致肾阴衰败，阴虚则相火动，相火之系，上系于心为君火，感物而动，动则相火翕然而随，虽不交会而精已离其位，即客于阴器间矣。夜卧时，当所寄之相火一遇，与接内时与阴气相合，故卧而即梦，梦而即遗也。"论述了肾阴亏虚，相火妄动，扰乱精室，引起梦遗滑泄的病机。《杂病源流犀烛•前阴后阴病源流》又曰："一曰阴纵，亦名阴挺，由前阴受热，则玉茎挺长不收，或肿胀而痿，或与股相磨难行，甚于两胁气逆上，手足倦弱。""前阴受热"，可能为肾阴不足，阳亢火热而致，说明男子阳强易举的病机与阴虚阳亢有关。治法宜滋阴补肾，泻火止遗。方药选用《医宗金鉴》三才汤合封髓丹（人参、天冬、熟地、砂仁、黄柏、炙甘草）。

Literature Review of Vacuity-Related Reproductive Hyperactivity

📖 *Jǐng Yuè Quán Shū* ("Jǐng-Yuè's Complete Compendium"), "Regular Patterns of Women: Women's Dreaming of Intercourse with Ghosts"

"Since this disease is engendered internally, it leaves no physical traces on the outside. Nevertheless, frequent encounters in her dreams cause emissions as well as symptoms like abstraction and turbid vaginal discharge. Also, this condition resembles dream emission in men and their pathomechanisms are identical. It is only that women are mostly unwilling to talk about it...

"If this disease is not regulated but endures without cure, essence-blood vanquishes by the day, and true yīn is reduced by the day. This leads to tidal heat and heat effusion, fatigued spirit and limbs, daily decreasing intake of food and drink, daily desiccation of menstrual flow, whittling of the flesh which gradually turns into taxation detriment, and a tight rapid pulse. In most cases, the disease can not be stemmed."

This quotation explains how kidney yīn depletion and yáng hyperactivity due to yīn vacuity lead to sexual dreams in women.

📖 *Yī Guàn* ("Thorough Knowledge of Medicine"), "Dream Emission and Seminal Efflux"

"If kidney yīn is vacuous, essence is not stored; if liver yáng is strong, fire is not tight. Now when fire that is not tight coincides with essence that is not stored, the patient suffers from seminal discharge, whether with dreams or without."

This quotation discusses how kidney yīn depletion and internally exuberant vacuity fire lead to dream emissions.

📖 *Biàn Zhèng Lù* ("Records on Pattern Differentiation"), "Section on Dream Emission"

"When people in the dead of night subjectively feel heat as if from fire in the spine and heart and therefore have dream emissions, they assume that this is the 'river cart fire' burning. Who is aware that actually this is caused by the desiccation of kidney water? Now, the path of the river cart is identical with the spinal vertebrae. Since the path of the kidney runs along the spine, this is the path of kidney fire. When water and fire help each other, the path of the river cart is quieted. However, when water and fire overcome each other, the path of the river cart is stopped. And when the path is stopped, there is no water to pour into it or to flow through it. As a result, fire qì flames upward and forms heat. In that case, how could the spine and heart be cool? When fire flames upward, water naturally flows downward.

> "In treating this condition, to stem the upward flaming of fire you must first replenish the desiccated water below. When water is sufficient, fire will cease, and the yellow river can once again run counterflow. For a formula, use *wǎn liú tāng* (Rescue the Flow Decoction): 2 *liǎng* of *shú dì huáng* (Rehmanniae Radix Praeparata), 1 *liǎng* of *shān yào* (Dioscoreae Rhizoma), 1 *liǎng* of *bái zhú* (Atractylodis Macrocephalae Rhizoma), 3 *qián* of *zé xiè* (Alismatis Rhizoma), 1 *liǎng* of *xuán shēn* (Scrophulariae Radix), 2 *qián* of *běi wǔ wèi zǐ* (Schisandrae Chinensis Fructus), and 5 *qián* of *shān zhū yú* (Corni Fructus)."

This quotation indicates the pathomechanism by which kidney yīn depletion and depleted water and flaming fire form dream emission.

文献评述

《景岳全书•妇人规•妇人梦与鬼交》曰："病由内生者，外无形迹，不过于梦寐间常有所遇，以致遗失，及为恍惚带浊等证，亦如男子之梦遗，其机一也，但在女子多不肯言耳。...若失于调理，久之不愈，则精血日败，真阴日损，乃致潮热发热，神疲体倦，饮食日减，经水日枯，肌肉消削，渐成劳损，脉见紧数，多致不救矣。"论述了 肾阴亏损，阴虚则阳亢，女子梦交的病机变化。

《医贯•梦遗并滑精》曰："肾之阴虚则精不藏，肝之阳强则火不秘，以不秘之火加临不藏之精，有不梦，梦即泄矣。"论述了肾阴亏虚，虚火内盛，导致梦遗的病机改变。

《辨证录•梦遗门》曰："人有至夜脊心自觉如火之热，因而梦遗，人以为河车火烧也，谁知是肾水之涸乎。夫河车之路，即脊骨之椎也。肾之路走夹脊者，乃肾火之路也。水火相济，而河车之路安，水火相胜，而河车之路塞。路塞者，无水以灌注之也。无水相通，则火气上炎而成热，脊心安得清凉哉?火炎于上，自然水流于下矣。治法救在上之火炎，必先沛在下之水涸，水足火息，黄河始可逆流也。方用挽流汤：熟地二两、 山药一两、白术一两、泽泻三钱、玄参一两、北五味二钱、山茱萸五钱。"指出肾阴亏损，水亏火炎，而成梦遗的病机。

Summary of Vacuity-Related Reproductive Hyperactivity
1. Reproductive Hyperfunction Persistent and frequent erection, erection that will not wane; in severe cases, spontaneous discharge of semen at any time; increased sexual desire in women. 2. Vacuity Fire Harassing Essence Frenetic dreaming and seminal emission. 3. Loss of Enrichment in the Formal Body Limp aching lower back and knees, emaciation. 4. Vacuity Fire Stirring Harassingly Night sweating during sleep, steaming bone tidal heat. 5. Yīn Vacuity Internal Heat Red tongue with scant fur and no liquid, fine rapid left cubit pulse.

生殖虚亢
生殖亢进—阳强易举，举而不衰，甚者不时精液自出，女子性欲增强 虚火扰精—妄梦遗精 形体失滋—腰膝酸软，形体消瘦 虚火扰动—夜寐盗汗，骨蒸潮热 阴虚内热—舌红少苔乏津，左尺脉细数

3.6 Vacuity Heat Arising Internally

Yīn and yáng are the root of the human body. Yīn governs cold, and yáng governs heat. When yīn and yáng are balanced, yīn is calm and yáng is sound. This is the necessary precondition for the normal performance of every single vital activity in the body. A variety of pathogenic factors such as constitutional insufficiency, debility in old age, lack of or inappropriate treatment, and enduring or severe disease can lead to consumption of kidney yīn. Yīn and yáng lose their balance, yīn fails to restrain yáng, and yīn vacuity results in yáng hyperactivity. This can manifest in the pathomechanical changes of vacuity heat arising internally.

Thus the "Treatise on Regulating the Channels" in the *Sù Wèn* ("Plain Questions") points out: "Yīn vacuity results in internal heat."

The chapter, "Vacuity Detriment" in the *Jǐng Yuè Quán Shū* ("Jǐng-Yuè's Complete Compendium"), "Schema of Miscellaneous Patterns" further details:

> "Yīn vacuity means increased heat, because water fails to help fire, and yīn vacuity therefore engenders heat. This disease is mostly contracted due to predilection for liquor and sexual intercourse, or due to anger, evil thoughts roving, and manic taxation, which stir fire in the five viscera. Patients with insufficiency of earlier heaven original yīn are particularly prone to this disease. Whenever patients are troubled by vacuity detriment and by increased heat and dryness, hot foods are inappropriate. These are the signs of yīn vacuity."

This quotation clearly explains the pathomechanical changes and processes of kidney yīn vacuity engendering internal heat.

The chapter, "Vacuity Detriment Consumption" in the *Yī Biǎn* ("Lancing Stones of Medicine") also states:

> "Among damage to any of the five viscera, damage to the kidney is the most severe. Kidney vacuity results in steaming bone tidal heat and in tidal heat after noon or midnight, with spontaneous and night sweating, emaciation, dry mouth and throat, hoarse voice or muteness, dispersion thirst and strangury-turbidity, seminal emission and blood loss, irascibility, dry cough with phlegm, sleeplessness with vexation and agitation, and abstraction and fearful throbbing. All these are caused by water vacuity and fire flaming."

This passage points out the numerous clinical manifestations that can result from yīn vacuity internal heat.

Because internally arising vacuity heat can bring about different pathomechanical trends and clinical manifestations, we can further divide this pathomechanism into eight types: yīn vacuity internal heat, vacuity heat steaming bones, vacuity heat forcing sweat, vacuity heat invading the lung, vacuity heat harassing the teeth, vacuity heat harassing the throat, vacuity heat disturbing urination, and vacuity heat dispersion-thirst.

虚热内生

阴阳为人身之根本，阴主寒而阳主热，阴阳平衡、阴平阳秘，人体各项生命活动才能得以正常进行。如因禀赋不足、年老体衰、失治误治、久病重病等多种致病因素引起肾阴亏耗，阴阳失衡，阴不制阳，阴虚则阳盛，就会出现虚热内生的病机变化。故《素问•调经论》指出："阴虚则内热。"《景岳全书•杂证谟•虚损》进一步阐述到："阴虚者多热，以水不济火而阴虚生热也。此病多得于酒色嗜欲，或愤怒邪思，流荡狂劳，以动五脏之火，而先天元阴不足者，尤多此病。凡患虚损而多热多燥，不宜热食者，便是阴虚之候。”清楚地说明了肾阴虚生内热的病机变化过程。《医碥•虚损痨瘵》亦曰：“五脏之伤，肾最为重，肾虚则骨蒸潮热，或午后或子后潮热，自汗盗汗，形体消瘦，口干咽燥，声嘶音哑，消渴淋浊，遗精失血，易生嗔（音恨之意）怒，干咳痰嗽，不眠烦躁，恍惚怔忡，皆水虚火炎所致。”指出阴虚内热可引起多种临床表现。由于虚热内生引起不同临床表现的病机趋势有别，此病机又可进一步分为阴虚内热、虚热蒸骨、虚热迫汗、虚热犯肺、虚热扰齿、虚热扰咽、虚热扰溺、虚热消渴等八种类型。

3.6.1 Yīn Vacuity Internal Heat

Yīn vacuity indicates a lack of fundamental substances that are ascribed to yīn by nature, such as liquid and humor or essence-blood. The special characteristic of this pathomechanism lies in the fact that yīn humor is insufficient and that the functions of enriching and moistening are impaired. If this reaches the point of yīn failing to restrain yáng, yáng qì becomes abnormally exuberant, and locations where yáng qì accumulates are affected by a superabundance of qì and the manifestation of heat arising. When kidney yīn is insufficient and kidney yáng becomes abnormally hyperactive, vacuity fire arises internally. This can manifest in the pathomechanism of yīn vacuity internal heat.

The foot lesser yīn kidney channel runs through the sole of the foot, and the hand lesser yīn heart channel runs through the center of the heart and the palm of the hand. When kidney yīn is depleted and vacuity heat arises internally, it can ascend and harass the heart channel, while vacuity fire blazes internally. The result is vexing heat in the five hearts, insomnia, and profuse dreaming.

The kidney channel runs upward along the throat, and the cheeks are ascribed to the kidney. When kidney yīn is depleted and vacuity fire harasses the upper body, the result is dry mouth and tongue, sore throat, and tidal reddening of the cheeks.

When kidney yīn depletion causes effulgent yīn vacuity fire, this can internally steam the bones and force liquid to spill to the outside. The result is steaming bone taxation heat, tidal heat, and night sweating.

The lower back is the house of the kidney. When kidney yīn is depleted, the lower back is deprived of enrichment. This results in aching lower back and knees.

Vacuity fire can also shift downward, causing reduced liquid and loss of enrichment. The result is yellow urine and dry stool.

Yīn vacuity internal heat results in a red tongue with scant fur, and a fine rapid pulse.

The chapter, "Vacuity Detriment" in the *Jǐng Yuè Quán Shū* ("Jǐng-Yuè's Complete Compendium"), "Schema of Miscellaneous Patterns" states: "Frequent agitation means that there is no yīn within yáng and that softness fails to help hardness... A searing sensation in the sole of the foot means that vacuity fire is scorching yīn and that the gushing spring is desiccated." When yīn fails to help yáng and vacuity heat harasses internally, the result is frequent agitation. Gushing Spring (*yǒng quán*, KI-1) is a source point of the kidney, and scalding heat in the sole of the foot also explains the pathomechanical changes resulting from kidney yīn vacuity and internal heat sweltering to the outside.

Furthermore, the chapter, "Yīn Vacuity Resulting in Heat" in the *Yīn Xū Zhèng Zhì* ("Yīn Vacuity Patterns and Treatment) states:

> "Yīn vacuity patterns are found in any of the five viscera, and each has a number of complications. In clinic we most commonly see liver or kidney yīn vacuity patterns. Among these, insufficiency of kidney yīn occupies a prominent place among the pathological mutations of yīn vacuity. Because the kidney is the root of yīn humor in the body, insufficiency of yīn humor and yīn failing to restrain yáng cause numerous manifestations of yīn vacuity internal heat, effulgent yīn vacuity fire, and yīn vacuity with yáng hyperactivity. Thus we see vexing heat in the five hearts and steaming bone tidal heat, accompanied by symptoms like emaciation, night sweating, dry mouth, red tongue, and a fine rapid pulse."

This quotation is a comprehensive summary of the pathomechanism and manifestations of yīn vacuity internal heat.

Yīn vacuity internal heat is treated by supplementing and boosting kidney yīn, and by enriching yīn and clearing heat. Recommended formulas are *zhī bǎi dì huáng wán* (Anemarrhena, Phellodendron, and Rehmannia Pill) from the *Yī Zōng Jīn Jiàn* ("The Golden Mirror of Medicine") or *zī yīn jiàng huǒ tāng* (Yīn-Enriching Fire-Downbearing Decoction) from the *Shòu Shì Bǎo Yuán* ("Prolonging Life and Preserving the Origin") with modifications.

Zhī Bǎi Dì Huáng Wán 知柏地黄丸 Anemarrhena, Phellodendron, and Rehmannia Pill
shú dì huáng (熟地黄 Rehmanniae Radix Praeparata, cooked rehmannia)
shān zhū yú (山茱萸 Corni Fructus, cornus)
shān yào (山药 Dioscoreae Rhizoma, dioscorea)
zé xiè (泽泻 Alismatis Rhizoma, alisma)
mǔ dān pí (牡丹皮 Moutan Cortex, moutan)
fú líng (茯苓 Poria, poria)
zhī mǔ (知母 Anemarrhenae Rhizoma, anemarrhena)
huáng bǎi (黄柏 Phellodendri Cortex, phellodendron)

Zī Yīn Jiàng Huǒ Tāng 滋阴降火汤 Yīn-Enriching Fire-Downbearing Decoction
dāng guī (当归 Angelicae Sinensis Radix, Chinese angelica)
chuān xiōng (川芎 Chuanxiong Rhizoma, chuanxiong)
huáng bǎi (黄柏 Phellodendri Cortex, phellodendron)
zhī mǔ (知母 Anemarrhenae Rhizoma, anemarrhena)
tiān huā fěn (天花粉 Trichosanthis Radix, trichosanthes root)
sháo yào (芍药 Paeoniae Radix, peony)
shú dì huáng (熟地黄 Rehmanniae Radix Praeparata, cooked rehmannia)
xuán shēn (玄参 Scrophulariae Radix, scrophularia)
jié gěng (桔梗 Platycodonis Radix, platycodon)
zhú lì (竹沥 Bambusae Succus, bamboo sap)
gān cǎo (甘草 Glycyrrhizae Radix, licorice)

阴虚内热

阴虚是指人体津液、精血等性质属阴的基本物质亏损。其病机特点为阴液不足，滋养、润泽功能失常，以及阴不制阳，阳气偏盛，阳气聚积之处，气盛有余而生热的表现。肾阴不足，肾阳偏亢，虚火内生，可出现阴虚内热的病机变化。足少阴肾经通足心，手少阴心经通心中和手心，肾阴亏虚，虚热内生，上扰心经，虚火内炽，则为五心烦热，失眠多梦；肾经上循咽喉，两颧属肾，肾阴亏虚，虚火上扰，则口干舌燥，咽喉疼痛，两颧潮红；肾阴亏虚，阴虚火旺，内蒸于骨，迫津外溢，则骨蒸劳热，潮热盗汗；腰为肾之府，肾阴亏虚，腰府失滋，则腰膝酸痛；虚火下移，津少失滋，则尿黄便干。阴虚内热，则舌红少苔，脉细数。如《景岳全书•杂证谟•虚损》曰："时多烦躁者，阳中无阴，柔不济刚也。...足心如烙者，虚火烁阴，涌泉涸竭也。"阴不济阳，虚热内扰，则时时烦躁，而涌泉穴为肾之原穴，足心烫热，说明了肾阴虚，内热熏蒸于外的病机改变。又如《阴虚证治•阴虚则热》云："阴虚之证，五脏具有，五脏之间亦每多兼挟，但就临床所见，一般以肝肾阴虚为主，其中又以肾阴不足在阴虚病理变化中占有重要地位。因为肾为人体阴液之本，阴液不足，阴不制阳，从而形成阴虚内热，阴虚火旺，阴虚阳亢等多种表现，而发生五心烦热，骨蒸潮热，伴见形体消瘦，盗汗，口干，舌红，脉细数等症。"对阴虚内热的病机和表现都作了全面总结。治法宜补益肾阴，滋阴清热。方药选用《医宗金鉴》知柏地黄丸（熟地黄、山萸肉、怀山药、泽泻、丹皮、茯苓、知母、黄柏），或选《寿世保元》滋阴降火汤（当归、川芎、黄柏、知母、天花粉、芍药、熟地、玄参、桔梗、竹沥、甘草）加减。

Literature Review of Yīn Vacuity Internal Heat

📖 *Zhū Bìng Yuán Hòu Lùn* ("Origin and Indicators of Disease"), "Symptoms of Vacuity Taxation Heat"

> "Heat that results from vacuity taxation means that yīn qì is insufficient and yáng qì is superabundant. Because of this, heat arises internally and externally. This is not evil qì from the outside arriving to exploit."

This quotation clearly indicates the pathomechanism of yīn vacuity causing internal engenderment of vacuity heat.

📖 *Shòu Shì Bǎo Yuán* ("Prolonging Life and Preserving the Origin"), "Heat Effusion"

> "One theory explains yīn-vacuity heat effusion as being caused by damage to yīn-blood, so that it is unable to restrain fire. Yáng qì ascends as internal heat, which is the same as yáng effulgence. Therefore, the pulse is rapid and forceless and ascribed to the heart and kidney."

This quotation analyzes in detail the pathomechanism of yīn vacuity (which includes kidney yīn vacuity) and internally arising vacuity heat.

📖 *Yī Biăn* ("Lancing Stones of Medicine"), "Miscellaneous Pathoconditions: Heat Effusion"

> "Yīn-vacuity heat effusion (the same as blood vacuity): Yīn vacuity means vacuity of kidney water. Fire by nature flames upward and manifests on the outside… If yīn is depleted and water vacuous, the firewood is dry and the fire so strong that its burning and scorching means disaster. (This condition can be caused by sexual desires reducing essence, by yīn collapse from diarrhea, or by dryness-heat damaging humor). This kind of fire blaze is in fact caused by vacuity of water and is different from the above-mentioned yáng hyperactivity without yīn debilitation."

This quotation clearly points out that the ordinarily referenced yīn-vacuity heat effusion is mostly related to the pathomechanism of kidney yīn insufficiency, depleted water and flaming fire, and vacuity fire scorching.

文献评述

《诸病源候论•虚劳热候》曰："虚劳而热者，是阴气不足，阳气有余，故内外生于热，非邪气从外来乘也。"明确指出阴虚不足，虚热内生的病机改变。

《寿世保元•发热》曰："一论阴虚发热，是阴血自伤，不能制火，阳气升腾内热，乃阳旺也。故其脉数而无力，属心肾。"对阴虚（包括肾阴虚）而内生虚热的病机变化进行了详细的分析。

《医碥•杂证•发热》曰："阴虚发热（血虚同）：阴虚，肾水虚也。火性本上炎而外现，…若阴亏水虚，则柴干火烈而焚灼为灾矣，（或由色欲损精，或由泻痢亡阴，或由燥热伤液，皆能致之也。）此之火炎，乃由水虚所致，与上条阳亢而阴未衰者不同。"明确提出一般所指的阴虚发热，其病机多为肾阴不足，水亏火炎，虚火焚灼。

Summary of Yīn Vacuity Internal Heat
1. Vacuity Fire Blazing Internally Vexing heat in the five hearts, insomnia and profuse dreaming.
2. Vacuity Fire Harassing the Upper Body Dry mouth and tongue, sore throat, tidal reddening of the cheeks.
3. Effulgent Yīn Vacuity Fire Steaming bone taxation heat, tidal heat, night sweating.
4. Loss of Enrichment in the Lower Back Aching lower back and knees.
5. Vacuity Fire Shifting Downward Yellow urine and dry stool.
6. Yīn Vacuity Internal Heat Red tongue with scant fur, fine rapid pulse.

阴虚内热
虚火内炽—为五心烦热，失眠多梦
虚火上扰—口干舌燥，咽喉疼痛，两颧潮红
阴虚火旺—骨蒸劳热，潮热盗汗
腰府失滋—腰膝酸痛
虚火下移—尿黄便干
阴虚内热—舌红少苔，脉细数

3.6.2 Vacuity Heat Steaming the Bones

The kidney stores essence, essence engenders marrow, and marrow nourishes the bones. As stated in the "Great Treatise on the Correspondences and Manifestations of Yīn and Yáng" in the *Sù Wèn* ("Plain Questions"), "The kidney engenders bone and marrow." When kidney essence is plentiful, it provides the source for the formation of bone and marrow. Only if this is the case can the skeleton maintain its normal physiological functions. Essence is yīn, and when kidney yīn is insufficient, yīn essence is unable to nourish the bones. This can bring about the pathomechanism of vacuity heat steaming bones.

When kidney yīn is depleted, there is a shortage of yīn essence. The bones are deprived of enrichment by yīn, and vacuity fire arises internally and deflagrates the bones. The result is steaming bone taxation heat, a subjective sensation of heat being thrust to the outside from inside the bones, and heart vexation that is difficult to bear.

When kidney yīn is depleted, vacuity heat internally harasses the entire body. This results in vexing heat in the five hearts, tidal heat, and night sweating.

The appearance of vacuity heat is not caused by a direct and absolute increase of yáng qì, but by a depletion of yīn humor and corresponding exuberance of yáng qì. Therefore, it normally manifests mostly with unabating prolonged low-grade fever.

When kidney yīn is depleted, yīn humor fails to nourish the formal body and the lower back and knees. The result is aching lower back, limp knees, and emaciation of the body.

Vacuity heat flaming upward causes reddening of the lips and cheeks.

Yīn vacuity internal heat results in a red tongue with scant liquid, and a fine rapid pulse.

The chapter, "The Various Symptoms of Vacuity Taxation Disease; Symptoms of Vacuity Taxation Steaming Bone" in the *Zhū Bìng Yuán Hòu Lùn* ("Origin and Indicators of Disease") states:

> "There are five kinds of steaming disease: The first is called steaming bone, and its root is in the kidney. It presents with an initially cool body at dawn, but heat effusion in the evening, and with vexation and agitation, inability to sleep quietly, inability to taste food, reddish or yellow urine, sudden vexation and derangement, fine feeble panting, lumbar pain, counterflow cold of the feet, and constant heat in the palms of the hands… All the steaming conditions are predominantly formed when patients after recovering from heat disease violate their health by eating beef or mutton or greasy and slimy foods, or by liquor or sexual activity."

This quotation describes how effulgent yīn vacuity fire leads to vacuity heat steaming bone.

The "Section on the Six Excesses; "Origin and Development of Fire Disease" in the *Zá Bìng Yuán Liú Xī Zhú* ("Incisive Light on the Source of Miscellaneous Disease") further states:

> "If you feel no heat when applying light pressure, and reach the bone when applying heavy pressure, and the heat burns the hand, this indicates heat of the kidney. These symptoms are particularly

> pronounced between 9 p.m. and 1 a.m. and arise together with a tingling feeling in the bones as if being assailed by worms, numbness in the bones because of the heat, and inability to get out of bed. *Zī shèn wán* (Kidney-Enriching Pill) is suitable."

This quotation analyzes the pathomechanism of kidney yīn depletion and vacuity heat steaming bones.

Vacuity heat steaming the bones is treated by enriching yīn and supplementing the kidney, and by clearing heat and abating steaming. The recommended formula is *qīng gŭ săn* (Bone-Clearing Powder) from the *Zhèng Zhì Huì Bŭ* ("Combined Supplements to Patterns and Treatment").

Qīng Gŭ Săn 清骨散 Bone-Clearing Powder
yín chái hú (银柴胡 Stellariae Radix, stellaria)
qīng hāo (青蒿 Artemisiae Annuae Herba, sweet wormwood)
dì gŭ pí (地骨皮 Lycii Cortex, lycium bark)
qín jiāo (秦艽 Gentianae Macrophyllae Radix, large gentian)
biē jiă (鳖甲 Trionycis Carapax, turtle shell)
zhī mŭ (知母 Anemarrhenae Rhizoma, anemarrhena)
hú huáng lián (胡黄连 Picrorhizae Rhizoma, picrorhiza)
gān căo (甘草 Glycyrrhizae Radix, licorice)

虚热蒸骨

肾藏精，精生髓，髓养骨。如《素问•阴阳应象大论》曰："肾生骨髓。"肾精充足，骨髓生化有源，骨骼才能保持正常的生理功能。精属阴，肾阴不足，阴精不能养骨，则会引起虚热蒸骨的病机。肾阴亏损，阴精匮乏，骨失阴滋，内生虚火，虚火焚骨，则为骨蒸劳热，自觉有热从骨中向外透发，心烦难忍；肾阴亏虚，虚热内扰全身，则五心烦热，潮热盗汗；虚热的出现不是阳气绝对值的增长，而是阴液亏损，阳气相对亢盛，所以一般多现低热，日久持续不退；肾阴亏虚，阴液不养形体、腰膝，则腰酸膝软，形体消瘦；虚热上炎，故唇红颧赤。阴虚内热，则舌红少津，脉细数。如《诸病源候论•虚劳病诸候•虚劳骨蒸候》曰："夫蒸病有五：一曰骨蒸，其根在肾，旦起体凉，日晚即热，烦躁，寝不能安，食无味，小便赤黄，忽忽烦乱，细喘无力，腰疼，两足逆冷，手心常热。…凡诸蒸患，多因热病患愈后，食牛羊肉及肥腻，或酒或房，触犯而成此疾。"阐述了阴虚火旺而致虚热蒸骨的病机变化。《杂病源流犀烛•六淫门•火病源流》又曰："如轻按不热，重按至骨，其热炙手，乃肾之热，亥子时尤甚，其症必兼骨苏苏然如虫蚀，其骨因热不仁，亦不能起于床，宜滋肾丸。"对肾阴亏虚，虚热蒸骨的病机改变进行了分析。治法宜滋阴补肾，清热退蒸。方药选用《证治准绳》清骨散（银柴胡、青蒿、地骨皮、秦艽、鳖甲、知母、胡黄连、甘草）。

Literature Review of Vacuity Heat Steaming Bones

📖 *Zhèng Zhì Huì Bǔ* ("Combined Supplements to Patterns and Treatment"), "Section on the External Body: Heat Effusion"

"Steaming bone heat effusion and steaming and scorching in the extremities as if from fire invariably means that yīn qì is vacuous and yáng qì exuberant. The extremities are the root of all yáng. When the two yáng contend and yīn qì is vacuous, scant water is unable to extinguish exuberant fire and yáng rules alone. Ruling alone, it is unable to engender and grow. Prevailing alone, it then merely stops.

"If the patient suffers a sensation like roasting and fire, this is the flesh being scorched. The external signs of this condition are dry mouth and thin body, reduced eating, and laziness and fatigue. These are particularly pronounced at night, but are not felt at dawn. *Qín jiāo sǎn* (Large Gentian and Turtle Shell Powder) is suitable to govern this condition."

This quotation describes the pathomechanism by which effulgent yīn vacuity fire brings about steaming bone heat effusion. Analyzing the treatment formula, it can be determined that what this text terms yīn vacuity should also include the pathomechanism of kidney yīn vacuity.

📖 *Yī Xué Rù Mén* ("The Gateway to Medicine"), "Vacuity: Heat Effusion"

"Bone heat is caused by qì being vacuous and unable to transform blood. When blood is dry, fire spontaneously seethes and soars up. This manifests in a sensation in the flesh as if stabbed by needles, heat in the bones and vexing pain, possibly heat in all the five hearts, or a sensation like fire in both rib-sides, and either corresponding sensations at midnight and noon or slight aversion to cold during the day but great heat at night. Although this condition is governed by the kidney channel, it shifts irregularly… Kidney pattern heat effusion is located in the

> bones and is most severe from 9 p.m. to 1 a.m., with a sensation like fire in the palms and soles. *Zī shèn wán* (Kidney-Enriching Pill) governs it."

The fact that we see evidence of yīn vacuity internal heat in kidney disease bone heat indicates that kidney yīn depletion and vacuity heat harassing internally lead to steaming bone heat effusion.

文献评述

《证治汇补•外体门•发热》曰："骨蒸发热，四肢蒸灼如火者，必阴气虚阳气盛。四肢者，诸阳之本也。两阳相搏而阴气虚少，少水不能灭盛火，而阳独治。独治者，不能生长也，独胜则止耳，如炙如火者，当肉烁也。外候口干体瘦，食少懒倦，遇夜尤甚，平旦不觉，宜秦艽鳖甲散主之。"论述阴虚火旺而致骨蒸发热的病机。此处阴虚，根据治疗所用处方分析，应包含肾阴虚的病机。

《医学入门•虚类•发热》曰："骨热因气虚不能化血，血干则火自沸腾，肉如针刺，骨热烦疼，或五心俱热，或两肋如火，或子午相应，或昼微恶寒而夜反大热。虽肾经所主，传变不常。…肾证发热，在骨，亥子时甚，两手足心如火，滋肾丸主之。"肾病骨热，见阴虚内热之征，即指肾阴亏损，虚热内扰，引起骨蒸发热。

Summary of Vacuity Heat Steaming Bones

1. Vacuity Fire Deflagrating Bone
   Steaming bone taxation heat, subjective sensation of heat being thrust to the outside from inside the bones, heart vexation that is difficult to bear.
2. Heat Harassing the Entire Body
   Vexing heat in the five hearts, tidal heat, night sweating.
3. Corresponding Exuberance of Yáng Qì
   Frequent low-grade fever that is prolonged over many days without abating.
4. Yīn Depletion and Loss of Enrichment
   Aching lower back and limp knees, emaciation.
5. Vacuity Heat Flaming Upward
   Reddening of the lips and cheeks.
6. Yīn Vacuity Internal Heat
   Red tongue with scant fur, fine rapid pulse.

虚热蒸骨
虚火焚骨—骨蒸劳热，自觉有热从骨中向外透发，心烦难忍
热扰全身—五心烦热，潮热盗汗
阳气相对亢盛—多现低热，日久持续不退
阴亏失滋—腰酸膝软，形体消瘦
虚热上炎—唇红颧赤
阴虚内热—舌红少津，脉细数

3.6.3 Vacuity Heat Forcing Sweat

Sweat is a product of transformation from the fluids. The chapter, "Miscellaneous Pathoconditions; Sweating" in the *Yī Biǎn* ("Lancing Stones of Medicine") states: "Stored internally, it is humor; bearing upward, it is liquid; descending, it is urine; and discharged to the outside, it is sweat." The distribution of the fluids is closely related to the kidney. Therefore, the kidney is of the greatest significance for the discharge of sweat.

Sleep is an important constituent among the vital activities of the body. When yáng enters yīn, sleep results. When yáng exits to the exterior, the person awakens. If kidney yīn is insufficient, yīn vacuity fire can become effulgent and force liquid to discharge outward. This manifests in the pathomechanical changes of vacuity heat forcing sweat.

When kidney yīn is insufficient and yīn is vacuous in the interior, vacuity fire distresses the fluids and forces them to discharge outward. During sleep, defensive yáng enters from the exterior into the interior. The defense of the exterior is vacuous, and the defensive exterior is difficult to secure. This results in sweating during sleep. After awakening, defensive yáng again moves to the exterior and the interstices of the flesh are secure and tight. As a result, the exterior is replete and sweating ceases spontaneously.

When vacuity heat harasses internally, and yáng fails to enter yīn, the spirit-mind cannot obtain quietude. The result is insomnia and profuse dreaming.

Depletion of kidney yīn causes yīn vacuity internal heat. This results in periodically occurring tidal heat and vexing heat in the five hearts.

Vacuity heat can scorch the lower body and damage yīn liquid. Stool and urine are deprived of enrichment, which results in dry bound stool and yellow or reddish urine.

Yīn vacuity internal heat results in a red tongue with scant fur and a fine rapid pulse.

The chapter, "Sweating" in the *Yī Biǎn* ("Lancing Stones of Medicine") states:

> "Sweat is water and is governed by the kidney... Night sweating, which is called "thief sweating," means that the person does not sweat when awake, but only when asleep, as if a thief entered while the person was soundly asleep. When a person is awake, qì moves in yáng; during sleep, it moves in yīn... When such a person suffers from yīn vacuity, they are especially easily stirred. When they awaken, yáng qì moves back to the exterior, and sweating stops spontaneously."

Sweat is governed by the kidney. Since yīn vacuity refers to kidney yīn vacuity, this quotation explains that insufficiency of kidney yīn can lead to night sweating by forcing liquid to discharge outward.

The chapter, "Sweating" in the *Shòu Shì Bǎo Yuán* ("Prolonging Life and Preserving the Origin") further points out:

> "Night sweating means that sweat is discharged during sleep, covering the entire body as if the person was bathed in it, and stops as soon as the person awakens. It is ascribed to yīn vacuity... Flaming yīn vacuity fire should be treated primarily by supplementing the kidney and strengthening water to dam the luster of yáng."

From the fact that this text recommends enriching and supplementing kidney yīn to treat night sweating we can deduce that by forcing liquid outward, kidney yīn vacuity and effulgent vacuity fire can lead to night sweating.

Vacuity heat forcing sweat is treated by enriching yīn and clearing heat, and by securing the exterior and checking sweating. The recommended formula is *dāng guī liù huáng tāng* (Chinese Angelica Six Yellows Decoction) from the *Lán Shì Mì Cáng* ("Secret Treasure of the Orchid Chamber"), with the addition of *shān zhū yú* (Corni Fructus) and *wǔ wèi zǐ* (Schisandrae Fructus).

Dāng Guī Liù Huáng Tāng 当归六黄汤 Chinese Angelica Six Yellows Decoction
dāng guī (当归 Angelicae Sinensis Radix, Chinese angelica)
shēng dì huáng (生地黄 Rehmanniae Radix, rehmannia)
shú dì huáng (熟地黄 Rehmanniae Radix Praeparata, cooked rehmannia)
huáng lián (黄连 Coptidis Rhizoma, coptis)
huáng qín (黄芩 Scutellariae Radix, scutellaria)
huáng bǎi (黄柏 Phellodendri Cortex, phellodendron)
huáng qí (黄其芪 Astragali Radix, astragalus)
Plus:
shān zhū yú (山茱萸 Corni Fructus, cornus)
wǔ wèi zǐ (五味子 Schisandrae Fructus, schisandra)

虚热迫汗

汗为津液所化，正如《医碥•杂症•汗》所云："内藏则为液，上升则为津，下降则为尿，外泄则为汗。"津液的输布与肾密切相关，故汗的排泄与肾有十分重要的联系。睡眠是人体生命活动中重要的组成部分，阳入于阴则寐，阳出于表则寤。如肾阴不足，阴虚火旺，迫津外泄，则出现虚热迫汗的病机变化。肾阴不足，阴虚于里，虚火从内逼迫津液外泄，睡时卫阳由表入里，表卫空虚，卫表难固，则睡中汗出，醒后卫阳复出于表，肌凑固密，则表实汗出自止，故引起睡眠盗汗; 虚热内扰，阳不入阴，神志不得安宁，则失眠多梦; 肾阴亏虚，阴虚内热，则潮热时作，五心烦热; 虚热下灼，损伤阴津，二便失滋，故大便干结，小便黄赤。阴虚内热，则舌质红少苔，脉细数。如《医碥•汗》云："汗者，水也，肾所主也。...盗汗者，寤时无汗，寐时汗即出，如盗乘人睡熟而入也。人寤则气行于阳，寐则气行于阴，...其人阴虚尤易动，及其醒觉，则阳气还出于表，而汗自止。"汗为肾所主，阴虚则为肾阴虚，说明肾阴不足，迫津外泄，可引起盗汗。《寿世保元•汗症》又指出："盗汗者，寐中出，通身如浴，觉来方止，属阴虚。...阴虚火炎者，法当补肾，壮水之主，以制阳光。"从滋补肾阴治疗盗汗，也可反证肾阴虚，虚火旺，迫津外出而致盗汗的病机。治法宜滋阴清热，固表止汗。方药选用《兰室秘藏》当归六黄汤（当归、生地、熟地、黄连、黄芩、黄柏、黄芪）加山茱萸，五味子。

Literature Review of Vacuity Heat Forcing Sweat

📖 *Jǐng Yuè Quán Shū* ("Jǐng-Yuè's Complete Compendium"), "Schema of Miscellaneous Patterns: Insomnia"

> "When true yīn and channel blood are insufficient, yīn and yáng fail to intermingle, and the spirit is disquieted in its chamber."

This quotation describes how kidney yīn depletion results in insomnia because yáng fails to enter yīn and harasses the spirit light instead.

📖 *Gū Sòng Yuán Yī Jìng* ("Gū Sòng-Yuán's Mirror of Medicine"), "Expounding Pathoconditions and Formulas: Sweating"

> "In night sweating, sweat is discharged stealthily during sleep, and the person only becomes aware of this upon awakening. When people with yīn vacuity fall asleep, defensive yáng from the outside exploits the vacuity and steps into yīn, and humor in the exterior loses its secure defense and is stolen. Upon wakening, yáng once again takes charge of its affairs, and defensive qì again exits from the exterior. The exterior is replete and sweating stops spontaneously. This condition is ascribed to yīn vacuity."

This quotation clearly indicates the pathomechanism by which yīn vacuity and yáng hyperactivity force liquid to discharge outward and thereby bring about night sweating.

文献评述

《景岳全书•杂证谟•不寐》曰："真阴经血之不足，阴阳不交，而神有不安其室耳"。描述了肾阴亏虚，阳不入阴，扰乱神明，引起失眠不寐的病机变化。

《顾松园医镜•症方发明•汗》曰："盗汗者，睡中盗出，至醒方知。盖阴虚之人，睡去则卫外之阳乘虚蹈入阴中，表液失去固卫而盗出，觉则阳复用事，卫气复出于表，表实而汗自止，此属阴虚。"明确指出了阴虚阳亢，迫津外泄，导致盗汗的病机。

Summary of Vacuity Heat Forcing Sweat
1. Vacuity Fire Forcing Liquid Night sweating during sleep.
2. Yáng Failing to Enter Yīn Insomnia and profuse dreaming.
3. Vacuity Heat Harassing Internally Periodically occurring tidal heat, vexing heat in the five hearts.
4. Vacuity Heat Scorching the Lower Body Dry bound stool, yellow or reddish urine.
5. Yīn Vacuity Internal Heat Red tongue with scant fur, fine rapid pulse.

虚热迫汗
虚火迫津—睡眠盗汗
阳不入阴—失眠多梦
虚热内扰—潮热时作，五心烦热
虚热下灼—大便干结，小便黄赤
阴虚内热—舌质红少苔，脉细数

3.6.4. Vacuity Heat Invading the Lung

The kidney belongs to water, and the lung belongs to metal. Metal engenders water; therefore the lung is the mother of the kidney. The foot lesser yīn kidney channel links with the spine, homes to the kidney, and nets the bladder, before it directly enters the lung. The chapter, "Transport Points" in the *Líng Shū* ("The Magic Pivot") states: "Lesser yīn homes to the kidney. The kidney is linked to the lung above." Through their channel connection in the upper body, the kidney has a containing impact on the lung. When the kidney as the child contracts a disease, this invariably sprouts and affects the mother, thereby impairing the normal physiological functions of the lung.

The treatise "On Cough" in the *Sù Wèn* ("Plain Questions") states: "The condition of kidney cough manifests with tautness and pain in the back and lower back, and in severe cases cough with drool." This quotation describes the pathomechanism by which disease in the kidney channel brings about impaired diffusion and downbearing of the lung.

If depletion of kidney yīn causes internally arising vacuity heat, the pathomechanical changes of vacuity heat invading the lung can appear.

When kidney yīn is insufficient, yīn vacuity fire flames, vacuity fire scorches liquid, and the lung is deprived of enrichment and moistening. The lobes of the lung dry out and wither, depuration breaks down, and lung qì ascends counterflow. This results in lung wilting with scorched lobes, and coughing and spitting turbid spittle and foamy drool.

When vacuity fire harasses the lung's network vessels above and forces blood to move frenetically, the result is cough with counterflow and expectoration of blood.

When kidney yīn is depleted, the lower back and knees are deprived of nourishment. The result is limp aching lower back and knees.

Owing to liquid depletion, the lung's irrigating function breaks down and the formal body is deprived of nourishment. The result is emaciation.

Yīn vacuity internal heat causes vacuity fire to stir and harass. This results in vexing heat in the five hearts, reddening of the cheeks, night sweating, and tinnitus and deafness.

Yīn vacuity internal heat results in a red tongue with scant fur and a surging and large cubit pulse.

The chapter, "Lung Wilting and Pulmonary Welling-Abscess" in the *Yī Mén Fă Lǜ* ("Axioms of Medicine") succinctly points out:

> "Lung wilting is cumulative and gradual and will not end in one day. The aversion to cold and heat effusion that are associated with it will not stop with only one extreme. It is always caused by a failure to move the fluids inside the kidney to the lung, so that the lung is deprived of nourishment and becomes dry. This is how this disease is formed."

This quotation discusses how insufficiency of kidney yīn and depleted water and flaming fire lead to vacuity heat invading the lung.

The chapter, "Internal Damage Cough; Kidney Channel Cough" in the *Zhèng Yīn Mài Zhì* ("Pathoconditions: Causes, Pulses, and Treatments") also states:

> "The cause of kidney channel cough is taxation damage to lung qì, as a result of which metal fails to engender water. It is possible that excessive sexual desire has caused the desiccation of true yīn. This results in vacuous water and effulgent fire, and in kidney fire tormenting metal. Alternatively, if true yáng is insufficient, water flooding can cause phlegm. As a result, the pathocondition of kidney channel cough occurs."

This quotation discusses the pathomechanical changes of insufficiency of kidney yīn and vacuity heat invading the lung.

Vacuity heat invading the lung is treated by downbearing fire and enriching yīn, and by cooling blood and stanching bleeding. The recommended formula is *dà bǔ yīn wán* (Major Yīn Supplementation Pill) from the *Dān Xī Xīn Fǎ* ("Dān Xī's Heart-Approach") in combination with *mài mén dōng tāng* (Ophiopogon Decoction) from the *Jīn Guì Yào Lüè* ("Essential Prescriptions of the Golden Coffer").

Dà Bǔ Yīn Wán 大补阴丸 Major Yīn Supplementation Pill
huáng bǎi (黄柏 Phellodendri Cortex, phellodendron)
zhī mǔ (知母 Anemarrhenae Rhizoma, anemarrhena)
shú dì huáng (熟地黄 Rehmanniae Radix Praeparata, cooked rehmannia)
guī bǎn (龟版 Testudinis Plastrum, tortoise plastron)

Mài Mén Dōng Tāng 麦门冬汤 Ophiopogon Decoction
rén shēn (人参 Ginseng Radix, ginseng)
mài dōng (麦冬 Ophiopogonis Radix, ophiopogon)
bàn xià (半夏 Pinelliae Rhizoma, pinellia)
jīng mǐ (粳米 Oryzae Semen, non-glutinous rice)
dà zǎo (大枣 Jujubae Fructus, jujube)
gān cǎo (甘草 Glycyrrhizae Radix, licorice)

虚热犯肺

肾属水，肺属金，金生水，故肺为肾之母。足少阴肾经之脉，贯脊属肾络膀胱，其直者入肺中，故《灵枢•本输》曰："少阴属肾，肾上连肺。"肾在经脉连属上对肺有统摄关系，肾子染疾，必秧及于母，使肺脏的正常生理功能受到影响。《素问•咳论》曰："肾咳之状，咳则腰背相引而痛，甚则咳涎。"对肾经病变导致肺失宣降的病机进行了论述。若肾阴亏损，虚热内生，则可出现虚热犯肺的病机变化。肾阴不足，阴虚火炎，虚火灼津，肺失滋润，肺叶枯萎，清肃失职，肺气上逆，则为肺痿叶焦，咳吐浊唾涎沫；虚火上扰肺络，迫血妄行，则为咳逆咯血；肾阴亏损，腰膝失养，则腰膝酸软；津亏肺之灌溉功能失职，形体失养，则形体消瘦；阴虚内热，虚火扰动，则五心烦热，颧红盗汗，耳鸣耳聋。阴虚内热，则舌红苔少，尺脉洪大。如《医门法律•肺痿肺痈门》明确指出："肺痿者，其积渐已非一日，其寒热不止一端，总由肾中津液不输于肺，肺失所养，转枯转燥，然后成之。"论述了肾阴不足，水亏火炎导致虚热犯肺的病机改变。《症因脉治•内伤咳嗽•肾经咳嗽》也云："肾经咳嗽之因有劳伤肺气，则金不生水；有色欲过度，则真阴涸竭，水虚火旺，肾火刑金；有真阳不足，水泛为痰，则肾经咳嗽之症作矣。"论述了肾阴不足，虚热犯肺的病机变化。治法宜降火滋阴，凉血止血。方药选用《丹溪心法》大补阴丸（黄柏、知母、熟地黄、龟板）合《金匮要略》麦门冬汤（人参、麦冬、半夏、粳米、大枣、甘草）.

Literature Review of Vacuity Heat Invading the Lung

📖 *Zá Bìng Yuán Liú Xī Zhú* ("Incisive Light on the Source of Miscellaneous Disease"), "The Origin and Development of the Various Blood Diseases"

> "In coughing of blood, fire has taken over the position of metal, and the lung network vessels have been damaged; therefore, blood is discharged with cough. If the patient first expectorates phlegm and you see red afterwards, this means that accumulated phlegm has engendered heat. Treat this urgently by downbearing phlegm-fire. If you first see red and afterwards phlegm-cough, this means yīn vacuity stirring fire, which is preventing phlegm from downbearing. Treat this by enriching yīn and downbearing fire."

This quotation unambiguously recognizes the pathomechanism by which effulgent yīn vacuity fire (which also includes kidney yīn vacuity) leads to coughing of blood.

📖 *Shòu Shì Bǎo Yuán* ("Prolonging Life and Preserving the Origin"), "Consumption"

> "Yīn vacuity stirring fire is a disease of taxation consumption. It is created by ministerial fire ascending and overwhelming lung metal. Damage to a person's essence results in yīn vacuity and stirring fire. Wearing of blood results in hyperactivity of fire and depletion of metal…

> "As soon as kidney water is vacuous, ministerial fire stirs frenetically. When it flames upward, it smokes and restrains lung-metal. Owing to the fact that the lung is restrained by fire, we see productive and non-productive cough, phlegm, rapid panting, night sweating, blood ejection, nosebleed, bloody stool, bloody urine, fatigued limbs, vexing heat in the five hearts, dry throat and muteness, tinnitus and flowery vision, seminal emission and turbid urine, *gǔ* distention and fullness, and all sorts of other symptoms difficult to describe."

This quotation describes in detail how kidney yīn depletion, water failing to help fire, and hyperactivity of fire with depletion of metal lead to cough, panting, and blood ejection.

文献评述

《杂病源流犀烛•诸血源流》曰："咳血者，火乘金位，肺络受伤，故血从咳嗽出也。先痰嗽而后见红者，是积痰生热，宜急降痰火；先见红而后痰嗽者，是阴虚火动，痰不下降，宜滋阴降火"。对阴虚火旺（亦包括肾阴虚），引起咳血的病机有清楚的认识。

《寿世保元•痨瘵》曰："夫阴虚火动，劳瘵之疾，盖由相火上乘肺金而成之也。伤其精，则阴虚而火动。耗其血，则火亢而金亏。…盖肾水一虚，则相火妄动。相火上炎，熏克肺金。肺受火邪所克，所以为咳、为嗽、为痰，为喘急，为盗汗，为吐血、衄血，为便血、尿血，为四肢倦怠，为五心烦热，为咽干声哑，为耳鸣眼花，为遗精便浊，为蛊胀肿满，为一切难状之症。"详细描述了肾阴亏虚，水不制火，火亢金亏，而致咳喘吐血的病机变化。

Summary of Vacuity Heat Invading the Lung

1. Vacuity Fire Flaming Upward

   Lung wilting with scorched lobes, coughing and spitting of turbid spittle and foamy drool, cough and counterflow with ejection of blood.

2. Yīn Liquid Deprived of Nourishment

   Limp aching lower back and knees, emaciation.

3. Vacuity Heat Harassing Internally

   Vexing heat in the five hearts, reddening of the cheeks and night sweating, tinnitus and deafness.

4. Yīn Vacuity Internal Heat

   Red tongue with scant fur, surging large cubit pulse.

虚热犯肺
虚火上炎—肺痿叶焦，咳吐浊唾涎沫，咳逆咯血
阴津失养—腰膝酸软，形体消瘦
虚热内扰—五心烦热，颧红盗汗，耳鸣耳聋
阴虚内热—舌红苔少，尺脉洪大

3.6.5 Vacuity Fire Harassing the Teeth

The kidney governs the bones, and the teeth are the surplus of the bone. Yīn essence in the kidney is able to ascend and nourish the teeth. Factors such as weak health in old age or damage to yīn from enduring illness can cause insufficiency of kidney yīn and effulgent yīn vacuity fire. When vacuity fire flames upward, it scorches the teeth, resulting in the pathomechanism of vacuity fire harassing the teeth.

When kidney yīn is vacuous, yīn is vacuous and deprived of enrichment, and the teeth are deprived of nourishment. The result is dry gums, desiccated appearance, gingival atrophy, and loosening of the teeth.

When vacuity fire harasses the upper body, the blood network vessels in the gums are stopped. The result is red gums and toothache that persists for years without abatement.

Effulgent yīn vacuity fire results in a red tongue with scant fur, and a fine sunken rapid pulse.

The chapter, "Teeth" in the *Jǐng Yuè Quán Shū* ("Jǐng-Yuè's Complete Compendium") states:

> "There are three disease patterns that affect the teeth: The first is fire, the second is worms, and the third is kidney vacuity… When the kidney is vacuous, the teeth are not secure, and either loosen or become brittle and protrude. Although you should supplement the kidney as your key concern, you must also identify whether it is a heat or cold condition. In all cases, *yòu guī wán* (Right-Restoring [Life Gate] Pill) and *liù wèi wán* (Six-Ingredient Pill) can invigorate yīn in the kidney."

This quotation clearly indicates the pathomechanism by which kidney yīn vacuity can bring about toothache.

The chapter, "Vacuity Fire Toothache" in the *Yīn Xū Zhèng Zhì* ("Yīn Vacuity Patterns and Treatment) also states:

> "Toothache refers to pain in the gums and roots of the teeth. The teeth are the surplus of the bone, and the gums are the network vessels of the

> teeth. Vacuity fire toothache is mostly caused by constitutional insufficiency, which results in effulgent yīn vacuity fire flaming upward and scorching…
>
> "Its symptoms are dull toothache, floating roots of the teeth, red cheeks and lips, dry throat, limp aching lumbar spine, vacuity vexation and insomnia, red tongue with scant fur, and mostly a fine rapid pulse. Treat this by enriching yīn and extinguishing fire. Administer *zuǒ guī wán* (Left-Restoring [Kidney Yīn] Pill) with modifications."

This is a rather comprehensive summary of the pathomechanical changes of kidney yīn depletion and vacuity fire harassing the teeth.

Vacuity fire harassing the teeth is treated by enriching yīn and clearing heat, and by downbearing fire and returning it to the kidney. Recommended formulas are *yòu guī wán* (Right-Restoring [Life Gate] Pill) from the *Jǐng Yuè Quán Shū* ("Jǐng-Yuè's Complete Compendium") or *jiàng huǒ guī shèn fāng* (Downbear Fire and Return Qi to the Kidney Formula) from Yè Tiān-Shì's *Lín Zhèng Zhǐ Nán Yī Àn* ("A Clinical Guide with Case Histories").

Zuǒ Guī Wán 左归丸
Left-Restoring [Kidney Yīn] Pill

shú dì huáng (熟地黄 Rehmanniae Radix Praeparata, cooked rehmannia)
shān yào (山药 Dioscoreae Rhizoma, dioscorea)
gǒu qǐ zǐ (枸杞子 Lycii Fructus, lycium)
niú xī (牛膝 Achyranthis Bidentatae Radix, achyranthes)
lù jiǎo (鹿角 Cervi Cornu, deerhorn)
guī bǎn (龟版 Testudinis Plastrum, tortoise plastron)
shān zhū yú (山茱萸 Corni Fructus, cornus)
tù sī zǐ (菟丝子 Cuscutae Semen, cuscuta)

Jiàng Huǒ Guī Shèn Fāng 降火归肾方
Downbear Fire and Return Qi to the Kidney Formula

shān zhū yú (山茱萸 Corni Fructus, cornus)
wǔ wèi zǐ (五味子 Schisandrae Fructus, schisandra)
niú xī (牛膝 Achyranthis Bidentatae Radix, achyranthes)
nǚ zhēn zǐ (女贞子 Ligustri Lucidi Fructus, ligustrum)
mò hàn lián (墨旱莲 Ecliptae Herba, eclipta)
yán (盐 Sal, salt)

虚火扰齿

肾主骨，齿为骨之余，肾中阴精能上养牙齿。年老体弱，或久病伤阴等因素导致肾阴虚不足，阴虚火旺，虚火上炎，灼伤牙齿，则可引起虚火扰齿的病机变化。肾阴虚，阴虚失滋，牙齿失养，则牙龈干燥，形色枯槁，牙龈萎缩，牙齿动摇；虚火上扰，齿龈血络不通，则牙龈红赤，齿痛经年不愈；肾阴不足，形体、腰膝失滋，则腰膝酸软，形体消瘦；阴虚内热，则五心烦热，潮热盗汗。阴虚火旺，则舌红少苔，脉沉细数。如《景岳全书•齿牙》曰："齿牙之病有三证：一曰火，二曰虫，三曰肾虚。...肾虚牙齿不固，或摇动，或脆弱浮突者，虽宜以补肾为主，然亦当辨其寒热。凡左归丸、六味丸，可壮肾中之阴。"明确指出了肾阴虚可致牙齿疼痛的病机。《阴虚证治•虚火牙痛》也云："牙痛，是指牙龈、牙根疼痛而言。齿为骨之余，龈为齿之络。虚火牙痛，多因禀赋不足，阴虚火旺，虚火上炎，灼烁致病。...其证牙齿隐痛，牙根浮动，颧红唇赤，咽干而燥，腰脊酸软，虚烦不寐，舌红少苔，脉多细数。治宜滋阴熄火，当予左归丸加减。"较为全面总结肾阴亏虚，虚火扰齿的病机变化。治法宜滋阴清热，降火归肾。方药选用《景岳全书》左归丸（熟地、山药、枸杞子、川牛膝、鹿胶、龟胶、山茱萸、菟丝子），或选用叶天士《临证指南医案》降火归肾方（山萸肉、五味子、牛膝、女贞子、旱莲草、盐）。

Literature Review of Vacuity Fire Harassing the Teeth

📖 *Zá Bìng Yuán Liú Xī Zhú* ("Incisive Light on the Source of Miscellaneous Disease"), "The Origin and Development of Disease in the Mouth, Teeth, Lips, and Tongue"

> "The teeth are the tip of the kidney and the root of bone… Cases that present with painful swollen gums and no swelling of the head and face, or with swelling of the head and face, but not too severe redness and swelling in the gums are all related to vacuity fire. It happens that in people with constitutional yīn depletion the qì of warm evil surges upward and causes toothache connecting to the vertex."

This quotation discusses how yīn vacuity (kidney yīn vacuity) and vacuity fire flaming upward bring about toothache.

📖 *Yī Biǎn* (“Lancing Stones of Medicine”), “Miscellaneous Pathoconditions: Teeth”

> “In kidney vacuity, when the teeth rise and extend and wobble to the point of falling out, *liù wèi wán* (Six-Ingredient Pill) is recommended.”

This quotation expresses the notion that insufficiency of kidney yīn and vacuity fire harassing the teeth can cause loosening of the teeth.

文献评述

《杂病源流犀烛•口齿唇舌病源流》曰：“齿者，肾之标，骨之本也。...有牙龈肿痛，头面不肿，或头面肿，牙龈反不甚红肿者，皆虚火也。...有阴亏体质，被温邪之气上冲、齿痛连头巅者。”论述了阴虚（包括肾阴虚），虚火上炎而致牙齿疼痛的病机变化。

《医碥•杂症•齿》曰：“肾虚牙浮长，动摇欲脱者，六味丸。”示意肾阴不足，虚火扰齿，可致牙齿动摇。

Summary of Vacuity Fire Harassing the Teeth

1. Teeth Deprived of Nourishment

   Dry gums, desiccated appearance, gingival atrophy, loosening of the teeth.

2. Vacuity Fire Harassing the Upper Body

   Red gums, toothache that persists for years without recovery.

3. Loss of Enrichment to the Formal Body and Lower Back and Knees

   Limp aching lower back and knees, emaciation.

4. Yīn Vacuity Internal Heat

   Vexing heat in the five hearts, tidal heat, night sweating.

5. Effulgent Yīn Vacuity Fire

   Red tongue with scant fur, fine sunken rapid pulse.

虚火扰齿

牙齿失养—牙龈干燥，形色枯槁，牙龈萎缩，牙齿动摇

虚火上扰—牙龈红赤，齿痛经年不愈

形体、腰膝失滋—腰膝酸软，形体消瘦

阴虚内热—五心烦热，潮热盗汗

阴虚火旺—舌红少苔，脉沉细数

3.6.6 Vacuity Heat Harassing the Throat

The kidney channel runs along the mouth, tongue, and throat. In "Treatise on Strange Diseases" in the *Sù Wèn* ("Plain Questions") it states: "The foot lesser yīn vessel passes through the kidney and ties to the root of the tongue." The kidney's yīn essence has a nourishing and moistening effect on the throat. If kidney yīn is depleted, yīn liquid is unable to bear upward to the throat, and vacuity fire flames upward instead. This can cause the pathomechanism of vacuity heat harassing the throat.

When kidney yīn is insufficient, liquid becomes scant and is deprived of enrichment, and the throat is deprived of nourishment. The result is dry itchy throat and dry mouth and tongue.

When vacuity fire surges upward and flames the throat, qì and blood are depressed and bind, putrefying flesh and vanquishing blood. The result is tenderness, redness, pain, and putrefaction in the pharynx, mouth and tongue sores, cough and counterflow, and hoarse voice.

Vacuity fire concentrates liquid into phlegm, which binds in the throat. The result is phlegm in the throat that cannot be ejected.

Effulgent yīn vacuity fire results in a red tongue with scant fur and lack of liquid, and a fine rapid pulse.

The treatise "On Heat" in the *Líng Shū* ("The Magic Pivot") points out: "On the fifth day of cold damage, it is contracted by lesser yīn. Since the lesser yīn vessel passes through the kidney, nets the lung, and ties to the root of the tongue, the result is dry mouth and tongue, and thirst." This states that on the fifth day of cold damage, lesser yīn has caught the disease. Consequently, kidney yīn is depleted and vacuity fire ascends and steams the throat. Therefore, the pathomechanism of dry mouth and tongue appears.

The chapter, "The Throat" in *Jǐng Yuè Quán Shū* ("Jǐng-Yuè's Complete Compendium"), "Schema of Miscellaneous Patterns" further states:

> "Throat impediment is ascribed to all channels. Lesser yáng, yáng brightness, reverting yīn, and lesser yīn are all affected by this pattern... The reverting yīn channel nets the pubic bone, ends at the epiglottis, and ties to the root of the tongue. Whenever yīn fire surges upward in counterflow, it mostly constitutes throat impediment...
>
> "If excesses of drink and sex have caused true yīn depletion, this is a pattern of vacuity fire within the kidney, and cannot be dealt with in any other way than by invigorating water...
>
> "The signs of yīn vacuity throat impediment are also internal heat, thirst, dry throat, as well as possibly reddening of the lips and cheeks, phlegm-

> drool congestion, and invariably a cubit pulse that lacks spirit, or possibly a rapid but floating, soft, and forceless pulse in all six pulses. If inspection additionally reveals excesses of liquor and sex or a constitutional insufficiency of yīn qì with increased fatigue and reduced strength, these signs all indicate depletion of kidney yīn and water failing to restrain fire."

This quotation clearly indicates the pathomechanism by which kidney yīn depletion, water failing to restrain fire, and vacuity fire flaming upward bring about a sore swollen throat.

Vacuity heat harassing the throat is treated by enriching yīn and clearing fire, and by disinhibiting the throat and relieving pain. Recommended formulas are *zhī bǎi dì huáng tāng* (Anemarrhena, Phellodendron, and Rehmannia Decoction) from the *Yī Zōng Jīn Jiàn* ("The Golden Mirror of Medicine") or *zī yīn qīng yān tāng* (Nourish Yin Throat-Clearing Decoction) from Yè Tiān-Shì's *Lín Zhèng Zhǐ Nán Yī Àn* ("A Clinical Guide with Case Histories").

Zhī Bǎi Dì Huáng Tāng 知柏地黄汤 Anemarrhena, Phellodendron, and Rehmannia Decoction
zhī mǔ (知母 Anemarrhenae Rhizoma, anemarrhena)
huáng bǎi (黄柏 Phellodendri Cortex, phellodendron)
shēng dì huáng (生地黄 Rehmanniae Radix, rehmannia)
shān zhū yú (山茱萸 Corni Fructus, cornus)
shān yào (山药 Dioscoreae Rhizoma, dioscorea)
mǔ dān pí (牡丹皮 Moutan Cortex, moutan)
fú líng (茯苓 Poria, poria)
zé xiè (泽泻 Alismatis Rhizoma, alisma)

Zī Yīn Qīng Yān Tāng 滋阴清咽汤 Nourish Yin Throat-Clearing Decoction
shēng dì huáng (生地黄 Rehmanniae Radix, rehmannia)
xuán shēn (玄参 Scrophulariae Radix, scrophularia)
rén zhōng bái (人中白 Hominis Urinae Sedimentum, urine sediment)
nuò dào gēn xū (糯稻根须 Oryzae Glutinosae Radix, glutinous rice root)
gān cǎo (甘草 Glycyrrhizae Radix, licorice)
jī zǐ huáng (鸡子黄 Galli Vitellus, egg yolk)

虚热扰咽

肾经经脉循行于口舌咽喉，如《素问•奇病论》曰："足少阴之脉，贯肾系舌本。"肾之阴精对咽喉有滋养、濡润的作用。如肾阴亏虚，阴津不能上承咽喉，虚火上炎，可出现虚热扰咽的病机改变。肾阴不足，津少失滋，咽喉失养，则咽干喉痒，口舌干燥; 虚火上冲，熏于咽喉，气血郁结，腐肉败血，则咽部嫩红，咽痛腐烂，口舌生疮，咳逆声嘶; 虚火炼津为痰，结于咽喉，则咽中有痰，吐之不出。阴虚火旺，则舌红少苔乏津，脉细数。如《灵枢•热论》指出："伤寒五日，少阴受之，少阴脉贯肾络于肺，系舌本，故口燥舌干而渴。"伤寒五日，少阴已病，肾阴亏虚，虚火上蒸咽喉，故出现口燥舌干的病机。又如《景岳全书•杂证谟•咽喉》曰："喉痹所属诸经，凡少阳、阳明、厥阴、少阴皆有此证，...少阴之脉络于横骨，终于会厌，系于舌本，凡阴火逆冲于上，多为喉痹。...若因酒色过度，以致真阴亏损者，此肾中之虚火证也，非壮水不可。...阴虚喉痹，其证亦内热口渴喉干，或唇红颊赤，痰涎壅盛，然必尺脉无神，或六脉虽数而浮软无力，但察其过于酒色，或素禀阴气不足，多倦少力者，是皆肾阴亏损，水不制火而然。"明确指出了肾阴亏损，水不制火，虚火上炎引起咽喉肿痛的病机变化。治法宜滋阴清火，利咽止痛。方药选用《医宗金鉴》知柏地黄汤（知母、黄柏、生地黄、山茱萸、怀山药、丹皮、茯苓、泽泻），或选用叶天士《临证指南医案》滋阴清咽汤（大生地、玄参、人中白、糯稻根须、生甘草、大鸡子黄）。

Literature Review of Vacuity Heat Harassing the Throat

📖 *Líng Shū* ("The Magic Pivot"), "Channel Vessels"

> "Disease engendered in the kidney foot lesser yīn channel manifests in heat in the mouth and dry tongue, swollen throat and qì ascent, and dry and painful throat."

This quotation describes the pathomechanical changes in the mouth, tongue, and throat that arise from pathology in the kidney channel.

📖 *Zá Bìng Yuán Liú Xī Zhú* ("Incisive Light on the Source of Miscellaneous Disease"), "Origin and Development of Diseases of the Throat and Voice"

> "Conditions of the throat all mean fire disease. Both the sovereign and ministerial fires of the lesser yīn and lesser yáng channels connect with the throat... Vacuity fire that is caused by excessive drinking,

irascibility, or excessive liking for sex results in phlegm fire attacking upward, dry throat and tongue, dry stool, a rapid vacuous heart pulse, and a faint kidney pulse. These signs indicate water failing to overcome fire, and should be treated by enriching yīn and downbearing fire."

This quotation describes how effulgent kidney yīn depletion fire leads to vacuity heat harassing the throat.

📖 *Yī Biǎn* ("Lancing Stones of Medicine"), "Miscellaneous Pathoconditions: Throat"

"Vacuity fire is due to taxation of the heart from sexual overindulgence and seven-affect internal damage, which leads to depletion of kidney water and upward flaming of fire. If the pain is aggravated in the afternoon, you should enrich yīn and downbear fire. This pattern begins by an initial sensation of dryness in the throat, as if it was irritated or blocked by something hard like hair or grass, with slight redness, swelling and pain. In enduring severe cases, the throat turns dark purple, rather like the color of frozen pomegranate. This is followed by breaking and putrefaction with the rotten coatings piling up like dried baby shrimp, hoarse voice, a putrid smell, and extensive erosion that hampers eating and drinking. *Zhī bǎi dì huáng tāng* (Anemarrhena, Phellodendron, and Rehmannia Decoction) is suitable."

This quotation discusses the pathomechanism of kidney yīn depletion detriment, vacuity fire flaming upward, and sore swollen throat.

文献评述

《灵枢•经脉》曰："肾足少阴也，是所生病，口热舌干，咽肿上气，嗌干及痛。"对肾经病变导致口舌咽喉疾患的病机变化进行了阐述。

《杂病源流犀烛•咽喉音声病源流》曰："咽喉症，皆火病也。少阴少阳君相二火经脉，并系咽喉。…虚火因过饮，或善怒，或好色，痰火上攻，喉舌干燥，便涩，心脉虚数，肾脉微，此水不胜火，宜滋阴降火。"阐述了肾阴亏火旺引起虚热扰咽的病机变化。

《医碥•杂症•咽喉》曰："虚火由劳心好色，七情内伤，以致肾水亏损，火上炎。午后痛甚者，宜滋阴降火。此证初起有觉咽喉干燥，如毛草硬物刺梗，微红肿痛，甚者日久紫暗不鲜，颇似冻榴子色，其后破烂，腐衣叠若虾皮，声音雌哑，臭腐延蚀，妨碍饮食，宜知柏地黄汤。"论述了肾阴亏虚损，虚火上炎，咽喉肿痛的病机。

Summary of Vacuity Heat Harassing the Throat
1. Throat Deprived of Nourishment Dry itchy throat, dry mouth and tongue.
2. Vacuity Fire Surging into the Throat Tenderness and redness in the throat, sore putrid pharynx, mouth and tongue sores, cough and counterflow, hoarse voice.
3. Vacuity Fire Condensing Phlegm Phlegm in the throat, which cannot be ejected outward.
4. Effulgent Yīn Vacuity Fire Red tongue with scant fur and no liquid, fine rapid pulse.

虚热扰咽
咽喉失养—咽干喉痒，口舌干燥
虚火冲咽—咽部嫩红，咽痛腐烂，口舌生疮，咳逆声嘶
虚火炼痰—咽中有痰，吐之不出
阴虚火旺—舌红少苔乏津，脉细数

3.6.7 Vacuity Heat Disturbing Urination

The kidney governs water and manages stool and urine. Yīn humor in the kidney and the kidney's qì transformation are both related to the formation and elimination of urine. Kidney yīn depletion and impaired enrichment or effulgent yīn vacuity fire interferes with the normal opening and closing function of the urinary orifice. As a result, the pathomechanical changes of vacuity heat disturbing urination can appear.

When kidney yīn is insufficient, the source of transformation is insufficient and therefore unable to engender urine. The result is scant yellow or reddish urine.

Depleted water and effulgent fire cause vacuity heat to harass the urinary orifice below and forces blood to move frenetically. The result is bloody and hot scorching urine, and possibly blood strangury.

Distressed by vacuity fire, the elimination of urine is inhibited. This results in dribbling and inhibited urination and in pain in the urethra.

When vacuity heat harasses internally, bladder qì transformation breaks down. This results in dribbling urinary block.

When kidney yīn is depleted, yīn liquid is deprived of nourishment. The result is dizzy head, lack of strength, and limp aching lower back and knees.

Yīn vacuity internal heat results in a red tongue with thin yellow fur, and a fine rapid pulse.

The chapter, "Strangury-Turbidity" in the *Jǐng Yuè Quán Shū* ("Jǐng-Yuè's Complete Compendium"), "Schema of Miscellaneous Patterns" states:

> "In the pattern of red turbidity, patients either have red-colored urine or urine that carries blood with it and is reddened by this... If excessive damage from taxation fatigue, enduring illness, damage to true yīn from liquor and sex, or habitual consumption of cooling substances causes urine to be continuously more red and more scant, but there is no pain or inhibition, this is related to water depletion and desiccation of humor, and not at all comparable to red turbidity."

This quotation indicates how kidney yīn insufficiency leads to vacuity heat internally harassing the urinary orifice and consequently to strangury-turbidity.

The chapter, "Strangury" in the *Yī Biǎn* ("Lancing Stones of Medicine"), "Miscellaneous Pathoconditions" also states:

> "The pathocondition of strangury generally means kidney vacuity and bladder heat. Kidney vacuity results in fire stirring, constant desire to discharge, and inability to store, which causes frequent urination. Heat in the bladder results in dryness of the waterways, which causes inhibited and stagnant exudation, urinary frequency and heat, pain in the penis, and incessant dribbling. Therefore it is called strangury."

Kidney vacuity stirring fire refers precisely to kidney yīn depletion and vacuity fire stirring frenetically. When vacuity heat harasses the urinary orifice, this causes dribbling urination.

Vacuity heat disturbing urination is treated by supplementing the kidney and nourishing yīn, and by clearing fire and freeing strangury. The recommended formula is *huà yīn jiān* (Yīn-Forming Brew) from the *Jǐng Yuè Quán Shū* ("Jǐng-Yuè's Complete Compendium").

Huà Yīn Jiān 化阴煎 Yīn-Forming Brew
shēng dì huáng (生地黄 Rehmanniae Radix, rehmannia)
shú dì huáng (熟地黄 Rehmanniae Radix Praeparata, cooked rehmannia)
niú xī (牛膝 Achyranthis Bidentatae Radix, achyranthes)
zhū líng (猪苓 Polyporus, polyporus)
zé xiè (泽泻 Alismatis Rhizoma, alisma)
huáng bǎi (黄柏 Phellodendri Cortex, phellodendron)
zhī mǔ (知母 Anemarrhenae Rhizoma, anemarrhena)
lóng dǎn cǎo (龙胆草 Gentianae Radix, gentian)
chē qián zǐ (车前子 Plantaginis Semen, plantago seed)
lǜ dòu (绿豆 Phaseoli Radiati Semen, mung bean)

虚热扰溺

肾主水，司二便。肾中阴液，肾的气化，均与小便的生成和排泄有关。如肾阴亏损，失于滋养，或阴虚火旺，干扰溺窍的正常开合功能，则可出现虚热扰溺的病机变化。肾阴不足，化源匮乏，不能化生小便，则尿少黄赤; 水亏火旺，虚热下扰溺窍，迫血妄行，则尿血灼热，或见血淋; 虚火逼迫，排尿不畅，则小便淋涩，尿道疼痛; 虚热内扰，膀胱气化不行，则小便癃闭。肾阴亏损，阴津失养，则头晕乏力，腰膝酸软。阴虚内热，则舌红苔薄黄，脉细数。如《景岳全书•杂证谟•淋浊》曰："赤浊之证，有溺之赤色者，有带血而赤者。...若或以劳倦过伤，或以久病，或以酒色耗伤真阴，或以素服清凉等药，愈服愈赤，愈见短少，而且无痛涩等证者，此系水亏液涸，全非赤浊之比。"指明了肾阴不足导致虚热内扰溺窍，引起小便淋浊的病机变化。《医碥•杂证•淋》也曰："淋症大概肾虚膀胱热，肾虚则火动，常欲泄而不能藏，故数。膀胱热则水道枯涩，故渗出涩滞，数而且热，茎中痛，淋沥不尽，故谓之淋。"肾虚火动，即指肾阴亏损，虚火妄动，虚热扰动尿窍，则为小便淋漓。治法宜补肾养阴，清火通淋。方药选用《景岳全书》化阴煎（生地黄、熟地黄、牛膝、猪苓、泽泻、黄柏、知母、龙胆草，车前子、绿豆）。

Literature Review of Vacuity Heat Disturbing Urination

📖 *Jǐng Yuè Quán Shū* ("Jǐng-Yuè's Complete Compendium"), "Schema of Miscellaneous Patterns: Vacuity Detriment"

> "When urine is yellow, inhibited, and dribbling, it means that true yīn is exhausted and that qì fails to transform water."

This quotation indicates the pathomechanism by which depletion of true yīn and vacuity heat harassing urination lead to strangury-turbidity.

📖 *Bǐ Huā Yī Jìng* ("Bǐ-Huā's Medical Mirror"), "Kidney Section"

> "When there is heat in the kidney, water is desiccated. This occurs in cold damage conditions but is rarely seen among the miscellaneous pathoconditions. The left and right cubit pulses are invariably sunken and rapid or floating and vacuous, and the tongue is black and without fluid. Symptoms include dry mouth and throat, dim vision, inhibited urination, turbid urine, discharge of blood in the urine, and constipation."

The above statement, "water is desiccated," explains the pathomechanism by which kidney yīn depletion and vacuity heat harassing the urinary orifice below lead to strangury-turbidity and inhibited urination.

文献评述

《景岳全书•杂证谟•虚损》曰："小水黄涩淋沥者，真阴亏竭，气不化水也。"指出了真阴亏损，虚热扰溺，而致小便淋浊的病机变化。

《笔花医镜•肾部》曰："肾之热，水将涸也，伤寒门有之，而杂症罕见，左尺右尺必沉数，或浮而空，舌黑无液，其症为口燥咽干，为目不明，为小便不利，为小便浊，为小便出血，为大便秘。""水将涸"，说明了肾阴亏损，虚热下扰溺窍，引起小便淋浊，小便不利的病机。

Summary of Vacuity Heat Disturbing Urination
1. Deficiency in the Source of Transformation Voidings of scant yellow or reddish urine.
2. Blood Forced to Move Frenetically Bloody and scorching hot urine, possibly blood strangury.
3. Vacuity Fire Distressing Dribbling and inhibited urination, pain in the urethra.
4. Breakdown of Qì Transformation Dribbling urinary block.
5. Yīn Liquid Failing to Nourish Dizzy head, lack of strength, limp aching lower back and knees.
6. Effulgent Yīn Vacuity Fire Red tongue with thin yellow fur, fine rapid pulse.

虚热扰溺
化源匮乏—尿少黄赤
迫血妄行—尿血灼热，或见血淋
虚火逼迫—小便淋涩，尿道疼痛
气化不行—小便癃闭
阴津失养—头晕乏力，腰膝酸软
阴虚火旺—舌红苔薄黄，脉细数

3.6.8. Vacuity Heat Dispersion-Thirst

The kidney stores original yīn, which has a nourishing and moistening effect on all the viscera, bowels, and organs throughout the body. Constitutional yīn vacuity or damage to yīn essence from immoderate sexual intercourse and taxation from excessive desires can make kidney yīn insufficient. This can cause yīn heat to arise internally and steam up into the lung and the stomach. When vacuity heat scorches liquid, dispersion-thirst arises.

Dispersion-thirst has the special characteristic of manifesting with increased drinking, increased eating, increased urination, emaciation, and possibly turbid urine and urine with a sweet flavor.

The disease term first occurred in the *Nèi Jīng* ("The Inner Canon"), as for example in the chapter, "The Five Transmutations" in the *Líng Shū* ("The Magic Pivot"): "When the five viscera are all soft and weak, it is most likely the disease of pure-heat dispersion-thirst." This passage explains that the pathomechanism of dispersion-thirst is based on vacuity.

The condition of dispersion-thirst can be divided into upper, center, and lower dispersion thirst. Insufficiency of kidney yīn with liquid damage, dryness, and thirst manifests mostly in the pathomechanism of lower dispersion.

When kidney yīn is depleted, kidney qì is deprived of nourishment and the bladder loses its ability to retain. The result is frequent and profuse urination.

When kidney yīn is depleted and yīn fails to transform qì, kidney qì loses its security and the subtle essence of grain and water pours downward. This results in turbid unctuous urine with a sweet flavor.

Owing to yīn vacuity internal heat, the formal body and the lower back are deprived of nourishment. This results in vexing heat in the five hearts and emaciation.

When kidney yīn depletion causes vacuity heat to scorch liquid, the offices and orifices are deprived of nourishment. This causes dry mouth, throat, nose, and lips, and dry bound stool.

Vacuity heat scorching liquid results in a red tongue with scant liquid, and a fine sunken rapid pulse.

The "Treatise on Dispersion-Thirst, Including Formulas for Treatment" in the *Gǔ Jīn Lù Yàn* ("Ancient and Present Records Verified") explains:

> "The source of dispersion-thirst is found in kidney vacuity... Thirst with inability to drink large amounts of water, but with swelling in the legs, prior thinness of the feet, impotence, and frequent urination constitutes the disease of kidney dispersion. Particularly avoid sexual taxation."

This quotation clearly indicates the pathomechanism by which sexual taxation damaging kidney yīn, kidney yīn depletion, and vacuity heat scorching liquid brings about kidney dispersion.

Elsewhere, the "Section on the Three Dispersion-Thirsts" in the *Dān Tái Yuàn Àn* ("Elixirs from the Jade Table") states:

> "Dispersion means that something is easy to disperse. When evil fire scorches internally, true yīn is desiccated and the person is prone to thirst and hunger, but is unable to nourish the skin and flesh. As food

> and drink enter the stomach, they are instantly and completely dispersed, which is why this condition is called dispersion…
>
> "This is a pathocondition of fire in the heart, spleen, and kidney channels, and the heat in both the heart and spleen channels is caused by kidney vacuity. The kidney governs water, and when true water is not exhausted, it is naturally sufficient for nourishing the spleen and for interacting with the heart above.
>
> "How could there be a disease of dryness dispersion-thirst? It is only when kidney water is vacuous that there is nothing to control fire. Fire becomes effulgent, cannot be extinguished, and boils the viscera and bowels. Due to water exhaustion, fire increases in strength; due to fire strength, water increases in dryness. This pathocondition is formed as a result of exuberant yáng and debilitated yīn, and the diseases of the three dispersion-thirsts begin to flare up."

This quotation describe how kidney yīn depletion and vacuity fire scorching liquid comprise the basic pathomechanism that forms dispersion-thirst.

Vacuity heat dispersion-thirst is treated by enriching yīn and securing the kidney. The recommended formula is *liù wèi dì huáng wán* (Six-Ingredient Rehmannia Pill) from the *Xiǎo Ér Yào Zhèng Zhí Jué* ("Key to Diagnosis and Treatment of Children's Diseases"), with heavy use of *shān yào* (Dioscoreae Rhizoma) and *shān zhū yú* (Corni Fructus) and the addition of *tiān huā fěn* (Trichosanthis Radix), *shā shēn* (Adenophorae seu Glehniae Radix), and *wǔ wèi zǐ* (Schisandrae Fructus).

Liù Wèi Dì Huáng Wán 六味地黄丸
Six-Ingredient Rehmannia Pill

- *shēng dì huáng* (生地黄 Rehmanniae Radix, rehmannia)
- *shān yào* (山药 Dioscoreae Rhizoma, dioscorea)
- *shān zhū yú* (山茱萸 Corni Fructus, cornus)
- *zé xiè* (泽泻 Alismatis Rhizoma, alisma)
- *fú líng* (茯苓 Poria, poria)
- *mǔ dān pí* (牡丹皮 Moutan Cortex, moutan)

Plus:

- *tiān huā fěn* (天花粉 Trichosanthis Radix, trichosanthes root)
- *shā shēn* (沙参 Adenophorae seu Glehniae Radix, adenophora/glehnia)
- *wǔ wèi zǐ* (五味子 Schisandrae Fructus, schisandra)

虚热消渴

肾藏元阴，具有滋养滋润全身脏腑器官的作用。如素体阴虚，复因房室不节，劳欲过度，损耗阴精，肾阴不足，导致阴热内生，上蒸肺胃，虚热灼津，而发为消渴。消渴以多饮，多食，多尿，身体消瘦，或尿浊、尿有甜味为其特征。其病名首见于《内经》，如《灵枢•五变》说："五脏皆柔弱者，善病消瘅。"说明消渴的病机以"虚"为基础。消渴之患，分为上、中、下三消，肾阴不足，津伤燥渴多表现为下消的病机变化。肾阴亏虚，肾气失养，膀胱失约，则小便频数而量多; 肾阴亏虚，阴不化气，肾气失固，水谷精微下注，则小便混浊如膏，有甜味; 阴虚内热，形体、腰府失养，则五心烦热，形体消瘦; 肾阴亏虚，虚热灼津，官窍失养，故口燥咽干，鼻干唇燥，大便干结。虚热灼津，则舌红少津，脉沉细数。如《古今录验方•消渴论及疗之方》说："消渴者，原其发动，此则肾虚所致。...渴饮水不能多，但腿肿，脚先瘦小，阴痿弱，数小便者，此是肾消病也。特忌房劳。"明确指出了房劳伤肾阴，肾阴亏虚，虚热灼津，而引起"肾消"的病机变化。再如《丹台玉案•三消门》曰："消者，易消之谓也。邪火内烁，真阴枯竭，善渴善饥，不能滋养肌肤，饮食入胃，顷刻消尽，故名消症。...乃心脾与肾三经之火症也。而心脾二经之热，又皆由于肾虚，盖肾之所主者水也，真水不竭，自足以滋养乎脾，而上交于心，何至有干枯消渴之病乎?惟肾水一虚，则无以制火，火旺不能扑灭，煎熬脏腑，火因水竭而益烈，水因火烈而益干，阳盛阴衰，构成此症，而三消之患始剧矣。"强调指出肾阴亏虚，虚火灼津是形成消渴的基本病机。治则为滋阴固肾。方药选用《小儿药证直诀》六味地黄丸（生地、山药、山茱萸、泽泻、茯苓、丹皮）重用山药、山茱萸加花粉、沙参、五味子。

Literature Review of Vacuity Heat Dispersion-Thirst

🕮 *Jǐng Yuè Quán Shū* ("Jǐng-Yuè's Complete Compendium"), "Schema of Miscellaneous Patterns: The Three Dispersion-Thirsts"

"The diseases of the three dispersion-thirsts mean that the three burners have contracted disease. ... Lower dispersion-thirst is a disease of the lower burner. It manifests with reddish or yellow urine, strangury or turbidity like paste or fat, black face and parched ears, and gradually increasing emaciation. The disease is located in the kidney and is therefore also called kidney dispersion-thirst… When water fails to help fire, fire fails to return to its source. Fire wanders into the lung causing upper dispersion, fire wanders into the stomach causing center dispersion, and fire scorches yīn essence causing lower dispersion. This is a pattern of dispersion-thirst due to insufficiency of true yīn and depletion of water in the lower body."

This quotation incisively discusses how kidney yīn depletion and vacuity fire scorching liquid form dispersion-thirst.

🕮 *Zá Bìng Yuán Liú Xī Zhú* ("Incisive Light on the Source of Miscellaneous Disease"), "The Origin and Development of the Three Dispersion-Thirsts"

"Lower dispersion refers to the kidney and is caused by kidney yīn vacuity or by latent fire in the lower burner… Because kidney water is depleted, the fluids are desiccated. Owing to depleted water, fire is effulgent and scorches lung-metal. Affected by fire evil, the lung is unable to engender the kidney. Therefore, lower dispersion-thirst is formed."

This quotation analyzes the pathomechanism by which insufficiency of kidney yīn and vacuity fire scorching liquid leads to dispersion-thirst.

文献评述

《景岳全书•杂证谟•三消》曰："三消之病，三焦受病也。…下消者下焦病也，小便黄赤，为淋为浊，如膏如脂，面黑耳焦，日渐消瘦，其病在肾，故又名肾消也。…盖水不济火，则火不归源，故有火游于肺而为上消者，有火游于胃而为中消者，有火烁阴精而为下消者，是真阴不足，水亏于下之消证也。"明确论述了肾阴亏虚，虚热灼津而成消渴的病机改变。

《杂病源流犀烛•三消源流》曰："下消肾也，由肾阴虚，或火伏下焦，…盖缘肾水亏虚，津液枯竭，水亏火旺，蒸烁肺金，肺被火邪，不能生肾，故成下消也。"对肾阴不足，虚热灼津而引起消渴的病机变化进行了阐述.

Summary of Vacuity Heat Dispersion-Thirst
1. Loss of Retention in the Bladder Profuse and frequent urination.
2. Subtle Essences Pouring Downward Turbid unctuous urine with a sweet flavor.
3. Formal Body and Lower Back Deprived of Nourishment Vexing heat in the five hearts, emaciation.
4. Offices and Orifices Deprived of Nourishment Dry mouth, throat, nose, and lips; dry bound stool.
5. Vacuity Heat Scorching Liquid Red tongue with scant liquid, fine sunken rapid pulse.

虚热消渴
膀胱失约—小便频数而量多
精微下注—小便混浊如膏，有甜味
形体、腰府失养—五心烦热，形体消瘦
官窍失养—口燥咽干，鼻干唇燥，大便干结
虚热灼津—舌红少津，脉沉细数

3.7 Vacuity Fire Floating Upward

The kidney governs water and stores original yīn and original yáng. If kidney yīn is depleted, yīn does not restrain yáng, and vacuity fire arises internally. Fire is a yáng evil and thus susceptible to upbearing and to stirring. Its nature is to flame upward. Therefore, it can bring about the pathomechanism of vacuity fire floating upward. Because of differences in this pathomechanism, we can further divide it into two types: dragon fire floating upward and fire failing to return to its source.

虚火上浮

肾主水，藏元阴元阳，如肾阴亏损，阴不制阳，虚火内生，火为阳邪，易升易动，其性上炎，故可引起虚火上浮的病机。因虚火上浮引起的病机有别，可进一步将其分为龙火上浮、火不归原二种类型。

3.7.1 Dragon Fire Floating Upward

The kidney belongs to water, and among the eight trigrams relates to *kǎn* (坎). Its image is the dragon, and the dragon lying submerged on the bottom of the sea is its physiology. When the dragon soars upward in flight, fire flames up along with it, and the state of illness arises. Because kidney fire is the same as life fire and depends on kidney water (yīn) to restrain it, it is only when water is able to moisten wood that it can maintain the state of water and fire helping each other, and of yīn and yáng being balanced.

Thus, in the *Yī Guàn* ("Thorough Knowledge of Medicine") Zhào Xiàn-Kě wrote: "The fire of the sovereign of the life gate is fire within water. These two are interdependent and must never depart from each other." This passage points to the state of balance between water and fire. If kidney water is depleted, dragon fire is without restraint, surges, and rises. This is exactly the pathomechanism of dragon fire not lying submerged, but floating astray upward.

The kidney is an important viscus. As soon as yīn humor is insufficient, vacuity fire ascends and becomes a force that is difficult to stem. In ancient China, the dragon was commonly depicted as soaring and the dragon's strength was considered to be exceptional. Thus when kidney yīn is depleted, the force of vacuity fire floating upward resembles a powerful and difficult to control dragon soaring upward in flight. Therefore, it is called dragon fire floating upward. Because this fire arises due to kidney yīn vacuity, it is also called "vacuity fire," "floating fire," and "rootless fire."

When kidney yīn is insufficient, yīn does not restrain yáng. Dragon fire floats upward, and vacuity heat accumulates, blocking the ears and causing heat congestion with blood stasis, and putrefied flesh and vanquished blood. The manifestation is pus and blood streaming from the ears and deafness.

When dragon fire soars and leaps up to harass the head and eyes, liquid is damaged and deprived of enrichment, and the blood network vessels in the face fill up. The result is dry mouth and throat, and red face and eyes.

Vacuity fire floating upward results in a red tongue with scant fur, and a fine sunken rapid pulse.

The chapter, "Fire; Vacuity Fire" in the *Yī Chún Shèng Yì* ("Enriching the Meaning of the Wine of Medicine") states:

> "Kidney fire is vacuity fire. The dragon ceases to hibernate and hide, and instead soars into the upper body. This manifests in dry mouth and throat, red face and eyes, pus and blood streaming from the ears, and deafness. *Jiā wèi shèn rè tāng* (Supplemented Kidney Heat Decoction) governs it."

This is a vivid description of the pathomechanism of kidney yīn vacuity and fire not being stored but floating astray into the upper body.

The chapter, "Origin and Development of Kidney Disease" in the *Zá Bìng Yuán Liú Xī Zhú* ("Incisive Light on the Source of Miscellaneous Disease") contains the following discussion:

> "Only the kidney has both water and fire in the form of true fire of the life gate and true water of hibernation. In the trigram *kǎn*, one yáng line is stored in the midst of two yīn lines; in the same way, the life gate fire is contained within true water. Initially it is not a case of fire being fire and water being water, with the two being separated from each other, but it is like the movement and tranquility of yīn and yáng in heaven and earth: When tranquility reaches its fullness, there is movement, and yáng is engendered within yīn. Consequently, it is able to bear yīn essence upward to attend to the heart ruler. This means upbearing *kǎn* to fill in *lí*. Water and fire thus help each other.
>
> "All this is a mystery of earlier heaven that cannot be comprehended rationally. The ancients said that in the kidney viscus, water resembles the sea, and fire resembles the dragon. When water is warm, the dragon is submerged; when water is cold, the dragon rises. This is what happens in the condition of kidney fire blazing, which is always caused by vacuity cold of kidney water."

This passage describes how water failing to help wood leads to the pathological state of dragon fire floating upward.

This condition is treated by enriching, replenishing, submerging, and restraining, and by supplementing water and downbearing fire. The recommended formula is *jiā wèi shèn rè tāng* (Supplemented Kidney Heat Decoction) from the *Yī Chún Shèng Yì* ("Enriching the Meaning of the Wine of Medicine").

Jiā Wèi Shèn Rè Tāng 加味肾热汤 Supplemented Kidney Heat Decoction
shēng dì huáng (生地黄 Rehmanniae Radix, rehmannia)
cōng bái (葱白 Allii Fistulosi Bulbus, scallion white)
cí shí (磁石 Magnetitum, loadstone)
mǔ lì (牡蛎 Ostreae Concha, oyster shell)
bái zhú (白朮 Atractylodis Macrocephalae Rhizoma, white atractylodes)
mài dōng (麦冬 Ophiopogonis Radix, ophiopogon)
sháo yào (芍药 Paeoniae Radix, peony)
dà zǎo (大枣 Jujubae Fructus, jujube)
gān cǎo (甘草 Glycyrrhizae Radix, licorice)

龙火上浮

肾属水，八卦属坎，在象为龙，龙潜海底，是其生理。龙腾飞跃，火随上炎，则生病况。因为肾火即命火，依赖肾水(阴)以制约，水能涵火，才能维持水火相济，阴阳平衡。赵献可说："命门君主之火，乃水中之火，相依而永不相离。"（《医贯•玄元肤论》）就是指水火相对平衡的状态。若肾水亏虚，龙火无制，冲跃而起，便是龙火不潜，向上浮越的病机。肾为要脏，一旦阴液不足，虚火上升，则成难以阻挡之势，古代中国以龙为图腾，认为龙的力量非常强大，肾阴亏损，虚火上浮之势有如龙之飞腾，不易控制，故称为龙火上浮。此火是因肾阴虚而起，故又有"虚火"、"浮游之火"、"无根之火"等称谓。肾阴不足，阴不制阳，龙火上浮，虚热聚积，耳窍闭塞，热壅血瘀，肉腐血败，则耳流脓血，不闻人声; 龙火腾跃，上扰头面，津伤失滋，面部血络充盈，则口燥咽干，面目红赤; 虚火上浮，则舌红少苔，脉沉细数。如《医醇剩义•火•肾火》云："肾火者，龙火也，龙不蛰藏，飞腾于上，口燥咽干，面红目赤，耳流脓血，不闻人声，加味肾热汤主之。"对肾阴虚而火不藏，浮越于上的病机进行了清晰的阐述。《杂病源流犀烛•肾病源流》论述到："独肾有水火两具，而命门真火，与蛰藏真水两相并见。然坎中一阳，要即藏于两阴之中，故命门之火，即涵于真水之内，初非火是火，水是水，截分为二者，殆如天地之阴阳动静然，静极而动，阳生阴中，遂能升阴精以上奉心主，此升坎填离，水火既济，皆先天之神妙，不可思议者也。先辈云：肾之脏，水犹海，火犹龙，水暖则龙潜，水寒则龙起，是肾火炎炽为患，皆由肾水虚寒。"论述水不济火，导致龙火上浮的病机变化。治法宜滋填潜纳，补水降火。方药选用《医醇剩义》加味肾热汤（生地黄汁、葱白、磁石、牡蛎、炒白术、麦冬、芍药、大枣、甘草）。

Literature Review of Dragon Fire Floating Upward

📖 *Yī Xué Zhèng Zhuàn* ("The Orthodox Tradition of Medicine"), "Ear Disease"

> "Lack of moderation in sensual desires, excessive taxation from overwork, or the after-effects of a major illness in the later half of a person's life can cause desiccation of kidney water and upflaming of yīn fire. Because of this, there is itching in the ear and tinnitus occurring every single day, like the singing of cicadas or the sounds of bells and drums, so severe as to be abominable. If not treated in the early stages, it will eventually turn into senility. What a great shame!"

This quotation deftly describes how kidney yīn vacuity and vacuity fire flaming upward and harassing the normal physiological functions of the ears can lead to tinnitus and deafness and when untreated to senility.

📖 *Zá Bìng Yuán Liú Xī Zhú* ("Incisive Light on the Source of Miscellaneous Disease"), "Origin and Development of Ear Disease"

> "The ears are ascribed to the foot lesser yīn channel and are the orifices entrusted to the kidney… Separately treat the stirring yīn vacuity fire that is causing the deafness. *Liù wèi wán* (Six-Ingredient Pill) is suitable, with the addition of *zhī mŭ* (Anemarrhenae Rhizoma), *huáng băi* (Phellodendri Cortex) *yuăn zhì* (Polygalae Radix), and *shí chāng pú* (Acori Tatarinowii Rhizoma), all stir-fried with brine."

This passage enumerates the medicinals that can treat deafness caused by yīn vacuity stirring fire.

📖 *Wàn Bìng Huí Chūn* ("Return-of-Spring for All Diseases"), "Ear Disease"

> "Enduring deafness is primarily the responsibility of the kidney. In fulminant disease [the pulse] is floating and surging; both cubit pulses are identical. If they are both rapid, it means that vacuity fire is surging upward."

In this quotation the cubit pulses give indication of how insufficiency of kidney yīn and dragon fire surging upward lead to deafness.

文献评述

《医学正传•耳病》曰：“其或嗜欲无节，劳役过度，或中年之后，大病之余，肾水枯涸，阴火上炎，故耳痒耳鸣，无日而不作也。或如蝉噪之声，或如钟鼓之响，甚为可恶，早而不治，渐而至于龙钟，良可叹哉!”明确论述了肾阴虚，虚火上炎，扰乱耳窍的正常生理功能引起耳鸣耳聋的病机变化。

《杂病源流犀烛•耳病源流》曰：“耳属足少阴，肾之寄窍也。…耳聋之其由阴虚火动别治。宜六味丸加知母、黄柏、远志、菖蒲，并盐水炒。”阴虚火动，即指肾阴亏虚，浮火扰动，可致耳聋。

《万病回春•耳病》曰：“久聋者，专于肾责。暴病浮洪，两尺相同;或两尺数，阴火上冲”。明确提出了肾阴不足，龙火上冲，而致耳聋的病机变化。

Summary of Dragon Fire Stirring

1. Dragon Fire Harassing the Ears

   Pus and blood streaming from the ears, deafness.

2. Dragon Fire Harassing the Head

   Dry mouth and throat, red face and eyes.

3. Vacuity Fire Floating Upward

   Red tongue with scant fur, fine sunken rapid pulse.

龙火欲动

龙火扰耳—耳流脓血，不闻人声

龙火扰头—口燥咽干，面目红赤

虚火上浮—舌红少苔，脉沉细数

3.7.2 Fire Failing to Return to its Source

The healthy performance of vital activities in the body is rooted in the balance of yīn and yáng. When yīn humor is insufficient, yáng qì manifests with a corresponding exuberance. In locations where yáng qì accumulates, superabundant qì becomes fire. Therefore, yīn vacuity forms fire, and vacuity heat arises internally. If yīn is vacuous, it is unable to subdue yáng, and dragon fire soars into the upper body without thinking of returning downward. This results in the pathomechanism of fire failing to return to its source.

When kidney yīn is insufficient and dragon fire soars upward without returning to its source, it can rise and harass the lung, so that lung qì fails to downbear. The symptoms of this are hasty panting, a dark purple facial complexion, and coughing and spitting of blood.

When dragon fire rises to harass the mouth and throat, it putrefies and erodes blood and flesh. The outcome is sore throat, hoarse voice, and oral putrescence and ulceration.

Yīn vacuity internal heat results in tidal heat and night sweating.

When vacuity fire harasses the upper body, it causes reduced liquid and loss of moistening in the upper body. The result is dry mouth and lips, or possibly dry mouth with no desire to drink water.

When kidney yīn is depleted, the dragon soars and fire ascends, while the fluids fail to descend, but collect in the mouth instead. The result is spittle and humor that is not reduced, but paradoxically increased.

Fire failing to return to its source results in red lips and scant tongue fur, and a stringlike pulse.

The "Treatise on the Pathomechanisms of the Viscera and Bowels" in the *Xuè Zhèng Lùn* ("On Blood Patterns") states,

> "When kidney water is plentiful, fire is stored within water, concealing its brightness and hiding its brilliance, and dragon thunder does not ascend. Therefore, sufficient qì means that respiration through the nose is subtle. If water is vacuous, fire fails to return to its source and the various signs of hasty panting and vacuity taxation all arise simultaneously. Thus we see sore pharynx, non-interaction of the heart and kidney, seminal emission and blood loss, swelling, fullness, cough, and counterflow, and phlegm panting and night sweating."

This quotation describes and lists the pathomechanical changes of "fire failing to return to its source."

The chapter, "Fire; Kidney Fire" in the *Yī Chún Shèng Yì* ("Enriching the Meaning of the Wine of Medicine") states:

> "Yáng fire can be drained, but yīn fire can not be drained. It is the dragon's nature to be difficult to tame, to move counterflow and change direction, and to wantonly surge and dash. Therefore, Dān-Xī's *zī shèn wán* (Kidney-Enriching Pill) adds the ingredient *ròu guì* (Cinnamomi Cortex) among yīn-enriching medicinals, to lead the dragon back to the sea. The method of co-acting treatment is most precise and appropriate."

From the angle of therapy, this quotation metaphorically explains the pathomechanical changes of yīn vacuity with yáng hyperactivity, and fire failing to return to the source.

Fire failing to return to its source is treated by enriching yīn and moistening yáng, and by returning fire to its source. The recommended formula is *qián lóng tāng* (Subdue the Dragon Decoction) from the *Yī Chún Shèng Yì* ("Enriching the Meaning of the Wine of Medicine").

Qián Lóng Tāng 潜龙汤 Subdue the Dragon Decoction
lóng chǐ (龙齿 Mastodi Dentis Fossilia, dragon tooth)
guī bǎn (龟版 Testudinis Plastrum, tortoise plastron)
shēng dì huáng (生地黄 Rehmanniae Radix, rehmannia)
lóng gǔ (龙骨 Mastodi Ossis Fossilia, dragon bone)
zhī mǔ (知母 Anemarrhenae Rhizoma, anemarrhena)
huáng bǎi (黄柏 Phellodendri Cortex, phellodendron)
rén shēn (人参 Ginseng Radix, ginseng)
xuán shēn (玄参 Scrophulariae Radix, scrophularia)
gé fěn (蛤粉 Meretricis seu Cyclinae Concha Pulverata, clamshell powder)
ròu guì (肉桂 Cinnamomi Cortex, cinnamon bark)
bào yú (鲍鱼, Haliotidis, abalone)

火不归原

阴阳平衡为人体生命活动正常进行之根本。阴液不足，阳气出现相对亢盛，阳气聚积之处，气有余便是火，是为阴虚化火，虚热内生。阴虚不能潜阳，龙火蒸腾于上，不思下还，则出现火不归原的病机变化。肾阴不足，龙火上腾，火不归原，上扰于肺，肺气不降，则呼吸喘促，面色紫暗，咳唾有血；上扰口咽，腐蚀血肉，则咽喉疼痛，声音嘶哑，口糜溃烂；阴虚内热，则潮热盗汗；虚火上扰，津亏失润，则口干唇燥，或口干不欲饮水；肾阴亏虚，龙腾火升，津液不降，停留口中，则唾液非减反多。火不归原，则唇红少苔，脉弦。如《血证论•脏腑病机论》曰："肾水充足，则火之藏于水中者，韬光匿彩，龙雷不升，是以气足而鼻息细微。若水虚则火不归原，喘促虚劳，诸证并作，咽痛声哑，心肾不交，遗精失血，肿满咳逆，痰喘盗汗。"明确指出了"火不归原"的病机变化。《医醇剩义•火•肾火》又曰："阳火可泻，阴火不可泻。况龙性难驯，逆而折之，反肆冲激，故丹溪滋肾丸，于滋阴药中，加肉桂一味，导龙归海，从治之法，最为精当。"从论治的角度说明了阴虚阳亢，火不归原的病机改变。治法宜滋阴涵阳，引火归原。方药选用《医醇剩义》潜龙汤（龙齿、龟板、生地、龙骨、知母、黄柏、人参、玄参、蛤粉、肉桂、鲍鱼）。

Literature Review of Fire Failing to Return to its Source

📖 *Jǐng Yuè Quán Shū* ("Jǐng-Yuè's Complete Compendium"), "Schema of Miscellaneous Patterns: Vacuity Detriment"

> "There are conditions characterized by a vacuity of yīn within yīn. Such a patient manifests with symptoms such as heat effusion and agitated vexation, red head and face, dry lips and tongue, sore pharynx and mouth sores, blood ejection and spontaneous external bleeding, bloody stool and urine, dry bound stool, and painful inhibited urination."

"Vacuity of yīn within yīn" refers to a vacuity of kidney yīn. This quotation sets forth the clinical manifestations resulting from kidney yīn vacuity, vacuity fire stirring frenetically, and fire failing to return to its source.

📖 *Zá Bìng Yuán Liú Xī Zhú* ("Incisive Light on the Source of Miscellaneous Disease"), "The Origin and Development of Kidney Disease"

> "The kidney is afflicted by both water and fire diseases. In fire disease, dragon fire soars intensely and, scorching upward, causes harm. Signs of this include heat in the mouth and dry throat, heart vexation, a sensation like suspension in the heart, huffing and panting, a lacquer-like facial complexion, and coughing and spitting of blood."

"Dragon fire soars intensely, and scorching upward causes harm" is an image that describes the pathomechanism of kidney yīn vacuity and fire failing to return to its source.

📖 *Zá Bìng Yuán Liú Xī Zhú* ("Incisive Light on the Source of Miscellaneous Disease"), "The Origin and Development of Disease in the Mouth, Teeth, Lips, and Tongue"

> "Mouth sores are always caused by fire, but fire must be divided into vacuity or repletion fire, differentiated by whether the color is pale or red. In vacuity fire, the color of the blood is pale white, and there are macules and speckles with minute indentations, and visible lines like on

> a tortoise-shell. The pulse is vacuous and there is no thirst. This condition is caused by excessive thought and vexation, by increased waking and reduced sleeping, and by vacuity fire stirring and erupting. It should be treated with *sì wù tāng* (Four Agents Decoction), with the addition of *zhī mǔ* (Anemarrhenae Rhizoma), *huáng bǎi* (Phellodendri Cortex), *mǔ dān pí* (Moutan Cortex), and *ròu guì* (Cinnamomi Cortex) to abduct it."

This quotation analyzes how yīn vacuity stirring fire and fire failing to return to its source is the pathogenesis of mouth sores, and gives the appropriate medicinal therapy.

文献评述

《景岳全书•杂证谟•虚损》曰："则有阴中之阴虚者，其病为发热躁烦，头红面赤，唇干舌燥，咽痛口疮，吐血衄血，便血尿血，大便燥结，小水痛涩等证。"其中阴中之阴虚，即指肾阴虚。论述了肾阴虚，虚火妄动，火不归原可引起多种临床表现。

《杂病源流犀烛•肾病源流》曰："肾家本有水火两病，火病者，龙火腾炽，上烁为害也。其症口热咽乾，烦心，心如悬，喝喝而喘，面如漆柴，咳唾有血等类。""龙火腾炽，上烁为害"，即是"火不归原"的别称，是对肾阴虚，火不归原病机的阐述。

《杂病源流犀烛•口齿唇舌病源流》曰："人之口破，皆由于火，而火必有虚实之分，色淡色红之别。虚火血色淡白，斑点细陷，露龟纹，脉虚不渴，此由思烦太甚，多醒少睡，虚火动而发也。宜四物汤，加知、柏、丹皮、肉桂以为引导。"详细分析了阴虚火动，火不归原而致口疮的病机变化。

Summary of Fire Failing to Return to its Source

1. Ascending to Harass the Lung

   Respiration marked by hasty panting, dark purple facial complexion, coughing and spitting of blood.

2. Ascending to Harass the Mouth and Throat

   Sore throat, hoarse voice, oral putrescence and ulceration.

3. Yīn Vacuity Internal Heat

   Tidal heat and night sweating.

<table>
<tr><td>4. Lack of Liquid and Loss of Moistening
Dry mouth and lips, possibly dry mouth with no desire to drink water.
5. Fluids Failing to Descend
Spittle and humor not reduced, but paradoxically increased.
6. Fire Failing to Return to its Source
Red lips, scant tongue fur, stringlike pulse.</td></tr>
<tr><td>火不归原</td></tr>
<tr><td>上扰于肺—呼吸喘促，面色紫暗，咳唾有血
上扰口咽—咽喉疼痛，声音嘶哑，口糜溃烂
阴虚内热—潮热盗汗
津亏失润—口干唇燥，或口干不欲饮水
津液不降—唾液非减反多
火不归原—唇红少苔，脉弦</td></tr>
</table>

3.8 Heat Damaging Kidney Yīn

The kidney is the water viscus, and yīn within the kidney is the root of yīn humor in the body. If a person contracts external disease like wind or cold and sweats excessively, yīn humor is greatly reduced and true yīn is exhausted. Alternatively, an invasion of warm or heat evil can cause heat to blaze exuberantly and consume yīn humor. When this saps kidney yīn, the pathomechanism of heat damaging kidney yīn appears.

The chapter, "The Lower Burner" in the *Wēn Bìng Tiáo Biàn* ("Systematized Identification of Warm Diseases") points out:

> "When enduring warm evil restrains the center burner, the yáng earth of the yáng brightness [channels] cannot restrain lesser *yīn guǐ* water. It either damages yīn after descending or it exhausts yīn before descending.
>
> "If repletion signs are in the majority, right qì has not yet reached the state of being vanquished. In that case, the pulse arrives sunken, replete, and forceful. This condition can still be precipitated, which in the *Shāng Hán Lùn* ("On Cold Damage") is called 'emergency precipitation to preserve liquid.'
>
> "If there is no bound stool in the center, there is less evil heat and more vacuity heat. In such a patient, the pulse must be vacuous. Since the center of the hands and feet governs the interior, heat must be more

> severe there than in the back of the hands and feet, which govern the exterior. If the heat has descended, this means that the person's liquid is exhausted and death will follow quickly."

This quotation describes in detail the pathomechanism of warm-heat evil damage affecting kidney yīn, which results in depletion of true yīn and the existence of vacuity heat inside the body.

Because of differences in the degree to which warm heat evil exuberates and in the depth to which kidney yīn is depleted, we can further differentiate between these pathomechanisms: Intense yīn vacuity fire, wear on true yīn, and yīn collapse with loss of water."

热伤肾阴

肾为水脏，肾中之阴为人体阴液之本。如遇外感风寒一类疾病，发汗太过，阴液大损，而真阴耗竭；或温热之邪侵袭，温热炽盛，耗伤阴液，下汲肾阴，则会出现热伤肾阴的病机变化。如《温病条辨•下焦篇》指出：“温邪久羁中焦，阳明阳土，未有不克少阴癸水者。或已下而阴伤，或未下而阴竭；若实证居多，正气未致溃败，脉来沉实有力，尚可假手于一下，即<伤寒论>中急下以存津液之谓。若中无结粪，邪热少而虚热多，其人脉必虚，手足心主里，其热必甚于手足背之主表也。若再下其热，是竭其津而速之死也。”详细论述了温热之邪伤及肾阴，导致真阴亏损，虚热存内的病机改变。因温热之邪亢盛的程度不同，肾阴亏虚的深浅有别，故可将其进一步分为阴虚火炽、真阴耗损、亡阴失水等三种病机类型。

3.8.1 Intense Yīn Vacuity Fire

The kidney stores original yīn. Debility in old age or enduring illness can damage yīn and cause a root depletion of kidney yīn. If this is further complicated by an invasion of warm heat evil, conditions like irresolvable high heat effusion will appear. Physicians whose pattern identification is incomplete limit their treatment to using effusing and dispersing medicinals to expel exterior evil and fail to take into account the constitutional yīn vacuity. Consequently, after they promote sweating, the external evil is still not terminated, but yīn humor is greatly damaged. This manifests in the pathomechanism of intense yīn vacuity fire.

When exuberant heat damages yīn kidney, yīn is depleted and vacuity heat harasses the inner body. This results in incessant heat vexation and unabating tidal heat.

When heat disease damages yīn, kidney yīn is depleted and therefore unable to ascend and nourish heart yīn. As a result, heart fire becomes abnormally hyperactive. Moreover, this is complicated by evil fire harassing the heart, which further exacerbates heart fire, so that it harasses the heart spirit. The result is heart vexation, agitation, and harassment, and fidgetiness whether lying or standing.

When yīn humor is damaged, its moistening function breaks down. The result is dry mouth with no thought of drinking, and emaciation.

Yīn vacuity internal heat results in a red tongue with scant fur, and a vacuous fine weak pulse.

"Treatise on Aversion to Cold that is not a Cold Disease and Aversion to Heat that is not a Heat Disease" in the *Gé Zhì Yú Lùn* ("Further Treatises on the Properties of Things") states:

> "Regarding yīn vacuity resulting in heat effusion, yáng is the defense of yīn on the outside, and yīn is the guard of yáng on the inside. If the essence-spirit is slack in the outer body, sensual desires lack moderation, yīn qì is dissipated, and yáng has no support. Consequently, it floats and disperses in the area of the fleshy exterior, which results in aversion to heat."

This quotation indicates the pathomechanism by which yīn vacuity can lead to heat vexation.

The chapter, "On the Lower Burner" in the *Wēn Bìng Tiáo Biàn* ("Systematized Identification of Warm Diseases") also states:

> "Heat vexation in the heart means that yáng evil together with heart yáng is alone hyperactive in the upper body, and that heart yīn has no place to be retained in. This causes vexation that is complex and unendurable. Inability to sleep is related to the fact that yáng is hyperactive and fails to enter yīn, and that yīn is vacuous and unable to absorb and take in. Although desiring sleep, how could the patient obtain it? In this pattern, yīn and yáng each go their different paths and do not interact with each other. Death is not far away."

This quotation describes how heat disease damaging yīn, liver-kidney yīn depletion, and vacuity fire harassing the upper body can lead to vacuity vexation and insomnia.

Intense yīn vacuity fire is treated by supplementing the kidney and engendering water, and by enriching yīn and clearing heat. The recommended formulas are *huáng lián ē jiāo tāng* (Coptis and Ass Hide

Glue Decoction) from the *Wēn Bìng Tiáo Biàn* ("Systematized Identification of Warm Diseases") or *yī yīn jiān* (All Yīn Brew) from the *Jǐng Yuè Quán Shū* ("Jǐng-Yuè's Complete Compendium").

Huáng Lián Ē Jiāo Tāng 黄连阿胶汤 Coptis and Ass Hide Glue Decoction
huáng lián (黄连 Coptidis Rhizoma, coptis)
huáng qín (黄芩 Scutellariae Radix, scutellaria)
ē jiāo (阿胶 Asini Corii Colla, ass hide glue)
bái sháo (白芍 Paeoniae Radix Alba, white peony)
jī zǐ huáng (鸡子黄 Galli Vitellus, egg yolk)

Yī Yīn Jiān 一阴煎 All Yīn Brew
shēng dì huáng (生地黄 Rehmanniae Radix, rehmannia)
shú dì huáng (熟地黄 Rehmanniae Radix Praeparata, cooked rehmannia)
sháo yào (芍药 Paeoniae Radix, peony)
mài dōng (麦冬 Ophiopogonis Radix, ophiopogon)
niú xī (牛膝 Achyranthis Bidentatae Radix, achyranthes)
dān shēn (丹参 Salviae Miltiorrhizae Radix, salvia)
gān cǎo (甘草 Glycyrrhizae Radix, licorice)

阴虚火炽

肾藏元阴，若年老体衰，或久病伤阴，肾阴本亏，又遇温热之邪侵袭，出现高热不解等症，医家辨证不全，尽用发散药驱逐外邪，未顾及阴虚体质，发汗之后，外邪未尽，阴液已大伤，表现为阴虚火炽的病机变化。热盛伤阴，肾阴亏损，虚热内扰，则烦热不止，潮热不退; 热病伤阴，肾阴亏损，不能上养心阴，心火偏亢，加之邪火扰心，心火更甚，扰乱心神，则心烦躁扰，卧起不安; 阴液损伤，失于滋润，则口干思饮，形体消瘦。阴虚内热，则舌红少苔，脉虚细弱。如《格致余论•恶寒非寒病恶热非热病论》曰："阴虚则发热，夫阳在外为阴之卫，阴在内为阳之守。精神外弛，嗜欲无节，阴气耗散，阳无所附，遂致浮散于肌表之间而恶热也。"指出了阴虚可致烦热的病机变化。《温病条辨•下焦篇》也曰："心中烦热，阳邪挟心阳独亢于上，心体之阴，无容留之地，故烦杂无耐。不得卧，阳亢不入阴，阴虚不能受纳，虽欲卧得乎？此证阴阳各自为道，不相交互，去死不远。"论述热病伤阴，肝肾阴亏，虚火上扰，可致虚烦不眠。治法宜补肾生水，养阴清热。方药选用《温病条辨》黄连阿胶汤（黄连、黄芩、阿胶、白芍、鸡子黄），或选用《景岳全书》一阴煎（生地、熟地、芍药、麦冬、牛膝、丹参、甘草）。

Literature Review of Intense Yīn Vacuity Fire

📖 *Wēn Rè Zòng Héng* ("A Comprehensive Review of Warm Heat"), "Warm Heat Disease: Effulgent Fire Damaging Yīn and Non-Interaction of the Heart and Kidney"

> "When the evil qì of warm heat blazes inside the body, it assists hand lesser yīn heart fire above and scorches foot lesser yīn kidney water below. This makes heart fire hyperactive in the upper body so that it is unable to interact with the kidney below, and makes kidney water depleted in the lower body so that it is unable to ascend and assist the heart. The more heart fire is hyperactive, the more the heart is damaged, yīn depleted, and fire intensified, to the point where the dynamic forms a vicious cycle. Damage to yīn from intense fire results in generalized heat and dry mouth. When the heart and kidney do not interact and yáng does not enter yīn, evil heat harasses the heart, which causes heart vexation, agitation, and sleeplessness."

This quotation describes in detail the pathomechanism of heat disease damaging yīn and intense yīn vacuity fire.

📖 *Wēn Bìng Xué* ("On Warm Diseases"), "Spring Warmth: Heat Scorching True Yīn"

> "When water and fire help each other and the heart and kidney interact usefully inside a person's body. Heart fire does not get excessively hyperactive and can be subdued. Thus, the person is able to wake and sleep. However, when kidney yīn is depleted and therefore unable to ascend and help heart fire, evil fire intensifies, which makes heart fire hyperactive in the upper body. Because yīn does not restrain yáng, yáng becomes yet more hyperactive, and because yáng hyperactivity damages yīn, yīn becomes yet more depleted. This is what Wú Jū-Tōng referred to as 'yáng being hyperactive and not entering yīn, and yīn being vacuous and not receiving from yáng.' Therefore, this condition manifests in generalized heat effusion, heart vexation, and sleeplessness."

This quotation describes the pathomechanism by which warm heat evil lying latent in kidney yīn and damaging yīn humor leads to intense yīn vacuity fire.

文献评述

《温热纵横•温热病•火旺伤阴心肾不交》曰：“温热邪气内炽，上助手少阴心火，下灼足少阴肾水，致使心火亢于上，而不能下交于肾；肾水亏于下，不能上济于心。心火亢而心愈伤，阴愈亏而火愈炽，势成恶性循环。火炽阴伤，则身热口干。心肾不交，阳不入阴，邪热扰心，故心烦躁不寐。”详细论述了热病伤阴，阴虚火炽的病机变化。

《温病学•春温•热灼真阴》曰：“人之一身，水火既济，心肾相交，则心火不致过亢而得以下潜，人能寤寐。今肾阴亏损，不能上济心火，邪火炽，则使心火亢于上。阴不制阳则阳愈亢，阳亢伤阴则阴愈亏，即吴鞠通所谓：’阳亢不入于阴，阴虚不受阳纳。’故表现为身热，心烦不得卧。”论述了温热之邪伏于肾阴，损伤阴液，导致阴虚火炽的病机变化。

Summary of Intense Yīn Vacuity Fire

1. Vacuity Heat Harassing the Inner Body
   Incessant vacuity heat, unabating tidal heat.
2. Non-Interaction of the Heart and Kidney
   Heart vexation, agitation, and harassment; fidgetiness whether lying or standing.
3. Yīn Humor Losing Enrichment
   Dry mouth and no thought of drinking, emaciation.
4. Yīn Vacuity Internal Heat
   Red tongue with scant fur, vacuous fine weak pulse.

阴虚火炽

虚热内扰—烦热不止，潮热不退。

心肾不交—心烦躁扰，卧起不安。

阴液失滋—口干思饮，形体消瘦。

阴虚内热—舌红少苔，脉虚细弱。

3.8.2 Wear on True Yīn

If warm disease persists for a long time and is drawn out without recovery, heat toxin lodges chronically and damages true yīn. When the vacuity is greater than the evil, the pathomechanism of wear on true yīn forms.

When liver-kidney yīn is depleted, water does not restrain fire, and vacuity heat arises internally. Therefore, we see constant low-grade generalized fever that persists without abating.

Wear on true yīn causes vacuity heat to arise internally. This heat invariably follows the yīn channels to effuse to the outside. Because the Palace of Toil (*láo gōng*, PC-8) of the hand reverting yīn pericardium channel is located in the palm of the hand, and the Gushing Spring (*yǒng quán*, KI-1) of the foot lesser yīn kidney channel in the sole of the foot, the patient feels greater heat in the palms and soles than in the back of the hands and feet.

When true yīn is worn, there is no liquid to bear upward. The result is dry mouth and tongue.

Since kidney water is unable to ascend and assist the heart, heart yīn becomes greatly depleted and the heart spirit is deprived of nourishment. This leads to heart palpitations, lassitude of the spirit and desire to sleep, and in severe cases to clouding of the spirit.

When kidney yīn is unable to ascend and assist the ears and eyes, the result is deafness and unclear vision.

If yīn damage is too severe, the tongue is deprived of nourishment. This can lead to stiffness of the tongue body.

Effulgent yīn depletion fire results in a red tongue with scant fur, and a large vacuous pulse similar to a scallion-stalk pulse, or a flaccid bound intermittent pulse.

The chapter, "On the Lower Burner" in the *Wēn Bìng Tiáo Biàn* ("Systematized Identification of Warm Diseases") points out:

> "In wind warmth, warm heat, warm epidemic, warm toxin, and winter warmth, the evil is located in yáng brightness and lodges there for a long time. Regardless of whether precipitation has already been used or not, if there is generalized heat effusion with a red face and dry mouth and tongue, in severe cases black teeth and cracked lips, and a replete sunken pulse, you can still precipitate. If you see a large vacuous pulse and greater heat in the palms and soles than in the back of the hands and feet, *jiā jiǎn fù mài tāng* (Pulse-Restorative Variant Decoction) governs it."

It also states:

> "If warm disease is mistaken for an exterior pattern and the fluids are robbed, the result is severe trembling in the heart, stiff tongue, and clouded spirit. The method of restoring the pulse is used to restore the fluids.
>
> "In warm disease with deafness, the disease is related to lesser yīn. If you administer *chái hú tāng* (Bupleurum Decoction), the patient will invariably die. After six or seven days, restoring the pulse will restore essence."

This quotation describes how warm heat damaging yīn and affecting heart yīn and kidney yīn, and wear on the fluids can lead to symptoms like heart palpitations, rigid tongue, deafness, and heat in the palms and soles.

Wear on true yīn is treated by enriching yīn, supplementing the kidney, and clearing heat. The recommended formula is *jiā jiǎn fù mài tāng* (Pulse-Restorative Variant Decoction) from the *Wēn Bìng Tiáo Biàn* ("Systematized Identification of Warm Diseases").

Jiā Jiǎn Fù Mài Tāng 加减复脉汤 Pulse-Restorative Variant Decoction
zhì gān cǎo (炙甘草 Glycyrrhizae Radix, mix-fried licorice)
shēng dì huáng (生地黄 Rehmanniae Radix, rehmannia)
bái sháo (白芍 Paeoniae Radix Alba, white peony)
mài dōng (麦冬 Ophiopogonis Radix, ophiopogon)
ē jiāo (阿胶 Asini Corii Colla, ass hide glue)
huǒ má rén (火麻仁 Cannabis Semen, cannabis seed)

真阴耗损

若温病日久，迁延不愈，热毒久羁，损伤真阴，虚多邪少，则可形成真阴耗损的病机变化。肝肾阴亏，水不制火，虚热内生，故身常低热，久留不退; 真阴耗损，虚热内生，热必循阴经而外发，因手厥阴心包经之劳宫穴在手心，足少阴肾经之涌泉穴在足心，则感手足心热甚于手足背; 真阴耗损，无津上承，则口干舌燥; 肾水不能上济于心，心阴大亏，心神失养，乃致心悸，神倦欲眠，甚则神昏; 肾阴不能上济于耳目，则耳聋，目视不清。若阴伤过甚，舌失所养，则可致舌体强硬。阴亏火旺，则舌红少苔，脉虚大，近似于芤，或脉迟缓结代。如《温病条辨•下焦篇》指出：“风温、温热、温疫、温毒、冬温，邪在阳明久羁，或已下，或未下，身热面赤，口干舌燥，甚则齿黑唇裂，脉沉实者，仍可下之。脉虚大，手足心热甚于手足背者，加减复脉汤主之。”又曰：“温病误表，津液被劫，心中震震，舌强神昏，宜复脉法复其津液。”又曰：“温病耳聋，病系少阴，与柴胡汤者必死。六七日以后，宜复脉辈复其精。”论述了温热伤阴，伤及心阴、肾阴，津液耗伤，可导致心悸、舌强、耳聋、手足心热等症状。治法宜滋阴补肾清热。方药用《温病条辨》加减复脉汤（炙甘草、干地黄、生白芍、麦冬、阿胶、麻仁）。

Literature Review of Wear on True Yīn

📖 *Wēn Rè Jīng Wěi* ("Warp and Weft of Warm Heat"), "On Warm Heat Disease by Xuē Shēng-Bái"

> "A damp-heat pattern after more than ten days manifests with a rapid cubit pulse, diarrhea, and possibly sore throat, thirst, heart vexation, and insufficiency of urine. This is a pattern where heat evil directly invades lesser yīn."

In the same text, the commentary in the section on dampness in "Damp Heat Patterns" on the pathomechanical changes of yīn of lesser yīn states:

> "Fluids exit from below the Ridge Spring (*lián quán*, CV-23) on the lesser yīn channel below the tongue. Therefore, whenever lesser yīn contracts an evil, the fluids fail to bear upward, and this results in thirst."

This passage describes the pathomechanism by which wear on true yīn in the advanced stages of warm heat disease leads to thirst.

📖 *Wēn Bìng Zòng Héng* ("A Comprehensive Review On Warm Disease"), "Warm Heat Disease: Wear on True Yīn"

> "Deafness in warm disease is in fact caused by warm disease that has endured over many days to the point where heat evil has dispersed and scorched true yīn, so that kidney yīn is unable to ascend and luxuriate the ears. In addition to deafness, other visible symptoms necessarily include dry mouth and tongue, in severe cases black teeth and cracked lips, greater heat in the palms and soles than in the back of the hands and feet, and a large vacuous pulse. This pattern is caused by wear on true yīn and is associated with pathology of the foot lesser yīn channel."

This quotation summarizes the pathomechanism of warm heat damaging yīn and wear on true yīn.

文献评述

《温热经纬•薛生白温热病篇》曰："湿热证，十余日后，尺脉数，下利，或咽痛口渴心烦，下泉不足，热邪直犯少阴之证。"又在"湿热证"湿中少阴之阴的病机变化后批注到："津液出于舌下少阴经之廉泉穴，故凡少阴受邪，津液不升则渴也。"对温热后期，真阴耗损，口干舌燥的病机变化进行了论述。

《温病纵横•温热病•真阴耗损》曰："温病之耳聋，乃因温病迁延日久，热邪消灼真阴，肾阴不能上荣于耳所致。其见症除耳聋外，还必见口干舌燥，甚则齿黑唇裂，手足心热甚于手足背，脉虚大等症。其证乃因真阴耗损，属足少阴经之病变。"明确指出了温热伤阴，真阴耗损的病机.

Summary of Wear of True Yīn

1. Vacuity Heat Arising Internally
   Constant low-grade generalized fever that persists without abating.
2. Wear on True Yīn
   Greater heat in the palms and soles than in the back of the hands and feet.
3. Lack of Liquid to Bear Upward
   Dry mouth and tongue.
4. Great Depletion of Heart Yīn
   Heart palpitations, lassitude of the spirit and desire to sleep, in severe cases clouding of the spirit.
5. No Assistance to the Ears and Eyes
   Deafness, unclear vision.
6. Tongue Network Vessels Deprived of Nourishment
   Stiffness of the tongue body.
7. Effulgent Yīn Vacuity Fire
   Red tongue with scant fur, flaccid, bound, intermittent pulse.

真阴耗损
虚热内生—身常低热，久留不退
真阴耗损—手足心热甚于手足背
无津上承—口干舌燥
心阴大亏—心悸，神倦欲眠，甚则神昏
不济耳目—耳聋，目视不清
舌络失养—舌体强硬
阴虚火旺—舌红少苔，脉迟缓结代

3.8.3 Yīn Collapse with Loss of Water

The kidney is the water viscus. It has true yīn entrusted to it, and it governs the five humors. When warm heat disease persists for days and months, heat evil scorches liver blood and kidney yīn. Alternatively, frequent precipitation can cause a collapse of yīn and can gradually desiccate essence-blood and fluids in the entire body. Although the evil is also removed slowly, gradually there is great damage to kidney yīn, thus forming the pathomechanism of yīn collapse with loss of water. This is a very critical condition by nature. Although related to the heart and liver, the primary responsibility for it is found in the kidney.

If warm disease persists for a long time, kidney yīn suffers great damage, and the fluids become desiccated and unable to nourish and moisten the skin and flesh. As a result, we see emaciation, dry wrinkled skin, parched lips, and limp tongue.

The liver opens at the eyes, and kidney yīn also ascends and assists the eyes. When liver blood and kidney yīn are greatly damaged, the eyes are deprived of nourishment. The result is sunken eye sockets, dim vision, and confounded eyes.

The kidney governs the bones and engenders marrow. The teeth are the surplus of the bone. When kidney yīn is depleted, the teeth are deprived of enrichment and moistening. The result is teeth dry as desiccated bones.

When the fluids are desiccated, later heaven is deprived of nourishment. Stomach qì vanquishes and expires, turbid qì fumes upward, and qì moves counterflow and does not descend. The result is accumulation of grime on the teeth, hiccup, and faint voice.

When kidney yīn is depleted in the lower body, it forces yáng into the upper body, and vacuity fire harasses the forehead. This results in reddening of both cheeks.

Owing to yīn collapse with loss of water, the channels and vessels are desiccated. This inhibits the flow of blood and makes qì stagnant. Yīn and yáng qì do not join smoothly, and yáng qì is not outthrust to the extremities of the limbs. The result is reverse-flow of the limbs.

When kidney yīn is greatly depleted so that it is unable to ascend and assist the heart, heart yīn and heart qì are exhausted, and the heart is deprived of nourishment. As a result, we see great thudding of the heart. When the heart network vessels are deprived of nourishment, the cardiac muscle becomes hypertonic and contracts. This results in pain in the center of the heart. Spirit deprived of nourishment results in clouding of the spirit and somnolence.

When kidney yīn is greatly depleted, liver yīn can become insufficient since the liver and kidney are of the same source. In that case, the sinews are deprived of nourishment and become hypertonic. In mild cases, the result is wriggling of the extremities; in severe cases, convulsions. These are the pathomechanical changes of water failing to moisten wood and vacuity wind arising internally.

Yīn collapse with loss of water results in a crimson tongue with scant fur, or possibly a bare crimson tongue without any fur. The pulse is fine, rapid, and bound and intermittent, because fine indicates yīn depletion, rapid indicates vacuity heat, and bound and intermittent means yīn collapse with loss of water. This is due to the fact that blood is desiccated and flows only with inhibition and great difficulty. A faint pulse on the verge of expiry is a sign for yīn collapse with loss of water to the point where life is critically endangered.

The chapter, "Fire" in the *Zá Bìng Yuán Liú Xī Zhú* ("Incisive Light on the Source of Miscellaneous Disease") points out:

> "If a person does not know how to conserve and nurture, but depletes true yīn, yáng has no a support and strays upward. This fire is empty and effuses, using the body's qì to merge with yáng. When it merges with yáng, yáng becomes exuberant. This causes heat in the upper burner resulting in cough and engenderment of phlegm, and forcing blood to move upward. Symptoms of this condition are blood ejection and spontaneous external bleeding, vexation and agitation, headache,

inability to sleep, bone pain in the anterior chest, and dry mouth with a bitter taste. The more exuberant yáng is, the more yīn becomes vacuous. The more vacuous yīn is, the more you see vexing heat in the five hearts, tidal heat and steaming bone, seminal emission, wearing of the bones and lack of strength, and short voidings of reddish urine. Lack of warmth in the cinnabar field results in non-transformation of food and drink, diarrhea, and sudden collapse. These are its symptoms."

This quotation describes in detail the pathomechanical changes of true yīn depletion and yīn collapse with loss of water.

Yīn collapse with loss of water is treated by enriching the kidney and nourishing yīn, and by subduing yáng and extinguishing wind. Select from the following formulas according to the degree of severity and urgency of the particular condition:

1. In the initial stages of yīn collapse with loss of water, if you see vacuity wind stirring internally and only slight wriggling of the extremities, *èr jiă fù mài tāng* (Double-Armored Pulse-Restorative Decoction) from the *Wēn Bìng Tiáo Biàn* ("Systematized Identification of Warm Diseases") with the addition of *shēng mŭ lì* (Ostreae Concha Cruda) and *shēng biē jiă* (Trionycis Carapax Crudus) is recommended.

Èr Jiă Fù Mài Tāng 二甲复脉汤 Double-Armored Pulse-Restorative Decoction
zhì gān căo (炙甘草 Glycyrrhizae Radix, mix-fried licorice)
shēng dì huáng (生地黄 Rehmanniae Radix, rehmannia)
bái sháo (白芍 Paeoniae Radix Alba, white peony)
mài dōng (麦冬 Ophiopogonis Radix, ophiopogon)
huŏ má rén (火麻仁 Cannabis Semen, cannabis seed)
ē jiāo (阿胶 Asini Corii Colla, ass hide glue)
mŭ lì (牡蛎 Ostreae Concha, oyster shell)
vbiē jiă (鳖甲 Trionycis Carapax Crudus, raw turtle shell)

2. If you see great thudding in the heart, and in severe cases pain in the center of the heart, this is a sign that heart yīn and heart qì are greatly damaged. Treat this with *sān jiă fù mài tāng* (Triple-Armored Pulse-Restorative Decoction) from the *Wēn Bìng Tiáo Biàn* ("Systematized Identification of Warm Diseases") with the addition of *shèng guī băn* (Testudinis Plastrum Cruda).

Sān Jiă Fù Mài Tāng 三甲复脉汤 Triple-Armored Pulse-Restorative Decoction
zhì gān cǎo (炙甘草 Glycyrrhizae Radix, mix-fried licorice)
shēng dì huáng (生地黄 Rehmanniae Radix, rehmannia)
bái sháo (白芍 Paeoniae Radix Alba, white peony)
mài dōng (麦冬 Ophiopogonis Radix, ophiopogon)
huǒ má rén (火麻仁 Cannabis Semen, cannabis seed)
ē jiāo (阿胶 Asini Corii Colla, ass hide glue)
mŭ lì (牡蛎 Ostreae Concha, oyster shell)
biē jiă (鳖甲 Trionycis Carapax, turtle shell)
guī băn (龟版 Testudinis Plastrum, tortoise plastron)

3. If the patient presents with greatly conspicuous tugging of the extremities, this indicates a severe pattern of vacuity wind stirring internally. Treat this with *dà dìng fēng zhū* (Major Wind-Stabilizing Pill) from the *Wēn Bìng Tiáo Bian* ("Systematized Identification of Warm Diseases").

Dà Dìng Fēng Zhū 大定风珠 Major Wind-Stabilizing Pill
bái sháo (白芍 Paeoniae Radix Alba, white peony)
ē jiāo (阿胶 Asini Corii Colla, ass hide glue)
guī băn (龟版 Testudinis Plastrum, tortoise plastron)
shēng dì huáng (生地黄 Rehmanniae Radix, rehmannia)
huǒ má rén (火麻仁 Cannabis Semen, cannabis seed)
wŭ wèi zǐ (五味子 Schisandrae Fructus, schisandra)
mŭ lì (牡蛎 Ostreae Concha, oyster shell)
mài dōng (麦冬 Ophiopogonis Radix, ophiopogon)
jī zǐ huáng (鸡子黄 Galli Vitellus, egg yolk)
biē jiă (鳖甲 Trionycis Carapax, turtle shell)
zhì gān cǎo (炙甘草 Glycyrrhizae Radix, mix-fried licorice)

亡阴失水

肾为水脏，寄真阴而主五液，温热之病日深月久，热邪消耗肝血肾阴，或数下亡阴，全身精血津液日渐枯竭，而邪亦缓去，渐致肾阴大伤，形成亡阴失水的病机变化。此病情危重，虽与心肝有关，但主要责之于肾。温病日久，肾阴大伤，津液枯竭，不能润养肌肤，则见形体消瘦，皮肤干皱，唇焦舌痿; 肝开窍于目，肾阴亦上济于目，肝血肾阴大亏，目失所养，则目眶塌陷，目暗睛迷; 肾主骨生髓，齿为骨之余，肾阴亏损，齿失滋润，则牙齿干燥如枯骨; 津液枯竭，后天失养，胃气败绝，浊气上熏，气逆不降，则齿上积垢，呃逆声微; 肾阴亏于下，逼阳于上，虚火扰颜，则两颧红赤; 亡阴失水，经脉枯涸，血涩气滞，阴阳气不相顺接，阳气不达于四末，则四肢厥逆; 肾阴大亏，不能上济于心，则心阴、心气亦告竭，心失所养，则见心中憺憺大动; 如心络失养，心肌拘急挛缩，则致心中作痛; 神失所养，则神昏嗜睡; 肾阴大亏，肝肾同源，则肝阴不足，筋失其养，筋脉拘急，轻则手足蠕动，甚则瘛疭，是为水不润木，虚风内生之病机变化。亡阴水亏，则舌绛少苔或光绛无苔。脉细数而结代，因细主阴亏，数主虚热，结代为亡阴失水，血液干枯，流动涩滞艰难。脉细欲绝，是亡阴失水，生命垂危之兆。如《杂病源流犀烛•火》指出："苟不知摄养，亏损真阴，阳无所附，而发越上升，此火空则发，用身之气并于阳也。并于阳则阳盛，故上焦热而咳嗽生痰，迫血上行，而为吐衄，为烦躁，为头痛，为不得眠，为胸前骨痛，为口干舌苦，此其候也。阳愈盛，则阴虚，阴愈虚则为五心烦热，为潮热骨蒸，为遗精，为骨乏少力，为小水短赤，丹田不暖，则饮食不化，为泻泄，为卒僵仆，此其候也。"详细论述了真阴亏虚，亡阴失水的病机改变。治法宜滋肾养阴，潜阳熄风。方药可随症轻重缓急而选用以下方药：（1）若亡阴失水而初见虚风内动，手足略有蠕动之象，可用《温病条辨》二甲复脉汤（加减复脉汤内加生牡蛎、生鳖甲）。（2）若见心中憺憺大动，甚则心中痛，是心阴、心气大伤之兆，治用《温病条辨》三甲复脉汤(二甲复脉汤内加生龟板)。（3）若手足瘛疭大显，已成虚风内动之重证，治用《温病条辨》大定风珠(生白芍、阿胶、生龟板、干地黄、麻仁、五味子、生牡蛎、麦冬、鸡子黄、生鳖甲、炙甘草)。

Literature Review of Yīn Collapse with Loss of Water

🕮 *Wēn Yì Lùn* ("On Warm Epidemics"), "Frequent Precipitation and Collapse of Yīn"

> "In patterns treated by precipitation, when the evil is not completely eliminated despite frequent precipitation, ask whether there is increased dryness in the eyes, a dry dessicated tongue, liquid failing to reach the throat, and dry cracked lips and mouth. The reason is that such a person is endowed with a constitutional profusion of fire and yīn depletion in the yáng viscera, and is therefore now suffering from a severe collapse of fluids. It should be treated with *qīng zào yǎng róng tāng* (Clear Dryness Construction-Nourishing Decoction)."

This quotation describes how inappropriate use of precipitating formulas in cases where warm heat evil has invaded the body leads to great depletion of kidney yīn and severe collapse of yīn and liquid.

🕮 *Wēn Bìng Tiáo Biàn* ("Systematized Identification of Warm Diseases"), "The Lower Burner"

> "When heat evil has penetrated deeply into the lower burner, the pulse will be sunken and rapid, the tongue dry and the teeth black, and the hands and fingers will suffer from contractions. Urgently prevent tetanic reversal. *Èr jiǎ fù mài tāng* (Double-Armored Pulse-Restorative Decoction) governs it."

The passage continues:

> "Warm disease in the lower burner results in deep heat and severe reversal, a fine skipping pulse, great thudding of the heart, and in severe cases, pain in the center of the heart. *Sān jiǎ fù mài tāng* (Triple-Armored Pulse-Restorative Decoction) governs it."

It further states:

> "Heat evil can chronically lodge in the body and scorch true yīn, possibly because of inappropriate resolving of the exterior or because of rash offensive treatment. This condition manifests with lassitude of the spirit, tugging, vacuous vessel qì, crimson tongue with scant tongue fur, and frequent verging on desertion. *Dà dìng fēng zhū* (Major Wind-Stabilizing Pill) governs it. In this treatment, evil qì is 80 or 90 percent gone, and only 10 or 20 percent of true yīn remains. The condition can be recognized by the vacuous pulse and scant tongue fur. Therefore one must copiously use concentrated medicine to replenish yīn and fill in the cracks, while at the same time subduing yáng and settling and stabilizing."

This quotation details a number of pathological processes and indications that result from depletion of true yīn and yīn collapse with loss of water in the later stages of warm disease.

文献评述

《瘟疫论•数下亡阴》曰："下证以邪未尽，不得已而数下之，间有两目加涩，舌反枯干，津不到咽，唇口燥裂，缘其人所禀阳脏，素多火而阴亏，今重亡津液。宜清燥养荣汤。"对温热之邪侵犯人体，而误用下剂，导致肾阴大亏，重亡阴津的病机变化进行了阐述。

《温病条辨•下焦篇》曰："热邪深入下焦，脉沉数，舌干齿黑，手指但觉蠕动，急防痉厥，二甲复脉汤主之。"又曰："下焦温病，热深厥甚，脉细促，心中憺憺大动，甚则心中痛者，三甲复脉汤主之。"又曰"热邪久羁，吸烁真阴，或因误表，或因妄攻，神倦瘛疭，脉气虚弱，舌绛苔少，时时欲脱者，大定风珠主之。此邪气已去八九，真阴仅存一二之治也。观脉虚苔少可知，故以大队浓浊填阴塞隙，介属潜阳镇定。"详细分析了温病后期，真阴亏虚，亡阴失水所引起的一系列病机变化过程。

Summary of Yīn Collapse with Loss of Water

1. Desiccation of the Fluids
   Emaciation, dry wrinkled skin, parched lips, and limp tongue.
2. Eyes Deprived of Nourishment
   Sunken eye sockets, dim vision, and confounded eyes.
3. Teeth Deprived of Moistening
   Teeth dry as desiccated bones.
4. Expiry of Stomach Qì
   Desiccated teeth with accumulated grime, hiccup, and faint voice.
5. Vacuity Fire Harassing the Face
   Reddening of both cheeks.
6. Yáng Qì Failing to Outthrust
   Reverse-flow of the limbs.
7. Heart Deprived of Nourishment
   Great thudding of the heart, pain in the heart.

8. Spirit Deprived of Nourishment

    Clouded spirit and somnolence.

9. Yīn Vacuity Engendering Wind

    Tension of the sinews; in mild cases, wriggling of the extremities; in severe cases, convulsions.

10. Yīn Collapse with Loss of Water

    Crimson tongue with scant fur, or bare crimson tongue with no fur, fine, rapid, bound, and intermittent pulse, or a fine pulse on the verge of expiry.

亡阴失水

津液枯竭—形体消瘦，皮肤干皱，唇焦舌痿

目失所养—目眶塌陷，目暗睛迷

齿失滋润—干燥如枯骨

胃气败绝—齿枯积垢，呃逆声微

虚火扰颜—两颧红赤

阳气不达—四肢厥逆

心失所养—心中憺憺大动，心中作痛。

神失所养—神昏嗜睡

阴虚生风—筋脉拘急，轻则手足蠕动，甚则瘛疭

亡阴水亏—舌绛少苔或光绛无苔，脉细数而结代，或脉细欲绝

Chapter Four

Insufficiency of Kidney Essence

The kidney stores the essence of earlier heaven and governs growth, development, and reproduction. If the endowment of earlier heaven is insufficient and kidney essence is depleted, numerous disturbances of physiological functions like growth, development, and reproduction can follow. As a result, the pathomechanism of insufficiency of kidney essence appears.

While the term kidney essence as such is not explicitly mentioned in the *Nèi Jīng* ("The Inner Canon"), the "Treatise on the Six Periods and Visceral Manifestation" in the *Sù Wèn* ("Plain Questions") contains the following statement: "The kidney governs hibernation, is the root of storage, and the location of essence." The chapter, "The Spirit" in the *Líng Shū* ("The Magic Pivot") further points out: "The kidney stores essence, and essence houses the mind."

The "Treatise of Heavenly Truth from Remote Antiquity" in the *Sù Wèn* ("Plain Questions") also states:

> "The kidney governs water and receives and stores essence from the five viscera and six bowels. Therefore, it can only percolate when the five viscera are exuberant... Nowadays, people consume liquor as if it were water, are regularly frenzied or overexcited, and engage in sexual intercourse while intoxicated. With their desires, they exhaust their essence; with their consumption, they squander the true. Not knowing how retain fullness, they drive the spirit in an untimely manner, devote themselves to pleasing their desires, treat disease adversely with crude medicinals, wake and sleep without regularity, and in this fashion become debilitated in only fifty years."

This passage describes how inappropriate lifestyles and consumption drive the pathomechanism of insufficiency of kidney yīn resulting in premature debilitation.

In the chapter, "Deafness" in the *Zhū Bìng Yuán Hòu Lùn* ("Origin and Indicators of Disease"), the Suí dynasty author Cháo Yuán-Fāng further pointed out::

> "The kidney is ascribed to the foot lesser yīn channel and stores essence... If essential qì is harmonized, the kidney viscus is strong and exuberant and the ears perceive the five notes. If taxation damages qì and blood and this is further compounded by a contraction of wind evil, the result is detriment to the kidney and desertion of essence. Desertion of essence in turn results in deafness."

This quotation notes how pathomechanical manifestations like deafness can result from kidney essence depletion.

In "A Point-by-Point Discussion on the Pathomechanism" of "Dream Emission and Efflux of Essence" in the *Gǔ Jīn Yī Tǒng Dà Quán* ("The Complete Compendium of Medical Works, Ancient and Modern"), the Míng period author Xū Chūn-Fǔ wrote:

> "The *Nèi Jīng* ("The Inner Canon") states that essence is the root of the body, the source of vital qì, and the transformation of marrow... It further states that the kidney gathers essence from the five viscera and six bowels and stores it, and is the key meeting point of yīn and yáng. This means that essence is stored and made in the kidney, and governed by the heart."

This quotation pointed out that the kidney's storage of essence from the viscera and bowels makes it the key meeting point of yīn and yáng.

In the chapter, "Six Causes for Vacuity Pattern" in the *Lǐ Xū Yuán Jiàn* ("The Original Mirror of Rectifying Vacuity"), Wāng Qǐ-Shí stated:

> "The cause of [weakness of] earlier heaven points to the beginning of receiving qì, possibly an age-related debilitaton of the father and mother... When essence-blood is not effulgent, it causes the newborn child to die young or to be weak."

This quotation points out that the kidney is the root of earlier heaven and stores the essence of earlier heaven. Thus, insufficiency of the parents' essence-blood often leads to the pathomechanism of kidney vacuity in their offspring.

The "Discussion of Earlier Heaven True Water" in the Qīng period text *Lǚ Shuāng Jí* ("Records of Lǚ-Shuāng") points out:

> "The root of earlier heaven is the kidney... Therefore, when essence is sufficient, the hundred diseases do not arise, but when essence is exhausted, the myriad evils swarm like hornets."

This quotation describes the importance of sufficient kidney essence for the health of the organism.

The *Nèi Jīng* ("The Inner Canon") stated: "When essence is stored, spring does not cause warm disease." Wú Jū-Tōng used this statement as the basis for his discussion in the chapter, "Original Disease" in the *Zēng Bŭ Píng Zhù Wēn Bìng Tiáo Biàn* ("Supplemental Annotations On Warm Disease Differentiation"):

> "When a patient falls ill with warm disease, a prior vacuity of essence qì must exist. …In the warmth of spring qì, yáng qì rises and strays, and if yīn essence is insufficient for supporting it, this causes warm disease."

This quote offers a succint analysis of the dynamic of insufficiency of kidney essence and occurrence of warm disease.

Insufficiency of kidney essence arises as a result of factors like constitutional insufficiency of earlier heaven, debilitation in old age, excessive sexual taxation and childbirth, or damage from enduring illness. The special characteristic of this pathomechanism is the depletion of kidney essence, as a result of which kidney essence is unable to engender marrow, fill the brain, and fill the bones, the timely arrival of *tiān-guĭ* is affected, or signs of premature exhaustion appear.

Consequently, we can further divide this pathomechanism into ten categories: brain deprived of nourishment, skull deprived of nourishment, lower back deprived of nourishment, bone and marrow deprived of nourishment, retarded growth, decreased fertility, essence depletion causing impaired absorption, essence depletion causing scantness of blood, essence depletion causing vacuity taxation, and essence depletion causing premature debilitation.

肾精不足

肾藏先天之精，主生长、发育，生殖。如先天禀赋不足，肾精亏虚，则可导致生长、发育、生殖等多项生理功能障碍，出现肾精不足的病机变化。肾精一词，《内经》虽未明确提及，但《素问•六节藏象论》曰："肾者，主蛰，封藏之本，精之处也。"《灵枢•本神》又指出："肾藏精，精舍志。"《素问•上古天真论》又曰："肾者主水，受五脏六腑之精而藏之，故五脏盛乃能泻。…今时之人，以酒为浆，以妄为常，醉以入房，以欲竭其精，以耗散其真，不知持满，不时御神，务快其心，逆于生药，起居无节，故半百而衰也。"对生活饮食不规律引起的肾精不足的病机变化有了一定的认识。隋代巢元方《诸病源候论•耳聋候》进一步指出：“肾为足少阴之经，而藏精，…若精气调和，则肾脏强盛，耳闻五音。若劳伤血气，兼受风邪，损于肾藏而精脱，精脱者，则耳聋。”对肾精亏虚可导致耳聋等病机变化有了充分的认识。至明代，对此病机的认识有了进一步发展。徐春甫《古今医统大全•梦遗精滑门•病机叙论》指出：“<内经>曰：精者，身之本，生气之源，髓之化也。…又曰：肾主五脏六腑之精而藏之，阴阳之要会也。是精之藏制在肾，精之主宰在心。”强调肾对精的调节作用。汪绮石《理虚元鉴•虚证有六因》曰：“因先天者，指受气之初，父母或年已衰老，…精血不旺，致令所生之子夭弱。”论述了肾为先天之本，以藏先天之精，父母精血不足，多导致子女肾虚的病机变化。清代《履霜集•先天真水论》指出：“先天根本，肾也，…所以足于精者，百病不生，穷於精者，万邪蜂起。”对肾精充足则机体健康的重要性进行了阐述。而吴鞠通在《内经》：“藏于精者，春不病温”之说的基础上于《增补评注温病条辨•原病篇》提出了“病温者，精气先虚”、“春气温，阳气发越，阴精不足以承之，故为病温”的理论，是对肾精不足与温病发生之间相因关系的深刻阐述。

肾精不足病机的形成，责之先天禀赋不足、年老体弱、房劳产育过度、久病耗伤等。其病机特点为肾精亏虚，不能生髓充脑充骨，影响天癸的应时而至，或出现过早衰竭，从而进一步可分为脑海失养、头颅失养、腰府失养、骨髓失养、生长迟缓、生育减退、精亏失纳、精亏血少、精亏虚劳、精亏早衰等十种病机类型。

4.1 Brain Deprived of Nourishment

The kidney stores essence and is the root of earlier heaven. It governs bones, engenders marrow, and links up with the brain. Kidney essence is able to nourish the brain marrow and the skeleton. When kidney essence is plentiful, there is superabundance in the sea of marrow, which results in lightness, vigor, and strength. If kidney essence is insufficient, essence-marrow is empty and the brain is deprived of nourishment.

Already in the Spring and Autumn period (770-476 BCE), we find rudimentary descriptions of the marrow-engendering function of kidney essence. For example, the chapter, “Channel Vessels” in the *Líng Shū* (“The Magic Pivot”) states: “At the beginning of a person’s life, essence is formed first, and when essence is formed, brain marrow is engendered.” The treatise, “On Wilting” in the *Sù Wèn* (“Plain Questions”) further states: “The kidney governs the body’s bones and marrow.”

Factors like constitutional insufficiency, debility in old age, enduring disease affecting the kidney, or sexual taxation damaging the kidney make kidney essence insufficient. Consequently, essence does not engender marrow, and marrow does not fill the bones or nourish the brain. This can result in the pathomechanism of emptiness of essence-marrow, and brain deprived of nourishment.

If kidney essence is insufficient and does not engender marrow, brain marrow is empty and the head and eyes are deprived of nourishment. This manifests in empty pain in the head, dizzy head and vision, tinnitus and deafness, and loss of vision.

If kidney essence is insufficient, it is unable to nourish the spirit, so that the spirit does not keep to its abode. The result is insomnia, forgetfulness, listless essence-spirit, sluggishness, fatigue, and increased resting.

Insufficiency of kidney essence can cause loss of nourishment in the lower back and lower legs. The result is aching lower back and limpness in the lower legs.

Insufficiency of kidney essence results in a pale tongue body, thin white tongue fur, and a fine forceless pulse.

The treatise, "On Seas" in the *Líng Shū* ("The Magic Pivot") states: "Emptiness of the sea of marrow results in spinning brain and ringing ears, aching of the lower legs, veiling dizziness, loss of vision, and sluggishness, fatigue, and increased resting." This quotation clearly points out a series of pathologies that can result from insufficiency of kidney essence and emptiness of the brain.

The chapter, "Symptoms of Ear Disease; Deafness" in the *Zhū Bìng Yuán Hòu Lùn* ("Origin and Indicators of Disease") points out:

> "The kidney is ascribed to the foot lesser yīn channel and stores essence. Its qì flows to the ears. The ears are the gathering place of the ancestral vessels. If essential qì is harmonized, the kidney viscus is strong and exuberant and the ears perceive the five notes. If taxation damages qì and blood, and this is compounded by a contraction of wind evil, the result is detriment to the kidney and desertion of essence. Desertion of essence leads to deafness… The symptom of desertion of essence and deafness in kidney disease is black cheeks."

This quotation concisely describes how depletion of kidney essence and loss of nourishment in the sea of marrow lead to deafness.

Brain deprived of nourishment is treated by supplementing the kidney and increasing essence, and by boosting the brain and sharpening the hearing. The recommended formula is *tiān jīng yì shèn tāng* (Increase Essence Kidney-Boosting Decoction) from the *Shèn Bìng Zhèng Zhì Gài Yào* ("Essentials of Kidney Disease Patterns and Treatment").

Tiān Jīng Yì Shèn Tāng 添精益肾汤 Increase Essence Kidney-Boosting Decoction
shú dì huáng (熟地黄 Rehmanniae Radix Praeparata, cooked rehmannia)
nǚ zhēn zǐ (女贞子 Ligustri Lucidi Fructus, ligustrum)
gǒu qǐ zǐ (枸杞子 Lycii Fructus, lycium)
shān yào (山药 Dioscoreae Rhizoma, dioscorea)
bǔ gǔ zhī (补骨脂 Psoraleae Fructus, psoralea)
huáng qí (黄其芪 Astragali Radix, astragalus)
fú líng (茯苓 Poria, poria)
niú xī (牛膝 Achyranthis Bidentatae Radix, achyranthes)
yú piāo mò (鱼螵末 Pisces Os Pulveres, ground fish bone)

脑海失养

肾藏精，为先天之本，主骨生髓通于脑。肾精能滋养脑髓骨骼，肾精充足，髓海有余，则轻劲多力。肾精不足，精髓空虚，则脑海失养。早在春秋时期，对肾精生髓的生理功能就有初步的描述。如《灵枢•经脉》篇曰："人始生，先成精，精成而脑髓生。"《素问•痿论》又曰："肾主身之骨髓。"如因禀赋不足，年老体衰，或久病及肾，或房劳伤肾等因素，导致肾精不足，精不生髓，髓不充骨，髓不养脑，则可出现精髓空虚，脑海失养的病机变化。肾精不足，精不生髓，脑髓空虚，头目失养，则出现头脑空痛，头晕目眩，耳鸣耳聋，目无所见; 肾精不足，不能养神，神不守舍，则失眠健忘，精神萎靡，懈怠安卧; 肾精不足，腰胫失养，则腰酸胫软。肾精不足，则舌质淡，苔薄白，脉细无力。如《灵枢•海论》云："髓海空虚，则脑转耳鸣，胫酸眩冒，目无所见，懈怠安卧。"明确指出了肾精不足，脑海空虚的病机改变可能导致的一系列临床病变。《诸病源候论•耳病诸候•耳聋候》指出："肾为足少阴之经，而藏精，气通于耳。耳，宗脉之所聚也。若精气调和，则肾脏强盛，耳闻五音。若劳伤血气，兼受风邪，损伤肾脏而精脱，精脱者，耳聋。...其肾病精脱耳聋者，其候颊颧色黑。"准确地论述了肾精亏损，髓海失养，而致耳聋的病机变化。治法宜补肾添精，益脑聪耳。方药用《肾病证治概要》添精益肾汤（大熟地、女贞子、枸杞子、怀山药、补骨脂、黄芪、茯苓、怀牛膝、鱼鳔末）。

Literature Review of Brain Deprived of Nourishment

📖 *Líng Shū* ("The Magic Pivot"), "Understanding Qì"

> "Desertion of essence results in deafness… Humor desertion ….results in frequent ringing of the ears."

This quotation points out that insufficiency of kidney essence can lead to loss of acuity in the ears.

📖 *Rén Zhāi Zhí Zhǐ Fù Yí Fāng Lùn* "Supplement to 'Rén-Zhāi Clear Guidance Formulary'," "Ears"

> "The kidney is connected to the ears and governs essence. When kidney qì is abundant, the ears can hear and are sharp. If taxation damages qì and blood, and wind evil assails this vacuity, this causes desertion of essence and exhaustion of the kidney. As a result, the ears suffer deafness."

This passage describes how insufficiency of kidney qì prevents qì from securing essence, so that kidney essence is depleted and fails to nourish the ears, which leads to deafness.

📖 *Yī Xué Zhōng Zhōng Cān Xī Lù* ("Records of Chinese Medicine with Reference to Western Medicine"), "Dizziness"

> "Ultimately, the kidney is the mother of the liver and governs the storage of essence. When essence is vacuous, the brain is empty and the head is heavy. Therefore, the *Nèi Jīng* ("The Inner Canon") reasoned that kidney vacuity is related to insufficiency of the sea of marrow. When it mentions vacuity, it refers to the root of the disease; when it mentions repletion, it refers to the symptom of the disease. Thus, the symptom and the root are a single link."

This quotation describes the pathomechanism of kidney essence depletion and brain deprived of nourishment.

文献评述

《灵枢•决气》曰："精脱者，耳聋，…液脱者，…耳数鸣。"指出了肾精不足，可致耳窍不聪的病机变化。

《仁斋直指附遗方论•耳》曰："肾通乎耳，所主者精，肾气充足则耳闻而聪。若劳伤气血，风邪袭虚，使精脱肾惫则耳转而聋。"阐述了肾气不足，气不固精，肾精亏虚，精不养耳，导致耳聋的病机变化。

《医学从众录•眩晕》曰："究之肾为肝母，肾主藏精，精虚则脑海空虚而头重，故<内经>以肾虚及髓海不足立论也。其言虚者，言其病根，其言实者，言其病象，理本一贯"。对肾精亏虚，脑海失养的病机变化进行了论述。

Summary of Brain Deprived of Nourishment

1. Head and Eyes Deprived of Nourishment

   Empty pain in the head, dizzy head and vision, tinnitus and deafness, loss of vision.

2. Spirit Failing to Keep to its Abode

   Insomnia, forgetfulness, listlessness of the essence-spirit, sluggishness, fatigue, and increased resting.

3. Lower Back and Lower Legs Deprived of Nourishment

   Aching lower back and limp knees.

4. Insufficiency of Kidney Essence

   Pale tongue body, thin white tongue fur, fine forceless pulse.

脑海失养

头目失养—头脑空痛，头晕目眩，耳鸣耳聋，目无所见

神不守舍—失眠健忘，精神萎靡，懈怠安卧

腰胫失养—腰酸胫软

肾精不足—舌质淡，苔薄白，脉细无力

4.2 Skull Deprived of Nourishment

Kidney essence fills and nourishes brain marrow and manages the growth and development of the brain marrow and cranium. Insufficiency of earlier heaven or later heaven lack of nourishment can cause depletion of kidney essence. Consequently, the brain marrow is not abundant and the cranium is poorly developed. This leads to the pathomechanical changes of skull deprived of nourishment.

When kidney essence is insufficient, it is unable to luxuriate the skull. In children this leads to incomplete development of the skull, non-closure of the fontanel gate at its due time, gradual widening and opening, enlarged skull, lack of strength in the neck, enlarged head with thin neck, and bowed and unstable head.

When the skull is open, circulation of blood in the network vessels is obstructed, and qì and blood are unable to enrich the hair. The result is bare tense scalp and hair loss.

When kidney essence is insufficient, marrow does not nourish the brain, and the brain marrow is not replete. The result is lowered intelligence and dull mental faculties.

Insufficiency of kidney essence manifests in a pale tongue, thin white tongue fur, and vacuous pulse.

The chapter, "Ununited Skull" in the *Zhāng Shì Yī Tōng* ("Zhang's Clear View of Medicine") states:

> "Ununited skull is engendered by non-closure of the fontanel gate below. Over time, it must lead to increased anxiety and reduced laughter, increased white in the eyes, a bright white faxial complexion, and emaciated limbs and body, all of which are related to kidney vacuity. Since the kidney governs the bones and marrow, and the brain is the sea of marrow, this condition is caused by the parents having insufficient essence-blood that hence cannot be secured and constrained. The recommended formula is *dì huáng wán* (Rehmannia Pill) with the addition of *wǔ wèi zǐ* (Schisandrae Fructus) and *lù róng* (Cervi Cornu Pantotrichum)."

This quotation points out that insufficiency of kidney essence-blood and skull deprived of nourishment are critical pathomechanisms that cause ununited skull.

The chapter, "Head, Nape, and Fontanel" in the *Yòu Yòu Jí Chéng* ("A Compendium of Pediatrics") further points out:

> "Ununited skull means that the cranial fissures are open instead of closed. This is caused by an insufficiency of blood and qì and by depletion of the earlier heaven origin in the kidney. The kidney governs brain marrow, and kidney depletion results in insufficiency of brain marrow, which causes opening of the fontanels. People without brain marrow are just like trees without roots. In less than a thousand days, it will destroy them. The symptoms of this condition are increased anxiety and reduced joy, increased white in the eyes, and a bright white faxial complexion. It is particularly ominous if this condition arises after an illness."

This quotation further details how depletion of earlier heaven kidney essence leads to ununited skull.

Skull deprived of nourishment is treated by supplementing the kidney and engendering marrow, and by nourishing the bones and closing the fontanels. The recommended formula is *bǔ shèn dì huáng tāng* (Supplement the Kidney Rehmannia Decoction) from the *Yī Zōng Jīn Jiàn* ("The Golden Mirror of Medicine") with modifications.

Bǔ Shèn Dì Huáng Tāng 补肾地黄汤 Supplement the Kidney Rehmannia Decoction
shú dì huáng (熟地黄 Rehmanniae Radix Praeparata, cooked rehmannia)
shān zhū yú (山茱萸 Corni Fructus, cornus)
fú líng (茯苓 Poria, poria)
shān yào (山药 Dioscoreae Rhizoma, dioscorea)
mǔ dān pí (牡丹皮 Moutan Cortex, moutan)
niú xī (牛膝 Achyranthis Bidentatae Radix, achyranthes)
lù róng (鹿茸 Cervi Cornu Pantotrichum, velvet deerhorn)

头颅失养

肾精充养脑髓，主持脑髓及颅骨的生长发育。如因先天不足，或后天失养，肾精亏损，脑髓不充，颅骨发育不良，则引起头颅失养的病机变化。肾精不足，不能荣养头颅骨骼，则小儿头颅发育不全，囟门逾期不合，逐渐加宽开解，头颅增大，颈项无力，头大颈细，头倾不定; 头颅开解，血络循环受阻，气血不能滋养头发，则头皮光急，头发脱落; 肾精不足，髓不养脑，脑髓不实，则智力下降，神识呆钝。肾精不足，则舌淡，苔薄白，脉虚。如《张氏医通•解颅》云："解颅者，生下囟门不合也。长必多愁少笑，目白睛多，面色白光白，肢体消瘦，皆属肾虚。按肾主骨髓，脑为髓海，因父母精血不足，不能固敛也。地黄丸加五味子、鹿茸。"指出肾之精血不足，头颅失养是形成解颅的重要病机。《幼幼集成•头项囟》又指出："解颅者，即头缝开解而不合也。是由血气不足，先天肾元大亏。肾主脑髓，肾亏则脑髓不足，故囟为之开解。然人无脑髓，犹树无根，不过千日，则成废人。其候多愁少喜，目白睛多，面白光色白。若成于病后者尤凶。"也阐述了先天肾精亏虚引起解颅的病机变化。治法宜补肾生髓，养骨愈囟。方药选用《医宗金鉴》补肾地黄汤加减（熟地、山茱萸、茯苓、山药、丹皮、牛膝、鹿茸）。

Literature Review of Skull Deprived of Nourishment

📖 *Zhū Bìng Yuán Hòu Lùn* ("Origin and Indicators of Disease"), "Various Symptoms of Miscellaneous Pediatric Diseases: Ununited Skull"

> "Ununited skull manifests in non-closure of the fontanel gate and opening of the cranial sutures in older children. It is caused by non-formation of kidney qì. The kidney governs the bones and marrow, and the brain is the sea of marrow. When kidney qì does not form, marrow in the brain is insufficient and cannot be bound. Therefore the skull opens."

Insufficiency of kidney qì also causes kidney essence to be depleted. While this passage ostensibly talks about depletion of kidney qì, in reality this also includes vacuity of kidney essence. Thus, it discusses how a lack of fullness in the sea of marrow causes the skull to be deprived of nourishment and remain open.

📖 *Yī Zōng Jīn Jiàn* ("The Golden Mirror of Medicine"), "Heart Approach to Pediatrics in Rhyme: Ununited Skull"

> "Ununited skull means that the cranial sutures in the fontanel do not close. The kidney engenders marrow, and the brain is the sea of marrow. When kidney qì is depleted, brain marrow is insufficient. This resembles a flower or tree without roots. It manifests in the following symptoms: a bright white facial complexion, emaciation and weakness of the formal body, increased white in the eyes, and increased anxiety and reduced laughter. In treatment, focus on supplementing and nourishing kidney qì. First, use *bǔ shèn dì huáng tāng* (Supplement the Kidney Rehmannia Decoction) to enrich and supplement its yīn, and then use *fú yuán sǎn* (Origin-Supporting Powder) to supplement and nourish its qì, while topically applying *fēng xìn sǎn* (Fontanel-Sealing Powder). This will cause essence-blood to be filled gradually and potentially the condition can be turned around from critical to safe."

The kidney's function of engendering marrow is in fact due to the accomplishment of kidney essence. Therefore, the pathomechanisms of insufficiency in the brain of marrow and ununited skull should be attributed to a depletion of kidney essence.

文献评述

《诸病源候论•小儿杂病诸候•解颅候》曰："解颅者，其状，小儿年大，囟应合而不合，头缝开解是也，由肾气不成故也。肾主骨髓，而脑为髓海。肾气不成，则髓脑不足，不能结成，故头颅开解也。"肾气不足，则肾精亦亏，虽明言肾气之亏，实质包含肾精之虚，论述了髓海不充，头颅失养而开解的病机改变。

《医宗金鉴•幼科心法杂病要诀•解颅》曰："解颅者，乃囟大骨缝不合也。盖肾生髓，脑为髓海，肾气有亏，脑髓不足，亦如花木无根。现证面色白光白，形体瘦弱，目多白睛，多愁少笑。治宜补养肾气为主。先以补肾地黄丸滋补其阴，再以扶元散补养其气，外用封囟散摊贴之，则精血稍充，或可转危为安也"。肾生髓之功能，实由肾精来完成，因此脑髓不足而解颅的病机变化应责之于肾精的亏虚。

Summary of Skull Deprived of Nourishment

1. Skull Deprived of Nourishment

   Poorly developed cranium, non-closure of the fontanel gate beyond its due time, gradual widening and opening, enlarged skull, lack of strength in the neck, enlarged head with thin neck, bowed and unstable head.

2. Obstruction of the Blood Network Vessels

   Bare tense scalp, hair loss.

3. Non-Repletion of Brain Marrow

   Dull mental facilities.

4. Insufficiency of Kidney Essence

   Pale tongue, thin white tongue fur, vacuous pulse.

头颅失养

头颅失养—颅骨发育不良，囟门逾期不合，逐渐加宽开解，头颅增大，颈项无力，头大颈细，头倾不定

血络受阻—头皮光急，头发脱落

髓脑不实—神识呆钝

肾精不足—舌淡，苔薄白，脉虚

4.3 Lower Back Deprived of Nourishment

The lower back is the house of the kidney, and the knees are the meeting point of the sinews. Both depend on being nourished by kidney essence for strength and unhindered activity. If kidney essence is insufficient, essence does not transform marrow to nourish the lower back, knees, and skeleton. As a result, the pathomechanism of insufficiency of kidney essence manifests as lower back and knees deprived of nourishment.

The chapter, "The Five Dribbling Urinary Stoppages and the Differences Between Liquid and Humor" in the *Líng Shū* ("The Magic Pivot") states:

> "The essence of the five grains combines with humor and forms a paste. This internally percolates into the empty spaces of the bones, supplements and boosts brain marrow, and flows down into the inguinal region. When yīn and yáng are not harmonious, humor spills and flows downward into the genitals, and marrow and humor are both reduced and descend. If they descend beyond their normal limit, this results in vacuity, which in turn causes lumbar pain and lower leg ache."

This quotation certainly recognizes the pathomechanism of kidney essence insufficiency manifesting as lower back and knees deprived of nourishment.

When kidney essence is insufficient, the lower back is deprived of nourishment, and the functions of the lower back and legs are impaired. The result is limpness and aching in the lumbar region, liking for being rubbed and pressed, and recurring limpness of knees and legs.

Taxation can easily consume essential qì. After activity, the damage to essence is therefore aggravated. The result is symptoms that are aggravated upon taxation and relieved by rest.

When kidney essence is insufficient, the formal body is deprived of nourishment. This results in a wan and haggard appearance.

When kidney essence is depleted, it is unable to raise and stiffen [the penis]. This causes seminal emission and yáng wilt.

Depletion of kidney essence manifests in a pale tongue with thin fur and a fine soft pulse.

The chapter, "Lumbar Pain" in the *Dān Tái Yù Àn* ("Cinnabar Platform and Jade Desk") states:

> "The kidney's abode inside the body corresponds externally to the lower back. Where the lower back is located is also where the kidney is located. Immoderate sexual taxation can exhaust a person's true essence. This results in vacuity of the kidney and thus disease of the lower back. When there is pain that is drawn-out and incessant, and a large pulse, this is it."

This quotation succinctly describes the pathomechanism by which depletion of kidney essence and lower back deprived of nourishment lead to lumbar pain.

The chapter, "Lumbar Pain and Aching" in the *Zhōng Yī Nèi Kē Zhì Liáo Dà Chéng* ("The Great Compendium of Chinese Internal Medicine Treatment") also states:

> "Constitutional insufficiency compounded by excessive fatigue, general vacuity after enduring illness, or debility in old age can lead to depletion of kidney essence. Consequently, there is nothing to nourish the sinews, and pain arises."

This quotation clearly points out that insufficiency of kidney essence and lower back deprived of nourishment can lead to the pathomechanism of lumbar pain.

Lower back deprived of nourishment is treated by supplementing and boosting kidney essence, and by strengthening the lower back and fortifying the bones. The recommended formula is *dāng guī dì huáng yǐn* (Chinese Angelica and Rehmannia Beverage) from the *Jǐng Yuè Quán Shū* ("Jǐng-Yuè's Complete Compendium"), with the addition of *gǒu qǐ zǐ* (Lycii Fructus), *guī bǎn jiāo* (Testudinis Carapacis et Plastri Gelatinum), *yú piāo jiāo* (fish bone gelatin), and *zǐ hé chē* (Hominis Placenta).

Dāng Guī Dì Huáng Yǐn 当归地黄饮 Chinese Angelica and Rehmannia Beverage
dāng guī (当归 Angelicae Sinensis Radix, Chinese angelica)
shú dì huáng (熟地黄 Rehmanniae Radix Praeparata, cooked rehmannia)
shān yào (山药 Dioscoreae Rhizoma, dioscorea)
dù zhòng (杜仲 Eucommiae Cortex, eucommia)
niú xī (牛膝 Achyranthis Bidentatae Radix, achyranthes)
shān zhū yú (山茱萸 Corni Fructus, cornus)
zhì gān cǎo (炙甘草 Glycyrrhizae Radix, mix-fried licorice)
Plus:
gǒu qǐ zǐ (枸杞子 Lycii Fructus, lycium)
guī bǎn jiāo (龟版胶 Testudinis Carapacis et Plastri Gelatinum, tortoise shell glue)
yú piāo jiāo (鱼螵胶 Pisces Os Gelatina, fish bone gelatin)
zǐ hé chē (紫河车 Hominis Placenta, placenta)

腰府失养

腰为肾府，膝为宗筋之会，赖肾精濡养，才强健有力，活动自如。若肾精不足，精不化髓以充养腰膝骨骼，则出现肾精不足，腰膝失养的病机变化。《灵枢•五癃津液别篇》曰："五谷之精液和合而为膏者，内渗入于骨空，补益脑髓，而下流于阴股。阴阳不和，则使液溢而下流于阴，髓液皆减而下，下过度则虚，虚故腰背痛而胫酸。"对肾精不足，腰膝失养的病机变化有一定的认识。肾精不足，腰失濡养，腰腿功能衰退，则腰部酸软，喜揉喜按，腿膝无力，反复发作; 劳作容易耗伤精气，活动后精伤加重，则遇劳加重，卧则减轻; 肾精不足，身形失养，则形容憔悴; 肾精亏虚，不能作强，故遗泄阳痿。肾精亏虚，则舌淡，苔薄，脉细软。如《丹台玉案•腰痛门》云："肾藏于内，外应乎腰，腰之所在，肾之所在也。惟房劳不节，竭其真精，则肾脏空虚而腰斯病矣。其痛悠悠不已，而脉大者是也。"对肾精亏损，腰府失养而引起腰痛的病机作了明确的论述。《中医内科治疗大成•腰痛腰酸》也云："素体禀赋不足，加之劳累太过，或久病体虚，或年老体衰，以致肾精亏损，无以濡养筋脉而发生疼痛。"明确提出肾精不足，腰失濡养，可致腰痛的病机。治法宜补益肾精，强腰健骨。方药选用《景岳全书》当归地黄饮（当归、熟地、山药、杜仲、牛膝、山茱萸、炙甘草）加枸杞、龟胶、鱼螵胶、紫河车。

Literature Review of Lower Back Deprived of Nourishment

🕮 *Jǐng Yuè Quán Shū* ("Jǐng-Yuè's Complete Compendium"), "Schema of Miscellaneous Patterns: Lumbar Pain"

> "In vacuity patterns with lumbar pain... whenever there is pain resulting from depletion of true yīn kidney water and debilitation of essence-blood, *dāng guī dì huáng yǐn* (Chinese Angelica and Rehmannia Beverage), as well as *zuǒ guī wán* (Left-Restoring [Kidney Yīn] Pill) and *yòu guī wán* (Right-Restoring [Life Gate] Pill) are best."

This passage summarizes how insufficiency of kidney essence and inability to nourish the lumbar region and the skeleton leads to lumbar pain from lower back deprived of nourishment.

🕮 *Zá Bìng Yuán Liú Xī Zhú* ("Incisive Light on the Source of Miscellaneous Disease"), "The Origin and Development of Lumbar and Umbilical Disease"

> "Lumbar pain is a disease caused by vacuity of essential qì and evil settling in... To summarize, whenever a person's essence is consumed and the kidney debilitated, bladder qì is also unable to be sufficient on

> its own. Therefore, evil can easily invade. Thus, kidney vacuity is its root, and wind, cold, dampness, heat, phlegm, rheum, qì stagnation, blood stasis, and wrenching and contusion are its tip.

This quotation sets forth the pathomechanism by which insufficiency of kidney essence can bring about lumbar pain.

文献评述

《景岳全书•杂证谟•腰痛》曰："腰痛之虚证，...凡肾水真阴亏损，精血衰少而痛者，宜当归地黄饮，及左归丸、右归丸为最。"也论述了肾精不足，不能充养腰部骨骼，导致腰府失养的病机变化。

《杂病源流犀烛•腰脐病源流》曰："腰痛，精气虚而邪客病也。...总之，凡人精耗肾衰，则膀胱之气亦不能独足，故邪易侵犯，则肾虚其本也。风寒湿热痰饮，气滞血瘀闪挫其标也，或从标，或从本，贵无失其宜而已。"明确指出了肾精不足可致腰痛的病机。

Summary of Lower Back Deprived of Nourishment

1. Lack of Nourishment from Essence
   Limpness and aching in the lumbar region, liking for being rubbed and pressed, limpness of knees and legs that occurs repeatedly.
2. Consumption of Essence Upon Taxation
   Symptoms aggravated upon taxation and relieved by rest.
3. Physical Body Deprived of Nourishment
   Wan and haggard appearance.
4. Inability to Raise and Stiffen
   Seminal emission and yáng wilt.
5. Depletion of Kidney Essence
   Thin tongue fur, fine pulse.

腰府失养

精失濡养—腰部酸软，喜揉喜按，腿膝无力，反复发作

劳作耗精—遇劳加重，卧则减轻

身形失养—形容憔悴

不能作强—遗泄阳痿

肾精亏虚—苔薄，脉细

4.4 Bone Marrow Deprived of Nourishment

The chapter, "On the Engenderment of the Five Viscera" in the *Sù Wèn* ("Plain Questions") states: "The kidney is connected with the bones." The "Great Treatise on the Correspondences and Manifestations of Yīn and Yáng" in the same text further states: "The kidney engenders bone and marrow." These passages explain the close physiological relationship between the kidney and the bones.

When kidney essencc is plentiful, bone marrow is also plentiful, and the skeleton is hard and strong. When kidney essence is insufficient, the bones and marrow lose their fullness and the skeleton falls ill. The treatise, "On Wilting" in the *Sù Wèn* ("Plain Questions") states: "When kidney qì is hot, the result is inability to lift the lumbar spine, desiccated bone, and reduced marrow, which erupts as bone disease."

When kidney essence is insufficient and unable to enrich the bones and marrow, the bones become desiccated and the marrow reduced, so that the person has no control over standing and walking. This results in sinew and bone wilting, lack of strength in the four limbs, and weakness and inability to walk.

The lower back is the house of the kidney. When kidney essence is deprived of nourishment, the result is limp aching lower back and knees, and inability to lift them.

When kidney essence is insufficient, essence is depleted and blood reduced. Thus, essence-blood is unable to nourish the flesh. This results in emaciation and withering of the flesh.

When kidney essence is insufficient, it is unable to nourish the teeth. This results in loose and desiccated teeth.

Insufficiency of kidney essence manifests in a pale tongue with white fur, and a fine sunken pulse.

The chapter, "Examples of the Five Wilting Patterns" in the *Sān Yīn Jí Yī Bìng Zhèng Fāng Lùn* ("A Unified Treatise on Diseases, Patterns, and Remedies According to the Three Causes") states:

> "When a patient suffers from kidney heat and there is inability to lift the lumbar spine, desiccated bone and reduced marrow, and a black complexion and desiccated teeth, this condition is called bone wilting. It can be caused by taxation fatigue after walking far distances, exposure to great heat and subsequent thirst, internal lack of yáng qì, and heat lodging in the kidney, preventing water from overcoming fire. This results in desiccation of the bone and vacuity of marrow. Therefore, the *Nèi Jīng* ("The Inner Canon") states that bone wilting is engendered by great heat."

This passage describes the pathomechanism by which heat damages kidney water, causes depletion of essence and vacuity of marrow, and forms bone wilting.

In a commentary to the chapter, "Wilting" in the *Lín Zhèng Zhǐ Nán Yī Àn* ("A Clinical Guide with Case Histories"), Zōu Zī-Jiǔ points out:

> "The kidney stores essence, and essence and blood engender each other. When essence is vacuous, it is insufficient to fill all the irrigation channels to their ends; when blood is vacuous, it is unable to supply nourishment to the sinews and bones… This is how the symptoms of inability to walk and wilting, weakness, and contraction of the sinews arise."

This quotation describes the pathomechanism of insufficiency of kidney essence manifesting as bone and marrow deprived of nourishment.

Bone marrow deprived of nourishment is treated by supplementing qì and engendering essence, and by enriching and nourishing sinews and bones. The recommended formula is *hǔ qián wán* (Hidden Tiger Pill) from the *Yī Fāng Jí Jiě* ("Medical Formulas Gathered and Explained"), formulated without *gān jiāng* (Zingiberis Rhizoma), and with *guī bǎn jiāo* (Testudinis Carapacis et Plastri Gelatinum) instead of *guī bǎn* (Testudinis Plastrum).

Hǔ Qián Wán 虎潜丸
Hidden Tiger Pill

shú dì huáng (熟地黄 Rehmanniae Radix Praeparata, cooked rehmannia)
bái sháo (白芍 Paeoniae Radix Alba, white peony)
dāng guī (当归 Angelicae Sinensis Radix, Chinese angelica)
niú xī (牛膝 Achyranthis Bidentatae Radix, achyranthes)
suǒ yáng (锁阳 Cynomorii Herba, cynomorium)
hǔ gǔ (虎骨 Tigris Os, tiger bone)
huáng bǎi (黄柏 Phellodendri Cortex, phellodendron)
zhī mǔ (知母 Anemarrhenae Rhizoma, anemarrhena)
yáng ròu (羊肉 Caprae seu Ovis Caro, goat meat)
chén pí (陈皮 Citri Reticulatae Pericarpium, tangerine peel)

Omitting:
gān jiāng (Zingiberis Rhizoma),
guī bǎn (龟版 Testudinis Plastrum, tortoise plastron)

Adding:
guī bǎn jiāo (龟版胶 Testudinis Carapacis et Plastri Gelatinum, tortoise shell glue)

骨髓失养

《素问•五脏生成》曰："肾之合骨也。"《素问•阴阳应象大论》又曰："肾生骨髓。"说明肾与骨在生理上有密切的联系。肾精充足，骨髓充足，则骨骼坚强。肾精不足，骨髓失充，则骨骼生病。如《素问•痿论》曰："肾气热，则腰脊不举，骨枯而髓减，发为骨病。"肾精不足，不能滋养骨髓，骨枯髓减，不任立行，则筋骨痿弱，四肢乏力，不能行走；腰为肾之府，肾精失养，则腰膝酸软不举；肾精不足，精亏血少，精血不能濡养肌肉，则形体消瘦，肌肉萎缩。肾精不足，不能养齿，则牙动齿槁。肾精不足，则舌淡苔白，脉沉细。如《三因极一病证方论•五痿证例》曰："病者肾热，腰脊不举，骨枯而髓减，其色黑而齿槁，名曰骨痿。因有所远行，劳倦，遇大热而渴，阳气内乏，热舍于肾，致水不胜火，则骨枯而髓虚，故<内经>曰：骨痿者，生于大热也。"指出热伤肾水，精亏髓虚，而成骨痿的病机。《临证指南医案•痿》邹滋九按指出："肾藏精，精血相生，精虚则不能灌溉诸末，血虚则不能营养筋骨。…此不能步履、痿弱筋缩之症作矣。"阐述了肾精不足，骨髓失养的病机变化。治法宜补气生精，滋养筋骨。方药选用《医方集解》虎潜丸（龟板、熟地黄、白芍、当归、牛膝、锁阳、虎骨、黄柏、知母、羊肉、陈皮、干姜）去干姜，龟板改用龟胶。

Literature Review of Bone Marrow Deprived of Nourishment

Sù Wèn ("Plain Questions"), "On Wilting"

> "Endless thinking, unfulfilled wishes, lascivious ideation, too much sexual intercourse …this is how sinew wilting arises… Taxation fatigue from walking long distances, encountering great heat and subsequent thirst …this is how bone wilting arises."

This quotation indicates that taxation fatigue and excessive sexual desires are among the causes of damage to essential qì in the kidney leading to sinews and bone deprived of nourishment and wilting patterns.

Jǐng Yuè Quán Shū ("Jǐng-Yuè's Complete Compendium"), "Wilting Patterns"

> "When original qì is vanquished, essence is vacuous and unable to irrigate, and blood is vacuous and unable to luxuriate and nourish. These conditions are not rare. Discussing this from the angle of fire, I fear that true yáng is vanquished, to the point where earth is debilitated

and water desiccated so that they are unable to sustain [the body]. Therefore, you must deliberate the depth of cold and heat and examine the urgency of vacuity and repletion, to carry out a treatment that will treat wilting comprehensively."

This quotation describes the pathomechanism of sinew and bone wilting caused by vanquishing of the essential qì of the kidney and by qì and blood failing to luxuriate.

🕮 *Zhèng Yīn Mài Zhì* ("Pathoconditions: Causes, Pulses, and Treatments"), "Internal Damage Impediment Conditions: Kidney Impediment"

"The pathocondition of kidney impediment is the same as bone impediment. It manifests in susceptibility to distention, lumbar pain, seminal emission, frequent change in the color of urine, hypertonicity of the feet and inability to stretch them, and bone wilting with inability to rise. These are the signs of kidney impediment…

"Possibly taxation fatigue after walking long distances, or exposure to great heat and subsequent thirst has prevented water from overcoming fire, the result of which is desiccation of bone and vacuity of marrow. Alternatively, lack of care regarding sexual taxation has exhausted essence and dried up blood, the result of which is sinews and bones deprived of nourishment, lumbar pain, and inability to rise. This is how the condition of kidney impediment arises.

"The pulse of kidney impediment is fine and rapid in both cubit positions, or possibly floating and large. The kidney pulse is originally deep, but in this condition turns agitated and racing because water is debilitated and fire stirs. This is the pulse of kidney impediment."

This quotation discusses how depletion of kidney essence and bone and marrow deprived of nourishment lead to kidney impediment.

文献评述

《素问•痿论》曰："思想无穷，所愿不得，意淫于外，入房太甚，…发为筋痿，…远行劳倦，逢大热而渴，…发为骨痿。"指出了劳倦色欲，伤及肾脏精气，导致筋骨失养，产生痿证的病机变化。

《景岳全书•痿证》曰："元气败伤则精虚不能灌溉，血虚不能营养者，亦不少矣。若概从火论，则恐真阳亏败，及土衰水涸者，有不能堪，故当酌寒热之浅深，审虚实之缓急，以施治疗，庶得治痿之全矣。"对肾之精气衰败，气血不荣引起的筋骨痿软的病机变化进行了论述。

《症因脉治•内伤痹症•肾痹》曰："肾痹之症，即骨痹也。善胀，腰痛，遗精，小便时时变色，足挛不能伸，骨痿不能起，此肾痹之症也。…或远行劳倦，逢大热而渴，水不胜火，则骨枯而髓虚; 或不慎房劳，精竭血燥，则筋骨失养，腰痛不举，而肾痹之症作矣。肾痹之脉两尺细数，或见浮大，肾脉本沉，今反躁疾，水衰火动，肾痹之脉。"论述了肾精亏虚，骨髓失养，导致肾痹的病机变化。

Summary of Bone and Marrow Deprived of Nourishment
1. Bone Marrow Deprived of Nourishment Weak wilting sinews and bones, lack of strength in the four limbs, inability to walk. 2. Lower Back Deprived of Nourishment Limp aching lower back and knees, inability to raise them. 3. Essence-blood Unable to Nourish the Flesh Emaciation, withering of the flesh. 4. Inability to Nourish the Teeth Loose and desiccated teeth. 5. Insufficiency of Kidney Essence Pale tongue, white tongue fur, fine sunken pulse.
骨髓失养
骨髓失养—筋骨痿弱，四肢乏力，不能行走 腰府失养—腰膝酸软不举 精血不能养肉—形体消瘦，肌肉萎缩 不能养齿—牙动齿槁 肾精不足—舌淡苔白，脉沉细

4.5 Retarded Growth

The kidney stores essential qì, which is the basic substance for originating and maintaining the growth and development of the body. Thus, the natural pattern of birth, growth, maturity, aging, and death is intimately related to the exuberance and debilitation of essential qì in the kidney. The "Treatise of the True Doctrine of the Golden Coffer" in the *Sù Wèn* ("Plain Questions") states: "Essence is the root of birth." If kidney essence is depleted, which can be caused by an insufficient endowment of earlier heaven or by later-heaven lack of nourishment, this restricts the birth, growth, and development of the body and can lead to retarded growth and development in small children.

This is recorded already in the *Zhū Bìng Yuán Hòu Lùn* ("Origin and Indicators of Disease") under the symptoms "Failure to Teethe," "Failure to Grow Hair," and "Inability to Speak at Four or Five Years of Age." However, this text does not specifically point out that insufficiency of kidney essence is the foundation of this pathomechanism.

It is later in the "Heart Approach to Pediatrics" in the *Yī Zōng Jīn Jiàn* ("The Golden Mirror of Medicine") that the various types of developmental retardation in small children are gathered, so that slowness to walk, slowness to stand, slowness to grow hair, slowness to teethe, and slowness to speak were combined into the "five slownesses."

Before the Sòng period, the "five limpnesses" were mostly mentioned in combination with the slownesses. For example, the chapter, "Slowness to Walk" in the *Xiǎo Ér Yào Zhèng Zhí Jué* ("Key to Diagnosis and Treatment of Children's Diseases") calls it "growing up without being able to walk, or walking but with limp legs."

The *Yīng Tóng Bǎi Wèn* ("A Hundred Questions About Infants and Children") was the first text to formally mention the "five limpnesses" by name. The chapter, "Five Limpnesses," stated: "The five limpnesses are limp head, limp neck, limp arms, limp legs, and limp flesh." This text suggested that the pathomechanism of the five limpnesses was based on a depletion of yáng qì.

Subsequently, the "Level-Line of Pediatrics" in the *Zhèng Zhì Zhǔn Shéng* ("The Level-Line of Pattern Identification and Treatment") pointed out:

> "The teeth are the end of the bones and are nourished by the marrow. If small children are supplied with insufficient kidney qì, they are unable to provide nourishment to the upper body, and marrow is vacuous and unable to fill the bones. Thus how could it reach up to the teeth? Therefore such children fail to teethe for a long time."

Marrow is engendered from essence. While this text does name the pathomechanism of "kidney essence depletion," its discussion of marrow vacuity and inability to fill the bones indicated the pathomechanical changes related to insufficiency of kidney essence.

When kidney essence is insufficient, it is unable to supply nourishment to the bones. The result is limpness of the celestial pillar, bowed and deviated head and nape, withering and limpness of the neck and nape, inability to lift and to rise, and delayed standing and walking.

When kidney essence is insufficient, essence fails to nourish the teeth. The result is long-term failure to teethe and loose, lusterless teeth.

Essence failing to nourish hair results in delayed hair growth, and hair that is sparse and falls out easily.

When essence is depleted, it is unable to enrich the head, face, and whole body. The result is withered and limp mouth, lips, and flesh, a lusterless facial complexion, tendency to fatigue, and generalized lack of strength.

Insufficiency of kidney essence manifests in a pale tongue with thin fur, and a fine soft pulse.

The chapter, "Five Limpnesses" in the *Huó Yòu Xīn Shū* ("Heart Text of Living Youth") states:

> "The pattern of the five limpnesses is called fetal timidity. It is inborn from an insufficiency of the father's essence or habitual debilitation of the mother's blood... Hence, after birth, essence and marrow are insufficient, resulting in wilting and weakness of the sinews and bones, debilitation of the flesh, and clouded and slow spirit. When to this is added an invasion of the six excesses, it further causes limpness of the head, neck, and extremities. This is called the five limpnesses."

This quotation clearly points out how the five limpnesses are related to insufficiency of kidney essence and developmental disturbances.

Retarded growth is treated by supplementing and boosting essence, and by engendering marrow and strengthening bone. The recommended formula is *liù wèi dì huáng wán* (Six-Ingredient Rehmannia Pill) from the *Xiǎo Ér Yào Zhèng Zhí Jué* ("Key to Diagnosis and Treatment of Children's Diseases"), with the addition of *lù jiǎo jiāo* (Cervi Cornus Gelatinum), *zǐ hé chē* (Hominis Placenta), *hé shǒu wū* (Polygoni Multiflori Radix), *gǒu qǐ zǐ* (Lycii Fructus), and *dù zhòng* (Eucommiae Cortex). For slowness to teethe, add *zǐ hé chē* (Hominis Placenta), *hé shǒu wū* (Polygoni Multiflori Radix), and *lóng gǔ* (Mastodi Ossis Fossilia). For limpness of the nape, add *gǒu qǐ zǐ* (Lycii Fructus), *tù sī zǐ* (Cuscutae Semen), and *bā jǐ* (Morindae Officinalis Radix). For slowness to stand, add *niú xī* (Achyranthis Bidentatae Radix) and *dù zhòng* (Eucommiae Cortex).

Liù Wèi Dì Huáng Wán 六味地黄丸
Six-Ingredient Rehmannia Pill

shú dì huáng (熟地黄 Rehmanniae Radix Praeparata, cooked rehmannia)
shān zhū yú (山茱萸 Corni Fructus, cornus)
shān yào (山药 Dioscoreae Rhizoma, dioscorea)
zé xiè (泽泻 Alismatis Rhizoma, alisma)
fú líng (茯苓 Poria, poria)
mǔ dān pí (牡丹皮 Moutan Cortex, moutan)

Plus:

lù jiǎo jiāo (Cervi Cornus Gelatinum),
zǐ hé chē (紫河车 Hominis Placenta, placenta)
hé shǒu wū (何首乌 Polygoni Multiflori Radix, flowery knotweed)
gǒu qǐ zǐ (枸杞子 Lycii Fructus, lycium)
dù zhòng (杜仲 Eucommiae Cortex, eucommia)

生长迟缓

肾藏精气，精气是构成和维持人体生长发育的基本物质，人体生、长、壮、老、已的自然规律，与肾中精气的盛衰有密切关系。《素问•金匮真言论》曰："夫精者，生之本也。"如肾精亏损，既可因先天禀赋不足，亦可因后天失养而致，使人体的生长发育受到制约，则可导致小儿生长发育迟缓的病机变化。早在《诸病源候论》中就有"齿不生候"、"头发不生候"、"四五岁不能语候"的记载，但未明确提出"肾精不足"是其病机基础。直到《医宗金鉴•幼科心法》才将小儿生长发育各类迟缓表现汇总，把行迟、立迟、发迟、齿迟、语迟归纳为"五迟"。五软宋代以前多与迟证并提，如《小儿药证直诀•行迟》指出："长大不行，行则脚软。"直至《婴童百问•五软》方正式提出"五软"的名称："五软者，头软、颈软、手软、脚软、肌肉软是也。"《保婴撮要•五软》认为五软的病机基础是阳气亏虚。《证治准绳•幼科准绳•幼科》则指出："齿者，骨之所终而髓之所养也。小儿禀受肾气不足，不能上营而髓虚不能充于骨，又安能及齿，故齿久不生也。"髓由精生，虽未明确提出"肾精亏虚"的病机名称，但髓虚不能充骨的论述已表明了肾精不足的病机变化。肾精不足，不能营养于骨，则天柱软弱，头项倾斜，颈项萎软，不能抬起，站立行走迟缓；肾精不足，精不养齿，则齿久不生，松动无光；精不养发，则头发生长迟慢，稀疏易脱；精亏不能滋养头面全身，则口唇、肌肉萎软，面色不华，容易疲乏，全身无力。肾精不足，则舌淡，苔薄，脉细软。如《活幼心书•五软》曰："五软证名胎怯，良由父精不足，母血素衰而得。...爰自降生之后，精髓不足，筋骨痿弱，肌肉虚衰，神色昏慢，才为六淫所侵，便致头项手足身软，是名五软。"明确指出五软的病机与肾精不足，生长发育障碍有关。治法宜补肾益精，生髓壮骨。方药选用《小儿药证直诀》六味地黄丸（熟地、山萸、山药、泽泻、茯苓、丹皮）加鹿角胶、紫河车、首乌、枸杞、杜仲; 齿迟加紫河车、首乌、龙骨; 项软加枸杞、菟丝、巴戟; 立迟加牛膝、杜仲。

Literature Review of Retarded Growth

🕮 *Yī Guàn* ("Thorough Knowledge of Medicine"), "On the Essentials of Earlier Heaven: On the Teeth"

> "The teeth are the tip of the bone. They are nourished by marrow. They are always related to the kidney... Whenever they are loose, bare, or fall out, whether with or without pain, and with or without bleeding, when they all look as if about to fall out, this condition is always related to the kidney... Whenever small children present with slowness to walk, slowness to speak, and slowness to teethe, as well as open fontanel, it is always related to an earlier heaven debilitation of the mother's kidney qì."

Kidney debilitation includes depletion of kidney essence. Therefore a failure of essence to nourish the bones and marrow can lead to the five slownesses and to dental disease in small children.

🕮 *Zhāng Shì Yī Tōng* ("Zhang's Clear View of Medicine"), "Five Slownesses. Five Limpnesses, Five Stiffnesses"

> "The five slownesses are slowness to stand, slowness to walk, slowness to teethe, slowness to grow hair, and slowness to speak. The kidney governs the bones. The teeth are the surplus of the bone, and hair is the luxuriance of the kidney. If the teeth fail to grow for a long time and grow insecurely when they do grow, and if hair fails to grow for a long time and is not black when it does grow, all of these signs mean fetal feebleness. They are inborn, due to an insufficiency of the parents' essence-blood, kidney qì vacuity, and inability to provide nourishment."

This quotation points out that insufficiency of the kidney's essence-blood and failure of essence to nourish the bones is one of the causes for the appearance of the pathomechanism of the five limpnesses.

📖 *Piàn Yù Xīn Shū* ("Jade Tablet of Heart Insights") "Section on Form and Sound"

> "What is the reason for the five slownesses? Bone is nourished by marrow, and when blood and qì are not full, marrow fails to fill the bones. This causes limpness and inability to walk. It is contracted as a result of dual vacuity of the kidney and liver. The liver governs the sinews, and when the sinews are weak, the child is unable to walk early. The kidney governs the bones, and when the bones are weak, there is no hardness. Thin legs mean insufficient endowment and no fullness of qì and blood. This causes thinness of the flesh, with all the joints showing, like the knees of cranes. This is also due to kidney vacuity and is called crane's-knee joint. *Jiā wèi dì huáng wán* (Supplemented Rehmannia Pill) governs it."

This quotation describes how kidney vacuity and scantness of marrow leads to slowness to walk.

文献评述

《医贯•先天要论•齿论》曰："齿者骨之标，髓之所养也，凡齿属肾。...凡动摇袒脱而痛，或不痛，或出血，或不出血，全具如欲落之状者，皆属肾。...凡小儿行迟语迟齿迟，及囟门开者，皆先天母气之肾衰。"肾衰，包括肾精亏虚，故精不养骨髓，可导致小儿五迟及齿病。

《张氏医通•五迟五软五硬》曰："五迟者，立迟行迟齿迟发迟语迟是也。肾主骨，齿者骨之余，发者肾之荣，若齿久不生，生而不固，发久不生，生则不黑，皆胎弱也。良由父母精血不足，肾气虚弱，不能荣养而然。"指出肾之精血不足，精不养骨，是出现"五迟"的病机之一。

《片玉心书•形声门》曰："行迟者何也？盖骨乃髓之所养，血气不充，则髓不满骨，故弱软不能行。此由肾与肝俱虚得之。盖肝主筋，筋弱不能早行; 肾主骨，骨弱而不坚，脚细者禀受不足，气血不充，故肌肉瘦薄，骨节俱露，如鹤之膝。此亦由肾虚，名鹤膝节，加味地黄丸主之。"对因肾虚髓少而致"行迟"的病机变化进行了阐述。

Summary of Retarded Growth
1. Essence Failing to Nourish Bone Limpness of the celestial pillar, bowed and deviated head and nape, withering and limpness of the neck and nape, inability to lift and to rise, delayed standing and walking. 2. Essence Failing to Nourish the Teeth Long-term failure to teethe; loose and lusterless teeth. 3. Essence Failing to Nourish Hair Delayed hair growth, hair that is sparse and falls out easily. 4. Essence Failing to Nourish the Head, Face, and Entire Body Withered and weak mouth, lips, and flesh; lusterless facial complexion, tendency to fatigue, generalized lack of strength. 4. Insufficiency of Kidney Essence Pale tongue with thin fur, fine soft pulse.

生长迟缓
精不养骨—天柱软弱，头项倾斜，颈项萎软，不能抬起，站立行走迟缓 精不养齿—齿久不生，松动无光 精不养发—头发生长迟慢，稀疏易脱 精不养头面全身—口唇、肌肉萎软，面色不华，容易疲乏，全身无力 肾精不足—舌淡，苔薄，脉细软

4.6 Decreased Fertility

The kidney stores essence and governs reproduction. The "Treatise of Heavenly Truth from Remote Antiquity" in the *Sù Wèn* ("Plain Questions") contains the following passage:

> "[In women,] at the age of two times seven, *tiān-guǐ* arrives, the controlling vessel flows, the great thoroughfare vessel exuberates, and the menses descend at their time. Therefore, they are able to bear children… [In men,] at the age of two times eight, kidney qì is exuberant, *tiān-guǐ* arrives, essential qì spills, and yīn and yáng mix. Therefore they are able to have children."

Depletion of kidney essence from an insufficiency of earlier heaven or a later heaven lack of nourishment can prevent reproductive essence from promoting the maturation of reproductive functions or cause their decline. As a result, the pathomechanism of decreased fertility appears.

When kidney essence is insufficient, the thoroughfare and controlling vessels are deprived of nourishment and therefore unable to congeal essence and form a pregnancy. This results in delayed menstruation, scant pale-colored menses, and inability to conceive in spite of long-term conjugality.

When kidney essence is insufficient, the sexual functions decline. This results in reduced sexual desire, yáng wilt and premature ejaculation, and thin semen.

When essence-blood is depleted, it is unable to luxuriate the upper body. The result is dizzy head, flowery vision, and heart palpitations.

When essence-blood is insufficient, the house of the kidney is deprived of nourishment. This results in aching pain in the lower back and legs.

If essence-blood is unable to moisten the skin and flesh, the result is a withered yellow facial complexion and lack of moisture in the skin.

Depletion of kidney essence manifests in a pale tongue with scant fur, and a fine sunken pulse.

The chapter, "Reproduction; Emaciation and Lack of Pregnancy" in the *Fù Qīng Zhǔ Nǚ Kē* ("Fù Qīng-Zhǔ's Gynecology") states:

> "In women with a thin and timid body stature, enduring lack of conception, and lying down ill all day immediately after sexual intercourse, it might be assumed that this is caused by qì vacuity. Who knows that the actual reason is blood vacuity! Some people say that since blood is stored in the liver and essence is moistened in the kidney, how could discharge of kidney essence that is contracted from sexual intercourse be connected to blood vacuity? They hardly realize that when liver qì fails to upbear, essence cannot be discharged, and that as soon as kidney essence is discharged, liver qì is also bound to be constrained. Since the kidney is the mother of the liver, as soon as the mother discharges essence, it is unable to divide some off to nourish her son, which results in wood being dry and lacking water. Moreover, fire moves secretly to scorch metal, further increasing kidney vacuity.
>
> "Now if a thin person has too much fire and in addition discharges their essence, then water is reduced even further and fire is intensified even further. In spite of the fact that water restrains fire, if kidney essence is depleted, it lacks the strength to assist in the formation of fire on top of water in the hexagram, and therefore we see fatigue and resting…

> "For a formula, use *yǎng jīng zhòng yù tāng* (Essence-Nourishing Jade-Planting Decoction)... The function of this formula is not limited to supplementing blood, but it is also useful for replenishing essence. When essence is full, the uterus can easily receive it, and when blood is sufficient, the uterus can easily contain matter. Both of these are the path to bearing children."

This quotation analyzes in detail how to understand and treat depletion of kidney essence and insufficiency of essence blood in regards to women's infertility.

The chapter, "Patterns of Kidney and Bladder Disease; Lack of Pregnancy" in the *Lín Chuáng Zhōng Yī Nèi Kē Xué* ("Clinical Chinese Internal Medicine") states:

> "The kidney governs the storage of essence. Kidney vacuity and essence depletion are the cause for inability to bear children, and for yáng wilt, premature ejaculation, and thin semen. Kidney vacuity results in lumbar pain, and essence depletion results in fatigued spirit"

This quotation describes the pathomechanism of depletion of kidney essence and lack of fertility.

Decreased fertility is treated by enriching the kidney and replenishing essence, and by regulating and supplementing the thoroughfare and controlling vessels. The recommended formula is *yǎng jīng zhòng yù tāng* (Essence-Nourishing Jade-Planting Decoction) from the *Fù Qīng Zhǔ Nǚ Kē* ("Fù Qīng-Zhǔ's Gynecology").

Yǎng Jīng Zhòng Yù Tāng 养精种玉汤 Essence-Nourishing Jade-Planting Decoction
shú dì huáng (熟地黄 Rehmanniae Radix Praeparata, cooked rehmannia)
dāng guī (当归 Angelicae Sinensis Radix, Chinese angelica)
bái sháo (白芍 Paeoniae Radix Alba, white peony)
shān zhū yú (山茱萸 Corni Fructus, cornus)

生育减退

肾藏精，主生殖。故《素问•上古天真论》有女子"二七而天癸至，任脉通，太冲脉盛，月事以时下，故有子。"男子"二八肾气盛，天癸至，精气溢泄，阴阳和，故能有子"之说。如先天不足，或后天失养，肾精亏虚，生殖之精不能促进生殖机能的成熟，或引起生殖机能的衰退，则会出现生育减退的病机变化。肾精不足，冲任失养，不能凝精成孕，则月经后期，量少色淡，婚久不孕; 肾精不足，性功能减弱，则性欲低下，阳痿早泄，精液稀薄; 精血亏少，不能上荣，则头晕眼花，心悸; 精血不足，肾府失养，则腰腿酸痛; 精血不能润养肌肤，则面色萎黄，皮肤不润。肾精亏损，则舌淡，苔少，脉沉细。如《傅青主女科•种子•身瘦不孕》曰："妇人有瘦怯身躯，久不孕育，一交男子，即卧病终朝，人以为气虚之故，谁知是血虚之故乎！或谓血藏于肝精涵于肾，交感乃泄肾之精，与血虚何与？殊不知肝气不升，则精不能泄，肾精既泄，则肝气亦不能舒; 以肾为肝之母，母既泄精，不能分润以养其子，则木燥乏水; 而火且暗动以烁金，则肾愈虚也。况瘦人多火而又泄其精，则水益少而火益炽，水虽制火，而肾精空乏，无力以济成火在水上之卦，所以倦怠而卧也。...方用养精种玉汤，...此方之用，不特补血而纯于填精，精满则子宫易于摄精，血足则子宫易于容物，皆有子之道也。"详细分析了肾精亏虚，精血不足导致妇女不孕的病机变化。《临床中医内科学•肾膀胱病证•不育症》云："肾主藏精，肾虚精亏，故生育不能，而阳痿、早泄、精液稀薄; 肾虚则腰痛，精亏则神疲。"论述肾精亏损，失于生育的病机。治法宜滋肾填精，调补冲任。方药选用《傅青主女科》养精种玉汤（大熟地，当归，白芍，山萸肉）。

Literature Review of Decreased Fertility

📖 *Zhū Bìng Yuán Hòu Lùn* ("Origin and Indicators of Disease"), "Symptoms of Vacuity Taxation Childlessness"

> "The signs of childlessness in the husband means that his semen is clear like water and cold like ice or iron. Furthermore, when during seminal discharge semen does not eject, but gathers in the penis, this also means childlessness… When men have a pulse that is faint, weak, and rough, this means childlessness and that essential qì is chilled."

This quotation illustrates the pathomechanical changes of insufficient kidney essence in regards to lack of or thin semen in men, and sterility and childlessness.

📖 *Zá Bìng Yuán Liú Xī Zhú* ("Incisive Light on the Source of Miscellaneous Disease"), "The Kidney: Disease of the Second Yáng [Channel]"

> "Disease of the second yáng refers to the pathocondition of blood vacuity and thin semen… That being so, how could second yáng

> disease not be caused by scantness of semen and debilitation of blood? The ancients ascribed this disease to blood taxation, and this is truly so. Women's failure to menstruate is caused by a blood disease. Since semen is blood, men's inability ejaculate is also a blood disease."

This quotation points out that thin semen and sterility stems from blood taxation and depletion of the kidney's essence-blood.

文献评述

《诸病源候论•虚劳无子候》曰："丈夫无子者，其精清如水，冷如泳铁，皆为无子之候。又，泄精精不射出，但聚于阴头，亦无子。...男子脉得微弱而涩，为无子，精气清冷也。"阐明了肾精不足，男子无精少精，不育无子的病机变化。

《杂病源流犀烛•肾•二阳病》曰："二阳病，血虚精少症也。...然则二阳之病，非由精少血衰而何。古人谓为症属血劳，洵有然也。盖以女于不月，因属血病。精即是血，男子不得隐曲，亦即血病也。"指出了肾之精血亏虚可导致精少不育的病机变化。

Summary of Decreased Fertility
1. Thoroughfare and Controlling Vessels Deprived of Nourishment Delayed menstruation, scant pale-colored menses, lack of pregnancy in spite of long-term marriage.
2. Decline of Sexual Functions Reduced sexual desire, yáng wilt and premature ejaculation, thin semen.
3. Depletion of Essence-Blood Clouded head and flowery vision, heart palpitations.
4. House of the Kidney Deprived of Nourishment Aching pain in the lower back and legs.
5. Failure to Nourish the Skin and Flesh Withered yellow facial complexion, lack of moisture in the skin.
6. Depletion of Kidney Essence Pale tongue with scant fur, fine sunken pulse.

生育减退
冲任失养—月经后期，量少色淡，婚久不孕
性功能减弱—性欲低下，阳痿早泄，精液稀薄
精血亏少—头晕眼花，心悸
肾府失养—腰腿酸痛
不养肌肤—面色萎黄，皮肤不润
肾精亏损—舌淡，苔少，脉沉细

4.7 Essence Depletion Causing Impaired Absorption

The lung governs the exhalation of qì; the kidney governs the absorption of qì. These two support and complement each other, and together accomplish the process of air exchange in the lung. In addition, the normal discharge and intake of inhaled and exhaled qì is also dependent on the abundance of kidney essence. If kidney essence is depleted, essence fails to transform qì. Kidney qì is insufficient and fails to absorb and contain. The lung's functions of diffusion and depuration are disturbed and original qì ascends counterflow. As a result, the pathomechanism of essence depletion causing impaired absorption can appear.

When kidney essence is depleted, kidney qì is insufficient and qì fails to return to its origin, but surges upward in counterflow instead. The result is shortness of breath resembling panting, hasty rapid breathing, and difficulty in inhalation and exhalation.

When original qì ascends counterflow and lung qì fails to downbear, it obstructs the key pathway in the throat. This manifests in obstruction and discomfort in the throat.

When kidney essence is depleted, essence-blood is insufficient and therefore unable to ascend and nourish the head. The result is clouded head and flowery vision.

When kidney essence is insufficient, the formal body and the lower back and knees are deprived of nourishment. The result is emaciation and limp aching lower back and knees.

When kidney essence is insufficient, qì and blood do not fill the vessel pathways. This manifests in a pale tongue with scant fur, and a faint fine spiritless or fine weak pulse.

The "Schema of Miscellaneous Patterns; Hasty Panting" in the *Jǐng Yuè Quán Shū* ("Jǐng-Yuè's Complete Compendium") states:

> "The lung is responsible for true panting, and the kidney is responsible for seeming panting. What do I mean by this? The lung is the governor of qì, and the kidney is the root of qì. The lung governs the skin and body hair and lives in the upper burner. Therefore, an invasion of evil qì results in qì congestion in the upper burner, which constitutes panting. This congestion and stagnation of qì should be cleared and broken up. The kidney governs essence and marrow and is located in the lower burner. If true yīn is depleted, essence fails to transform qì, and above and below fail to interact, which constitutes hasty breathing. Hastiness is the first step towards complete interruption. When short and hasty breathing is further aggravated by dispersing and scattering, this is said to be 'like pressing on eggs.'"

This quotation clearly points out that insufficiency of kidney essence prevents essence from transforming qì, and kidney qì from absorbing, which manifests in the pathomechanical changes of short hasty breathing that resembles panting.

Essence depletion causing impaired absorption is treated by boosting essence and nourishing blood, and by downbearing qì and calming panting. The recommended formula is *zhēn yuán yǐn* (True Origin Beverage) from the *Jǐng Yuè Quán Shū* ("Jǐng-Yuè's Complete Compendium") with the addition of *zǐ hé chē* (Hominis Placenta), *guī bǎn jiāo* (Testudinis Carapacis et Plastri Gelatinum), *hé táo ròu* (Juglandis Semen), *wǔ wèi zǐ* (Schisandrae Fructus), and *zǐ shí yīng* (Fluoritum). In cases with extreme qì vacuity and faint pulse, add *rén shēn* (Ginseng Radix).

Zhēn Yuán Yǐn 贞元饮 True Origin Beverage
shú dì huáng (熟地黄 Rehmanniae Radix Praeparata, cooked rehmannia)
zhì gān cǎo (炙甘草 Glycyrrhizae Radix, mix-fried licorice)
dāng guī (当归 Angelicae Sinensis Radix, Chinese angelica)
Plus:
zǐ hé chē (紫河车 Hominis Placenta, placenta)
guī bǎn jiāo (龟版胶 Testudinis Carapacis et Plastri Gelatinum, tortoise shell glue)

hé táo rén (胡桃仁 Juglandis Semen, walnut)
wǔ wèi zǐ (五味子 Schisandrae Fructus, schisandra)
zǐ shí yīng (紫石英 fluorite, Fluoritum)

精亏失纳

肺主呼气，肾主纳气，二者相辅相成，共同完成气体在肺部的交换过程。而呼吸之气的正常出入，又离不开肾精的充足。如肾精亏虚，精不化气，肾气不足，而失纳摄，肺之宣肃功能障碍，元气上逆，则可出现精亏失纳的病机变化。肾精亏虚，肾气不足，气不归元，冲逆向上，则气短似喘，呼吸促急，提之不能升，吞之不能降;元气上逆，肺气不降，阻于咽喉要道，表现为咽道阻塞不适; 肾精亏损，精血不足，不能上养于头，则头昏眼花; 肾精不足，形体、腰膝失养，则形体消瘦，腰膝酸软。肾精不足，气血不充脉道，则表现为舌淡，苔少，脉微细无神，或脉细弱。如《景岳全书•杂证谟•喘促》曰："真喘者其责在肺，似喘者其责在肾。何也?盖肺为气之主，肾为气之根。肺主皮毛而居上焦，故邪气犯之，则上焦气壅而为喘，气之壅滞者，宜清宜破也。肾主精髓而在下焦，若真阴亏损，精不化气，则下不上交而为促，促者断之基也，气既短促，而再加消散，如压卵矣。"明确指出了肾精不足，精不化气，肾气不纳，出现气短促似喘的病机变化。治法宜益精养血，降气平喘。方药选用《景岳全书》贞元饮（熟地黄、炙甘草、当归）加紫河车、龟板胶、核桃肉、五味子、紫石英。如气虚脉微至极者，加人参。

Literature Review of Essence Depletion Causing Impaired Absorption

📖 *Zhèng Yīn Mài Zhì* ("Pathoconditions: Causes, Pulses, and Treatments"), "On the Pathocondition of Panting: Yīn Vacuity Panting and Counterflow"

"The cause of yīn vacuity panting and counterflow is an insufficiency of yīn blood. The fire of the five minds in reverting yáng stirs the fire in the thoroughfare and controlling vessels and makes it surge upward from below. When yīn essence is insufficient, dragon and thunder fire surges straight into the upper burner, and both fires surge upward. All this is called yīn vacuity panting and counterflow… For cases with insufficiency of yīn essence, use *jiā mì tiān dì jiān* (Family Secret Heaven and Earth Brew) or *jiā mì gān shèn wán* (Family Secret Liver and Kidney Pill)."

While this passage focuses on discussing the disease cause and pathomechanism of yīn vacuity panting and counterflow, we can see from the fact that it mentions "insufficiency of kidney essence" that it also includes this factor. Thus, it explains the objective existence of the pathomechanism by which kidney essence failing to absorb leads to hasty panting.

📖 *Lín Zhèng Zhǐ Nán Yī Àn* ("A Clinical Guide with Case Histories"), "Panting" (a quotation by Shào Xīn-Fǔ)

> "The cause of panting is repletion when the lung is responsible, and vacuity when the kidney is responsible... Where vacuity is concerned, it can be divided into damage to essence and qì desertion. Replenish essence with concentrated formulas, and at the same time invariably settle containment.
>
> "To make a kidney qì [decoction], add *chén xiāng* (Aquilariae Lignum Resinatum), to make a qì-gathering [decoction], add *qīng qiān* (Minium) (identical to the Chinese medicinal *qiān dān* (Minium), which has the effect of settling fright and quieting the spirit, is toxic, and is presently mostly used in topical application). Differentiate between yīn and yáng conditions. In qì desertion, the root floats, and inhalation damages the sea of origin. This is a perilous condition for which there is no hope. Knowing that herbs and shrubs are indifferent, and that hard and soft measures will provide little succor, there are [nevertheless] medicinals like *rén shēn* (Ginseng Radix), *zǐ hé chē* (Hominis Placenta), *wǔ wèi zǐ* (Schisandrae Fructus), and *bái shí yīng* (Quartz Album), to rapidly rectify the true origin and instantly reverse the situation by supplementing the treatment of heaven, which was left unmentioned by the ancients."

This quotation clearly points out that insufficiency of kidney essence and essence depletion with kidney qì failing to absorb can lead to hasty panting. At the same time, it emphasizes that you should use concentrated medicinals in treatment to replenish and supplement kidney essence. Thus it explains that kidney essence depletion is one of the pathomechanisms that lead to panting.

文献评述

《症因脉治•喘症论•阴虚喘逆》曰："阴虚喘逆之因，阴血不足，五志厥阳之火，触动冲任之火，自下冲上，阴精不足，龙雷之火，直冲上焦，二火上冲，皆名阴虚喘逆之症。...阴精不足者，用家秘天地煎、家秘肝肾丸。”虽然以讨论阴虚喘逆的病因病机为主，但从“阴精不足”的提法中，可以看出肾精不足已包含其中，说明肾精失纳，引起喘促的病机客观存在。

《临证指南医案•喘》邵新甫曰：“喘症之因，在肺者实，在肾者虚。...虚者，有精伤、气脱之分，填精以浓厚之剂，必兼镇摄，肾气加沉香，都气入青铅(即是中药铅丹，有镇惊安神作用，有毒，现在多外用)，从阴从阳之异也。气脱则根浮，吸伤元海，危亡可力而待。思草木之无情，刚柔所难济，则又有人参、河车、五味、石英之属，急续真元，挽回顷刻，补天之治，古所未及。”明确指出肾精不足，精亏肾气失纳，可致喘促，并强调在治疗上应以浓厚之药，填补肾精，说明肾精亏损是引起气喘发作的病机之一。

Summary of Essence Depletion Causing Impaired Absorption
1. Kidney Vacuity and Lack of Absorption Shortness of breath resembling panting, hasty rapid breathing, lifting it without being able to upbear, and swallowing it without being able to downbear.
2. Upward Counterflow of Lung Qì Obstruction in the throat.
3. Essence Blood Deprived of Nourishment Clouded head and flowery vision.
4. Lower Back and Knees Deprived of Nourishment Emaciation, limp aching lower back and knees.
5. Insufficiency of Kidney Essence Pale tongue with scant fur, faint fine spiritless pulse.

精亏失纳
精虚不纳—气短似喘，呼吸促急，提之不能升，吞之不能降
肺气上逆—咽道阻塞
精血失养—头昏眼花
形体、腰膝失养—形体消瘦，腰膝酸软
肾精不足—舌淡，苔少，脉微细无神

4.8 Essence Depletion Causing Scantness of Blood

The kidney stores essence and is able to convert this into blood. Thus essence and blood engender each other. The "Treatise on Qì, Blood, Essence and Spirit" in the *Dú Yī Suí Bǐ* ("Informal Essays on Reading Medical Texts"), for example, states:

> "Why is it that essence is classified together with blood, liquid, and humor? The treatise, 'The Spirit' in the *Líng Shū* ("The Magic Pivot") says that the five viscera govern the storage of essence. Therefore it is summarily called essence. Blood is the essence of grain and water. Transformed through steaming by the life gate fire, it engenders and grows the flesh, skin, and body hair. All tangible aspects of the body's sinews and bones, flesh, skin, and hair are of the same type as blood. Essence is formed from the subtle essence of blood and is dependent on vital qì… Essence combines with the quintessence of blood and the fluids, is extremely clear and rich, and furthermore extremely wondrous. It is the abode of the spirit."

This quotation points out that essence-blood is the most fundamental substance of the body, and that when kidney essence is plentiful, qì and blood are abundant, the formal body is bountiful, and the essence-spirit is exuberant.

The chapter, "The Kidney" in "Separate Notes on The Internal Viscera and Bowels" from the *Yī Xué Rù Mén* ("The Gateway to Medicine") further states: "The whiskers, head hair, and face are all netted by the kidney vessel. When yáng essence exuberates and pours to the outside, the whiskers and head hair are luxuriant and the face is lustrous and moist." This quotation denotes that the whiskers, head hair, and face are all filled by essence-blood, and that when kidney essence is replete, qì and blood are exuberant, and the person glows with health.

In terms of pathology, when essence is vacuous, blood is also vacuous, and when blood is depleted, essence is also scant. An incidence of major bleeding, a history of chronic bleeding, or drunkenness during sexual intercourse can consume essence and discharge qì, so that essence is lost and qì is exhausted. Since essence fails to engender blood, this can lead to the pathomechanism of essence depletion causing scantness of blood.

When kidney essence is depleted, essence fails to transform blood. Essence-blood is insufficient, and the formal body is deprived of nourishment. The result is emaciation, fatigue of the essence-spirit, and desiccated body and head hair that has a tendency to fall out.

When essence is desiccated and blood scant, it is unable to ascend and nourish the head and eyes. This results in dizzy head and vision, and a haggard or drawn facial complexion.

When kidney essence is insufficient, qì and blood are depleted, and their movement lacks strength. Consequently, qì stagnation and blood stasis impede the movement of the qì dynamic in the chest and rib-side. This manifests in propping fullness in the chest and rib-side, and hampered eating and drinking.

Depletion of essence causes desiccated blood, which is retained inside the body and putrefies over a long period of time. This can cause a smelly fishy dry odor at the onset of the disease.

When static blood is retained internally and new blood is not engendered, static blood obstructs the network vessels, the network vessels break, and blood spills. This manifests in frequent spitting of blood, menstrual irregularities, flooding and spotting descent of blood, and frequent blood in the stool, which are the special characteristics of essence depletion causing blood stasis and bleeding.

Essence depletion and scantness of blood results in a pale white or dark pale tongue body with stasis speckles, and a fine rough pulse.

The chapter, "Blood Patterns" in the *Jǐng Yuè Quán Shū* ("Jǐng-Yuè's Complete Compendium"), "Schema of Miscellaneous Patterns" points out:

> "Essence is certainly the wellspring of the individual's life. Essence and blood seem to not be of the same category, yet the alchemists say that snivel, spittle, essence, liquid, sweat, blood, and humor are seven wondrous substances that all belong to yīn...
>
> "Blood belongs to essence. The essence stored in the kidney is not contained in profuse amounts; however, blood is abundant in the thoroughfare vessel. Essence and blood are steadily engendered by the spleen, managed by the heart, received by the liver, distributed by the lung, and discharged by the kidney. Essence and blood irrigate the channels of the entire body and reach everywhere. They animate the seven orifices, produce the movement of the limbs, the harmony and softness of sinew and bone, and the bounty of the flesh. Essence and blood enriche the viscera and bowels, quiet the spirit and the ethereal soul, moistens the facial complexion, and fill construction and defense. The fluids are able to be obtained and to move freely, and the two yīn are regulated and disinhibited. Wherever there is form and substance, it must be the effect of blood. For this reason, the fact that humans have a tangible form depends solely on blood."

This quotation discusses how kidney essence and blood are intimately related to the formal body, flesh, and countenance.

The chapter, "Various Symptoms of Vacuity Taxation Disease; Vacuity Taxation with Marked Emaciation" in the *Zhū Bìng Yuán Hòu Lùn* ("Origin and Indicators of Disease") also states:

> "Blood and qì are used to nourish the body. In patients with vacuity taxation, essence and marrow are withered and exhausted, and qì and blood are vacuous. Since they are unable to fill the skin and flesh, this causes marked emaciation."

This quotation points out how insufficiency of kidney essence and essence failing to engender blood cause vacuity of qì and blood, desiccated essence, and scant blood, so that they are unable to supply nourishment to the formal body, which leads to marked emaciation.

Essence depletion causing scantness of blood is treated by supplementing the kidney and boosting essence, and by supplementing and quickening blood. The recommended formula is *hé chē dà zào wán* (Placenta Great Creation Pill) from the *Yī Fāng Jí Jiě* ("Medical Formulas Gathered and Explained") in combination with *sì wū zéi yī lú rú wán* (Four of Cuttlefish to One of Madder Pill) from the *Sù Wèn* ("Plain Questions").

Hé Chē Dà Zào Wán 河车大造丸 Placenta Great Creation Pill
shú dì huáng (熟地黄 Rehmanniae Radix Praeparata, cooked rehmannia)
guī bǎn (龟版 Testudinis Plastrum, tortoise plastron)
zǐ hé chē (紫河车 Hominis Placenta, placenta)
rén shēn (人参 Ginseng Radix, ginseng)
tiān mén dōng (天门冬 asparagus, Asparagi Radix)
mài dōng (麦冬 Ophiopogonis Radix, ophiopogon)
dù zhòng (杜仲 Eucommiae Cortex, eucommia)
niú xī (牛膝 Achyranthis Bidentatae Radix, achyranthes)

Sì Wū Zéi Yī Lú Rú Wán 四乌贼一藘茹丸 Four of Cuttlefish to One of Madder Pill
wū zéi gǔ (乌贼骨 Sepiae Endoconcha, cuttlefish bone)
qiàn cǎo (茜草 Rubiae Radix, madder)
bào yú zhī (鲍鱼汁 Abalone Succus, abalone juice)

精亏血少

肾藏精，可转化为血，精血相互化生。如《读医随笔•气血精神论》曰："精之以精、血、津、液，列为四者，何也?<本神>曰：五脏主藏精者也，故统谓之精。夫血者，水谷之精微，得命门其火蒸化，以生长肌肉、皮毛者也。凡人身筋骨、肌肉、皮肤、毛发有形者，皆血类也。精者，血之精微所成，生气之所依也。...精者合血与津液之精华，极清极厚，而又极灵者也，是神之宅也。"认为精血为人体最基本的物质，肾精充足，则气血充沛，形体丰满，精神旺盛。《医学入门•脏腑条分•肾》又曰："须发颜面，皆肾脉所络，阳精盛注于外，则须发荣盛，面体光润。"指出须发颜面皆为精血所充，肾精充实，气血旺盛，则容光焕发。病理上，精虚则血亦虚，血亏则精亦少。如因有大出血或慢性失血病史，或醉入房中，耗精泄气，精去气竭，精不生血，则可引起精亏血少的病机变化。肾精亏损，精不化血，精血不足，形体失养，则形体消瘦，精神疲乏，毛发枯燥，容易脱落; 精枯血少，不能上养头目，则头目眩晕，面容憔悴; 肾精不足，气血亏损，运行无力，气滞血瘀，阻碍胸胁气机运行，则表现为胸胁支满，妨碍饮食; 精亏血枯，枯血留于体内，日久化腐，则可病至则先闻腥燥臭味; 瘀血留内，新血不生，瘀血阻络，络破血溢，出现时时唾血，月经不调，崩漏下血，时时便血等精亏血瘀出血的病变特点。精亏血少，则舌质淡白或暗淡，有瘀点，脉细涩。如《景岳全书•杂证谟•血证》指出："人之初生，必从精始，精之与血，若乎非类，而丹家曰：涕、唾、精、津、汗、血、液，七般灵物总属阴。...而血即精之属也，但精藏于肾，所蕴不多，而血富于冲，所至皆是。盖其源源而来，生化于脾，总统于心，藏受于肝，宣布于肺，施泄于肾，灌溉一身，无所不及。故凡为七窍之灵，为四肢之用，为筋骨之和柔，为肌肉之丰盛，以至滋脏腑，安神魂，润颜色，充营卫，津液得以通行，二阴得以调畅，凡形质所在，无非血之用也。是以人有此形，唯赖此血。"论述肾精和血与形体、肌肉、容颜有密切的关系。《诸病源候论•虚劳诸病候•虚劳羸瘦候》也指出："夫血气者，所以荣养其身也。虚劳之人，精髓萎竭，血气虚弱，不能充盛肌肤，此故羸瘦也。"指明了肾精不足，精不生血，气血虚弱，精枯血少，不能充养形体，导致机体羸瘦的病机改变。治法宜补肾益精，补血活血。方药选用《医方集解》河车大造丸（熟地黄、龟板、紫河车、人参、天门冬、麦门冬、杜仲、牛膝）合《素问》四乌贼一藘茹丸（乌贼骨、茜草、鲍鱼汁）。

Literature Review of Essence Depletion Causing Scantness of Blood

📖 *Jīn Guì Yào Lüè* ("Essential Prescriptions of the Golden Coffer"), "Pulse Symptoms and Treatments of Blood Impediment Vacuity Taxation"

> "When patients present with lesser abdominal tension, yīn head cold, dizzy vision, hair loss, and an extremely vacuous, scallion-stalk slow pulse, this means clear-food diarrhea, blood collapse, and seminal loss. Whenever the pulse is scallion-stalk, stirred, faint, and tight, this indicates seminal loss in men and dreaming of intercourse in women. *Guì zhī mǔ lì tāng* (Cinnamon Twig, Dragon Bone, and Oyster Shell Decoction) governs it."

This quotation describes how insufficiency of kidney essence presenting as lesser abdominal tension, yīn head cold, dizzy vision, hair loss, and slow vacuous pulse leads to clear-food diarrhea, blood collapse, and seminal loss.

📖 *Fù Rén Dà Quán Liáng Fāng* ("Compendium of Good Remedies for Women"), "On Formulas for Blood Desiccation"

> "Discussion of the Inside of the Abdomen: When a patient suffers from propping fullness in the chest and rib-side, hampered eating, a fishy or animal odor at the onset of the condition, discharge of clear humor from the nose, pain in the limbs, dizzy vision, and frequent anterior and posterior bleeding, this disease is called blood desiccation. It is caused by great blood desertion at a young age or drunkenness during sexual intercourse, either of which has depleted the kidney and liver."

This quotation describes the pathomechanism great blood desertion or drunkenness during intercourse deplete the kidney and liver and lead to blood desiccation and bleeding.

文献评述

《金匮要略•血痹虚劳病脉证并治》曰："夫失精家少腹弦急，阴头寒，目眩，发落，脉极虚芤迟，为清谷，亡血，失精。脉得诸芤动微紧，男子失精，女子梦交，桂枝龙骨牡蛎汤主之。"对肾精不足导致亡血的病机变化进行了论述。

《妇人良方大全•血枯方论》曰："腹中论曰，有病胸胁支满，妨于食，病至则先闻腥臊，鼻出清液，四肢痛。目眩，时时前后血出，病名曰血枯。此年少时，因大脱血，或醉而入房，亏损肾肝。"论述了房室不节，肾精大亏，导致血枯出血的病机变化。

Summary of Essence Depletion Causing Scantness of Blood
1. Formal Body Deprived of Nourishment Emaciation, fatigue of the essence-spirit, desiccated body and head hair that has a tendency to fall out.
2. Head and Face Deprived of Nourishment Dizzy head and vision, haggard or drawn facial complexion.
3. Qì Stagnation and Blood Stasis Propping fullness in the chest and rib-side, hampered eating and drinking.
4. Desiccated Blood Putrefying Smelly dry fishy odor at the onset of disease.
5. Blood Stasis and Bleeding Frequent spitting of blood, menstrual irregularities, flooding and spotting descent of blood, frequent bloody stool.
6. Depleted Essence and Scant Blood Pale white or dark pale tongue body with stasis speckles, fine rough pulse.

精亏血少
形体失养—形体消瘦，精神疲乏，毛发枯燥，容易脱落
头面失养—头目眩晕，面容憔悴
气滞血瘀—胸胁支满，妨碍饮食
枯血化腐—病至则先闻腥燥臭味
血瘀出血—时时唾血，月经不调，崩漏下血，时时便血
精亏血少—舌质淡白或暗淡，有瘀点，脉细涩

4.9 Essence Depletion Causing Vacuity Taxation

The "General Treatise on Vacuity and Repletion" in the *Sù Wèn* ("Plain Questions") states: "When essential qì is despoliated, there is vacuity." This is understood to mean that all patterns of vacuity taxation and insufficiency are related to depletion of kidney essence. The chapter, "Internal Causes; Vacuity Taxation" in the *Zá Bìng Guǎng Yào* ("Broad Essentials of Miscellaneous Disease") also explains:

> "People have essence and afterwards have spirit. When people suffer from vacuity detriment, this always comes from the heart and the kidney… The various vacuities and hundred detriments are all without exception caused by the heart and kidney."

The heart stores the spirit, and the kidney stores essence. When kidney essence is insufficient, the root of earlier heaven loses its ability to engender and nourish, and the functions and activities of the viscera and bowels in the entire body are weakened. This can lead to the pathomechanism of essence depletion causing vacuity taxation.

The *Jīn Guì Yào Lüè* ("Essential Prescriptions of the Golden Coffer") was the first text to mention "vacuity taxation" by name. The chapter, "Blood Impediment Vacuity Taxation" from this text points out:

> "Vacuity taxation with abdominal urgency, palpitations, spontaneous bleeding, pain in the abdomen, seminal loss while dreaming, aching pain in the limbs, heat vexation in the hands and feet, and dry throat and dry mouth are governed by *xiǎo jiàn zhōng tāng* (Minor Center-Fortifying Decoction)… Vacuity taxation with lumbar pain, hypertonicity in the lesser abdomen, and inhibited urination are governed by *bā wèi shèn qì wán* (Eight-Ingredient Kidney Qì Pill)."

This quotation describes the pathomechanism of insufficiency of kidney essence causing vacuity taxation with abdominal urgency and lesser abdominal tension and pain.

When kidney essence is depleted, essence fails to transform blood, and the head and face are deprived of nourishment. The result is a pale white and lusterless facial complexion.

When essence-blood is insufficient, original qì is vacuous and therefore unable to nourish the lung. The result is shortness of breath and shortage of qì.

When kidney essence is depleted, transformation of blood is insufficient. Consequently, blood fails to nourish the heart, and the heart spirit fails to keep its composure. The result is heart palpitations, disquietude, insomnia, and profuse dreaming.

When kidney essence is insufficient, it is unable to engender blood to nourish the flesh, and to engender marrow to nourish the bones. The result is withering of the major bones, wasting and sagging of the major masses of flesh, sacrum and coccyx carrying the heel [hypertonicity of the feet], and the spine carrying the head.

When essence-blood is depleted, the lesser abdomen is deprived of moistening, which causes qì stagnation and hypertonicity of the sinews.

The result is lesser abdominal fullness and distention, abdominal pain and hypertonicity, and painful defecation and urination.

Insufficiency of kidney essence manifests in a pale tongue with white tongue fur, and a vacuous sunken stringlike pulse.

The chapter, "Various Symptoms of Vacuity Taxation Disease; Vacuity Taxation" in the *Zhū Bìng Yuán Hòu Lùn* ("Origin and Indicators of Disease") points out:

> "Kidney taxation results in difficulty bending forward and backward, inhibited voidings of reddish yellow urine with residual dripping, pain in the penis, dampness in the genitals, heaviness in the scrotum, and lesser-abdominal fullness and tension... Kidney damage results in thin semen, lumbar and back pain, and reverse flow and cold in the lower body."

This passage describes the pathomechanical manifestations of depletion of kidney essence leading to kidney taxation.

The "General Treatise on Vacuity Taxation; Internal Damage Vacuity Taxation" in the *Zhèng Yīn Mài Zhì* ("Pathoconditions: Causes, Pulses, and Treatments") also states:

> "The pathocondition of essence vacuity taxation damage: Withering of the major bones, wasting and sagging of the major masses of flesh, sacrum and coccyx carrying the heel [hypertonicity of the feet], spine carrying the head, possibly steaming bone tidal heat, and painful defecation and urination. This is the pathocondition of essence vacuity taxation damage."

This quotation clearly indicates the pathomechanism and manifestations of kidney essence depletion and essence damage leading to vacuity taxation.

Essence vacuity taxation damage is treated by supplementing the kidney and replenishing essence, and by boosting qì and engendering blood. The recommended formula is *jì tián jīng shēng xuè fāng* (Salvation Formula for Replenishing Essence and Engendering Blood) from the *Shèn Bìng Zhèng Zhì Gài Yào* ("Essentials of Patterns and Treatment in Kidney Disease").

Jì Tián Jīng Shēng Xuè Fāng 济填精生血方 Salvation Formula for Replenishing Essence and Engendering Blood
nǚ zhēn zǐ (女贞子 Ligustri Lucidi Fructus, ligustrum)
mò hàn lián (墨旱莲 Ecliptae Herba, eclipta)
pó gù zhī (婆固脂 Psoraleae Fructus, psoralea)
hé táo rén (胡桃仁 Juglandis Semen, walnut)
yú piāo jiāo (鱼鳔胶 , Pisces Os Gelatina, fish bone gelatin)
zǐ hé chē (紫河车 Hominis Placenta, placenta)
shēng dì huáng (生地黄 Rehmanniae Radix, rehmannia)
shú dì huáng (熟地黄 Rehmanniae Radix Praeparata, cooked rehmannia)
dǎng shēn (党参 Codonopsis Radix, codonopsis)
gǒu qǐ zǐ (枸杞子 Lycii Fructus, lycium)
guī bǎn (龟版 Testudinis Plastrum, tortoise plastron)
lù jiǎo (鹿角 Cervi Cornu, deerhorn)

精亏虚劳

《素问•通评虚实论》曰："精气夺则虚。"说明一切虚劳不足的病证都与肾精亏损有关。《杂病广要•内因类•虚劳》也说："人有精而后有神，今人之虚损，皆出于心肾。...诸虚百损，莫不由心肾而然。"心藏神，肾藏精，肾精不足，先天之本失却滋生、濡养，全身脏腑功能活动衰减，则会发生精亏虚劳的病机变化。《金匮要略》首先提出了"虚劳"的病名。《金匮要略•血痹虚劳病》指出："虚劳里急，悸，衄，腹中痛，梦失精，四肢酸疼，手足烦热，咽干，口燥，小建中汤主之。...虚劳腰痛，少腹拘急，小便不利者，八味肾气丸主之。"对包括肾精不足在内的虚劳里急，少腹拘急疼痛的病机变化进行了描述。肾精亏虚，精不化血，头面失养，则面色淡白而无光泽; 精血不足，元气虚少，不能养肺，则少气短气; 肾精亏虚，化血不足，血不养心，心神失守，则心悸不安，失眠多梦; 肾精不足，不能生血养肉，不能生髓养骨，则大骨枯槁，大肉陷下，尻以代踵，脊以代头; 精血亏虚，少腹失濡，气滞筋挛，则少腹胀满，腹痛拘急，大小便牵引作痛。肾精不足，则舌淡，苔白，脉虚沉弦。如《诸病源候论•虚劳病诸候•虚劳候》指出："肾劳者，背难以俯仰，小便不利，色赤黄而有余沥，茎内痛，阴湿，囊生疮，小腹满急。...肾伤，少精，腰背痛，厥逆下冷。"描述了肾精亏损而致肾劳的病机改变。《症因脉治•虚劳总论•内伤虚劳》也云："精虚劳伤之症：大骨枯槁，大肉陷下，尻以代踵，脊以代头，或骨蒸潮热，大小便牵引作痛，此精伤虚劳之症作矣。"明确提出肾精亏损，精伤而致虚劳的病机及表现。治法宜补肾填精，益气生血。方药选用《肾病证治概要》既济填精生血方（女贞子、旱莲草、破故纸、胡桃肉、鱼螵胶、紫河车、生地、熟地、党参、枸杞子、龟胶、鹿胶）。

Literature Review of Essence Depletion Causing Vacuity Taxation

📖 *Yī Xué Rù Mén* ("The Gateway to Medicine"), "The Various Vacuities"

> "Kidney taxation with restraint of ambition and moral fortitude results in lumbar and bone pain, seminal emission and white turbidity, and in extreme cases grimy facial complexion and pain in the spine... If the original cause is vacuity in the bowels that leads to vacuity in the viscera, causing dual vacuity in the bowels and viscera, the result is debilitated sight and hearing, and inability to walk straight. This is called 'extreme of essence' and causes people to suffer from essence turbidity and weak penis with small testicles. Therefore, it is also called 'six extremes.' Extreme here refers to damage."

This quotation discusses how depletion of kidney essence, essence vacuity taxation damage, and dual bowel/viscera vacuity leads to "six extremes."

📖 "*Lǐ Xū Yuán Jiàn* ("The Original Mirror of Rectifying Vacuity"), "The Three Treatments for Vacuity"

> "There are six causes of vacuity patterns: The cause of earlier heaven, the cause of later heaven, the cause of disease after pox and papules, the cause of external contraction, and the cause of medicinals. The cause of earlier heaven points to the beginning of receiving qì, whether the father and mother were already debilitated by age, or were overwhelmed by taxation during sexual intercourse, or the pregnancy was irregular, or there was excessive sexual desire. All these factors prevent essence-blood from being effulgent and cause the new-born child to die young or to be weak."

This quotation discusses that the majority of causes among the earlier heaven factors in the disease of vacuity taxation are related to a lack of exuberant essence-blood. Thus it explains that depletion of kidney essence is a critical pathomechanism at the base of vacuity taxation.

📖 *Mì Chuán Zhèng Zhì Yào Jué* ("Secret Transmission of Essential Rhymes for Patterns and Treatment"), "Vacuity Detriment"

> "Although all five viscera can be affected by taxation, it is most common in the heart and kidney. The heart governs blood, and the kidney governs essence. When kidney is exhausted and blood desiccated, consumption arises."

This quotation explains that depletion of kidney essence and scantness of blood is a key pathomechanism that leads to vacuity taxation.

文献评述

《医学入门•诸虚》曰："肾劳矜持志节，则腰骨痛，遗精白浊，极则面垢脊痛。…若原因腑虚，以致脏虚，脏腑俱虚，视听已衰，行步不正，名曰'精极'，令人精浊，茎弱核小，故又曰'六极'。'极'，即伤也。"阐述了肾精亏虚，虚劳精极导致腰脊疼痛的病机变化。

《理虚元鉴•治虚有三》曰："虚证有六因：有先天之因，有后天之因，有痘疹及病后之因，有外感之因，有医药之因，因先天者，指受气之初，父母或年已衰老，或乘劳入房，或妊娠失调，或色欲过度，此皆精血不旺，致令所生之子夭弱。"论述引起虚劳病证的先天因素中，大部分原因为精血不旺。说明肾精亏虚是引起虚劳的重要病机之一。

《秘传证治要诀•虚损门》曰："五脏虽皆有劳，心肾为多，心主血，肾主精，精竭血燥而痨生。"说明肾精亏损，精亏血燥，是引起虚劳的重要病机。

Summary of Essence Depletion Causing Vacuity Taxation

1. Head and Face Deprived of Nourishment
   Pale white and lusterless facial complexion.
2. Vacuity of Original Qì
   Shortness of breath and shortage of qì.
3. Essence-Blood Failing to Nourish the Heart
   Heart palpitations and disquietude, insomnia and profuse dreaming.
4. Inability to Nourish the Flesh and Bones
   Withering of the major bones, wasting and sagging of the major masses of flesh, sacrum and coccyx carrying the heel [hypertonicity of the feet], spine carrying the head.
5. Lesser Abdomen Deprived of Moistening
   Lesser abdominal distention and fullness, abdominal pain and hypertonicity, painful defecation and urination.
6. Insufficiency of Kidney Essence
   Pale tongue with white tongue fur, vacuous sunken stringlike pulse.

精亏虚劳
头面失养—面色淡白而无光泽
元气虚少—少气短气
精血不养于心—心悸不安，失眠多梦
不能养肉养骨—大骨枯槁，大肉陷下，尻以代踵，脊以代头
少腹失濡—少腹胀满，腹痛拘急，大小便牵引作痛
肾精不足—舌淡，苔白，脉虚沉弦

4.10 Essence Depletion Causing Premature Debilitation

The kidney stores essence. The length of human life is therefore determined to a large extent by the exuberance or debilitation of essential qì in the kidney. Essence in the kidney decides a person's lifespan and provides the foundation for existence, by influencing the entire process of birth, growth, maturity, aging, and death.

As the "Treatise of Heavenly Truth from Remote Antiquity" in the *Sù Wèn* ("Plain Questions") states:

> "In women…at the age of six times seven, the three yáng vessels are debilitated in the upper body, the face is all parched, and the hair begins to turn gray. At the age of seven times seven, the controlling vessel is vacuous and the great thoroughfare vessel is debilitated. *Tiān-guǐ* is exhausted and menstruation stops. Therefore, the physical body spoils and she cannot bear children.
>
> "In men…at the age of five times eight, kidney qì is debilitated, the hair falls out, and the teeth are desiccated. At the age of six times eight, yáng qì is exhausted in the upper body, the face is parched, and the hair of the head and side-locks turn gray. At the age of seven times eight, liver qì is debilitated, the sinews are unable to move, *tiān-guǐ* is exhausted, semen is scant, the kidney is debilitated, and the body is extremely fatigued. At the age of eight times eight, the teeth and hair fall out."

This quotation clearly indicates that the decline of kidney essence is an important factor leading to age-related debilitation.

When kidney essence is depleted, it is unable to ascend and nourish the brain. The result is a dull spirit-affect, unsustained vitality, forgetfulness and abstraction, slowness of thought, and delayed reactions. When essence fails to nourish the spirit, thoughts are confused and the spirit is disquieted. The result is insomnia and profuse dreaming, slowness to fall asleep, waking up early, light sleep, and increased dozing.

Failure of essence to nourish the ears results in tinnitus, deafness, and impaired hearing.

When essence fails to nourish the teeth and hair, the result is premature graying of the whiskers and head hair, and hair loss and loose teeth.

When kidney essence is unable to govern the bones and marrow, essence-marrow is empty. The result is wilting and limpness of both legs, difficulty in walking, flaccid movements, and strained action.

Insufficiency of kidney essence manifests in a pale tongue and a fine weak pulse.

The chapter, "Living Out the Complete Number of One's Allotted Years" in the *Lǚ Shì Chūn Qiū* ("Lu's Spring and Autumn Annals") states:

> "The reason why flowing water does not putrefy and the door pivot does not rot is that they move. When the physical body does not move, essence does not flow; when essence does not flow, qì is depressed. If located in the head, it causes swelling and wind; if located in the ears, hardness of hearing and deafness; if located in the eyes, gum in the eyes and eye sockets, and blindness; if located in the nose, snivelling nose and nasal congestion; if located in the abdomen, distention and lesser-abdominal pain; if located in the legs, wilting and stumbling."

Essence failing to flow includes kidney essence. When kidney essence is depleted, qì does not flow and the whole body is deprived of nourishment. This creates numerous manifestations of aging.

The "Treatise on Nourishing the Aged" in the *Gé Zhì Yú Lùn* ("Further Treatises on the Properties of Things") states:

> "When people reach the age of sixty or seventy, essence and blood are both consumed… This results in dizzy head, eye discharge, itchy flesh, frequent urination, nasal mucus, loss of teeth, increased drool, reduced sleeping, weak legs, deafness, forgetfulness, dizziness, intestinal dryness, grimy facial complexion, hair loss, flowery vision, prolonged sitting with suddenly falling asleep, coldness even prior to exposure to wind, tendency to hunger after eating, and a tendency to tear when crying. The later years of life do not come without these."

This quotation further points out that age-related depletion of the kidney's essence-blood and impaired enrichment cause numerous manifestations of aging.

Essence depletion causing premature debilitation is treated by supplementing and boosting kidney essence, and by promoting longevity. For medicinals, select *shú dì huáng* (Rehmanniae Radix Praeparata), *gǒu qǐ zǐ* (Lycii Fructus), *shān zhū yú* (Corni Fructus), *hé shǒu wū* (Polygoni Multiflori Radix), *rén shēn* (Ginseng Radix), *ròu cōng róng* (Cistanches Herba), *yín yáng huò* (Epimedii Herba), and *tù sī zǐ* (Cuscutae Semen).

精亏早衰

肾藏精，人体寿命的长短，很大程度上决定于肾中精气的盛衰。肾中之精主宰人之寿命和生存基础，肾精影响人的生、长、壮、老、死的全过程。如《素问•上古天真论》曰：“女子…六七，三阳脉衰于上，面皆焦，发始白; 七七，任脉虚，太冲脉衰少，天癸竭，地道不通，故形坏而无子也。丈夫…五八，肾气衰，发堕齿槁; 六八，阳气衰竭于上，面焦，发鬓颁白; 七八，肝气衰，筋不能动，天癸竭，精少，肾脏衰，形体皆极; 八八，则齿发去。”明确指出肾精不足是引起早衰的重要病机。肾精亏损，不能上养于脑，则神情呆钝，精力不支，健忘恍惚，思维迟钝，反应缓慢; 精不养神，神思错乱，神不安宁，则失眠多梦，睡得迟，醒得早，睡得浅，打盹多; 不养于耳，则耳鸣耳聋，听力下降; 不养于齿发，则须发早白，发脱齿摇; 肾精不能主骨生髓，精髓空虚，则两足痿软，步履艰难，行动迟缓，动作吃力; 肾精不足，则舌淡，脉细弱。如《吕氏春秋•尽数》曰：“流水不腐，户枢不蠹，动也。形不动则精不流，精不流则气郁，处头则为肿为风，处耳则为挶（重听）为聋，处目则为蔑（指眼屎糊满眼眶）为盲，处鼻则为鼽（鼻流清涕）为窒（鼻塞），处腹则为张（同胀）为府（指小腹痛），处足则为痿为蹶。”精不流，是指精微物质，其中应包括肾精，肾精亏损，气不流行，全身失养，产生多种衰老的表现。《格致余论•养老论》曰：“人生至六十、七十以后，精血俱耗。…头晕目眵，肌痒溺数，鼻涕牙落，涎多寐少，足弱耳聩，健忘眩晕，肠燥面垢，发脱眼花，久坐兀睡，未风先寒，食则易饥，哭则有泪，但是老境，无不如此。”进一步指出，年老肾之精血亏损，失于滋养，出现各种衰老的表现。治宜补益肾精，益寿延年。药物可选熟地、枸杞、山茱萸、首乌、人参、苁蓉、淫羊藿、菟丝子。

Literature Review of Essence Depletion Causing Premature Debilitation

🕮 *Líng Shū* ("The Magic Pivot"), "Natural Lifespan"

> "At ninety years of age, kidney qì is parched, and the four visceral channels are empty. At a hundred years of age, the five viscera are all vacuous, spirit qì is all gone, and the skeleton merely lives out its end."

This quotation points out that exhaustion of the kidney's essential qì and vacuity of all five viscera occur with aging.

🕮 *Jǐng Yuè Quán Shū* ("Jǐng-Yuè's Complete Compendium"), "Record of Transmitting Loyalty: On Treating the Form"

> "It is said that movement, vision, and hearing cannot exist without this form; that pretty and ugly, good and malign cannot exist without this form; and that courage and timidity, stupidity and wisdom cannot exist without this form. Indeed life and death also only exist within this form! … In reality, the hidden meaning of the term 'form' consists of nothing but the two characters essence and blood."

The same text further states:

> "Essence and blood are exactly this form, and the form is exactly this essence and blood."

These remarks discuss how all aspects of life and aging are closely related to the exhaustion of essence and blood. This includes premature debilitation due to depletion of kidney essence.

🕮 *Shòu Qīn Yǎng Lǎo Xīn Shū* ("The New Book of Longevity"), "Prohibitions and Safeguards"

> "Humans are one of the myriad things and cannot escape the plan of heaven and earth. If *tiān-guǐ* is used up, essence-blood is exhausted and spirit qì becomes weak and floating, reverting to the state of infants."

This quotation expounds that all the changes of aging are rooted in the progressive debilitation of essence-blood.

文献评述

《灵枢•天年》曰："九十岁肾气焦，四脏经脉空虚。百岁，五脏皆虚，神气皆去，形骸独居而终矣。"指出肾之精气耗竭，五脏皆虚，可致衰老。

《景岳全书•传忠录•治形论》曰："言动视听非此形乎，俊丑美恶非此形乎，勇怯愚智非此形乎，生死安否非此形乎。...而形以阴言，实惟精血二字，足以尽之。"又曰："精血即形也，形即精血。"论述衰老与精血耗损有密切关系，其中包含肾之精亏而致早衰的病机。

《寿亲养老新书•戒忌保护》曰："人万物中一物也，不能逃天地之数，若天癸数穷，则精血耗竭，神气浮弱，返同小儿。"认识到衰老的各种变化的根源在于精血随着增龄而不断衰耗。

Summary of Essence Depletion Causing Premature Debilitation

1. Essence Failing to Nourish the Brain
   Dull spirit-affect, unsustained vitality, forgetfulness and abstraction, slowness of thought, delayed reactions.
2. Essence Failing to Nourish the Spirit
   Insomnia and profuse dreaming, slowness to fall asleep, waking up early, light sleep, increased dozing.
3. Failure to Nourish the Ears
   Tinnitus and deafness, impaired hearing.
4. Failure to Nourish the Teeth and Hair
   Premature graying of the whiskers and hair, hair loss, loose teeth.
5. Inability to Govern Bone and Marrow
   Wilting and limpness of both legs, difficulty in walking, flaccid movements, strained action.
6. Insufficiency of Kidney Essence
   Pale tongue, fine weak pulse.

精亏早衰

精不养脑—神情呆钝，精力不支，健忘恍惚，思维迟钝，反应缓慢

精不养神—失眠多梦，睡得迟，醒得早，睡得浅，打盹多

不养于耳—耳鸣耳聋，听力下降

不养于齿发—须发早白，发脱齿摇

不能主骨生髓—两足痿软，步履艰难，行动迟缓，动作吃力

肾精不足—舌淡，脉细弱

Chapter Five

Dual Vacuity of Kidney Yīn and Yáng

The human body is an organic whole that is permeated with the unity of the two opposites yīn and yáng. As the "Treatise on Treasuring [Heaven's] Mandate to Preserve the Body" in the *Sù Wèn* ("Plain Questions") explains: "The formal aspect of human life does not depart from yīn and yáng." "Treatise on Yīn and Yáng" in the *Yī Guàn* ("Thorough Knowledge of Medicine") also points out: "Yīn and yáng further constitute each other's root. Yáng is rooted in yīn, and yīn is rooted in yáng. Without yáng, yīn lacks that which it can engender. Without yīn, yáng lacks that which it can transform." The kidney is the root of earlier heaven and houses original yīn and original yáng. In physiology, kidney yīn and kidney yáng serve as each other's cause and effect. In pathology, they damage each other. If this situation endures, it forms the pathomechanism of dual vacuity of yīn and yáng.

The chapter, "Yin Vacuity Conditions are Tied to the Lung" in the *Lǐ Xū Yuán Jiàn* ("The Original Mirror of Rectifying Vacuity") points out: "When yáng vacuity endures, yīn also becomes vacuous... and when yīn vacuity endures, yáng also becomes vacuous."

In the *Zhèng Yīn Mài Zhì* ("Pathoconditions: Causes, Pulses, and Treatments"), Qín Jǐng-Míng noted that the "Treatise on Disease Causes and Specific Treatments of Yīn Vacuity and Yáng Vacuity in the *Nèi Jīng* ("The Inner Canon") and the *Jīn Guì Yào Lüè* ("Essential Prescriptions of the Golden Coffer")" described how excessive consumption of warming and supplementing formulas, as well as of yīn-enriching formulas, could lead to the pathomechanism of dual vacuity of kidney yīn and yáng. He stated:

> "If patients with an insufficiency of true yīn and the pathocondition of vacuity fire are prescribed yīn-enriching medicines, the condition will transmute into vacuity cold. If they take warming and supplementing

> medicinals, it will also transmute the vacuity fire. The reason for this is that whenever yīn water is exhausted, yáng fire is also vacuous. This is therefore a deathly condition that cannot bear enriching yīn."

The chapter, "Vacuity Detriment" in the *Jǐng Yuè Quán Shū* ("Jǐng-Yuè's Complete Compendium"), "Schema of Miscellaneous Patterns" also describes how yáng detriment can affect yīn and how yīn can cause detriment to yáng. It points out:

> "If the five detriments affect the kidney, the disease will consist of bone wilting and urinary incontinence. This is a situation where prior damage to yáng has afterwards affected yīn, so that yīn is exhausted in the lower body. Thus, solitary yáng exists alone."

The chapter, "Answering Liú Xī-Wén's Questions About the Seven Damages" in the *Yī Xué Zhōng Zhōng Cān Xī Lù* ("Records of Chinese Medicine with Reference to Western Medicine") further states:

> "Exerting oneself during sexual intercourse damages yīn; prolonged sitting on damp ground damages yáng. Dual damage to the kidney's true yīn and true yáng damages the kidney. Kidney damage results in inability to absorb qì and return it to the root during breathing, and therefore results in shortness of breath. The lower back is the house of the kidney, and kidney damage therefore causes lumbar pain. The bones are governed by the kidney, and kidney damage therefore causes pain in the leg bones. If the condition manifests with reverse flow and cold in the lower body, this indicates that the qì of water and fire in the kidney is unable to spread."

This quotation analyzes in detail the pathomechanism of dual vacuity of kidney yīn and kidney yáng.

Because of differences in the degree of pathology, we can further divide dual vacuity of kidney yīn and kidney yáng into two pathomechanisms: debilitation of both yīn and yáng, and detriment in all five viscera.

肾阴阳两虚

人体是一个有机的整体，充满着阴阳对立统一的关系。如《素问•宝命全形论》说："人生有形，不离阴阳。"《医贯•阴阳论》又指出："阴阳又各互为其根，阳根于阴，阴根于阳；无阳则阴无以生，无阴则阳无以化。"肾为先天之本，内舍元阴元阳，肾阴肾阳在生理上的互根互用，病理上相互损伤，久则形成阴阳两虚的病机变化。如《理虚元鉴•阴虚之症统于肺》指出："阳虚之久者，阴亦虚…，阴虚之久者，阳亦虚。”秦景明《症因脉治•论内经金匮阴虚阳虚症因个别治法不同》记载了过服温补及滋阴之剂，可导致肾阴阳两虚的病机变化，曰：“有真阴不足，虚火之症，服滋阴则变虚寒，服温补药又变虚火者，此阴水既竭，阳火亦虚，不耐滋阴之死症也。”《景岳全书•杂证谟•虚损》也描述了阳损及阴，阴又损阳的情况，指出：“五损及肾，则病为骨痿，小便不禁，此先伤于阳，而后及于阴，阴竭于下，则孤阳无以独存，不可为也。”《医学衷中参西录•答刘希文问七伤》又曰：“强力入房则伤阴，久坐湿地则伤阳，肾之真阴、真阳俱伤，所以伤肾。肾伤则呼吸之时，不能纳气归根，所以短气。腰者，肾之腑，肾伤所以腰疼。骨者肾所主，肾伤所以脚骨作疼。至于厥逆下冷，亦肾中水火之气，不能敷布之故也。”对肾阴肾阳俱虚的病机变化进行了详细的分析。肾阴阳两虚因病变程度不同，又可分为阴阳两衰、五脏俱损两种病机变化。

5.1 Debilitation of Both Yīn and Yáng

Yīn and yáng are rooted in each other and make use of each other. Thus unilateral exuberance is harmful. Yáng exuberance damages yīn, and yīn exuberance damages yáng. If enduring disease or debility in old age cause kidney yīn vacuity and this affects yáng, or causes kidney yáng vacuity and this affects yīn, then yīn and yáng damage each other. This situation forms the pathomechanism of debilitation of both yīn and yáng.

The "Treatise on the Natural Life Span" in the "Record of Transmitting Loyalty" from the *Jǐng Yuè Quán Shū* ("Jǐng-Yuè's Complete Compendium") states: "Qì is yáng, and yáng governs the spirit. Blood is yīn, and yīn governs the form. If blood and qì are debilitated, form and spirit are both vanquished. This means that every least bit of construction and defense must be carefully tended."

When kidney yáng is vacuous, yáng loses its ability to warm. The result is fear of cold and lack of warmth in the limbs.

When yáng qì is vacuous and therefore unable to nourish the heart spirit, spirit qì is insufficient. This results in clouded head and flowery vision, and devitalized essence-spirit.

Vacuity of kidney yīn causes yīn vacuity internal heat. The result is heat in the heart of the palms and soles, dry throat and tongue, tidal reddening of the cheeks, and steaming bone taxation heat.

The kidney's bloom is in the hair, which is the surplus of the blood. When kidney yīn and yáng are both debilitated, neither qì nor blood are engendered, and the hair is deprived of nourishment. This results in premature graying.

When yīn and yáng are both vacuous, blood and qì are vanquished, and the formal body is not nourished and filled by them. Emaciation results.

Dual vacuity of yīn and yáng results in a fat pale or dry emaciated tongue and a fine weak sunken pulse.

The chapter, "Vacuity Taxation Guest Heat" in the *Zhū Bìng Yuán Hòu Lùn* ("Origin and Indicators of Disease") points out: "In patients with vacuity taxation, qì and blood are weak and yīn and yáng are both vacuous. Taxation engenders heat; heat is engendered by taxation." This quotation indicates the special characteristic of the pathomechanism by which dual vacuity of yīn and yáng leads to vacuity taxation heat effusion.

The chapter, "Internal Damage; The Various Vacuities" in the *Yī Xué Rù Mén* ("The Gateway to Medicine") states:

> "The seven damages are originally caused only by extreme taxation: Prolonged use of the eyes damages the blood; prolonged resting damages qì; prolonged sitting damages the flesh; prolonged standing damages the bones; prolonged walking damages the liver; sexual taxation and thought and preoccupation damage the heart and kidney, making yīn blood vacuous; and taxation, overwork, hunger, and overeating damage the stomach, making yáng qì vacuous. These are the key factors in damage conditions.
>
> "Treat dual vacuity of yīn and yáng with *bā wù tāng* (Eight Agents Decoction), *gù zhēn yǐn zǐ(wán)* (True-Securing Drink (Pill)), *rén shēn yǎng róng tāng* (Ginseng Construction-Nourishing Decoction), or *shí quán dà bǔ tāng* (Perfect Major Supplementation Decoction) with the addition of *ròu cōng róng* (Cistanches Herba), *fù zǐ* (Aconiti Radix Lateralis Praeparata), *bàn xià* (Pinelliae Rhizoma), and *mài dōng* (Ophiopogonis Radix), or *bā wèi wán* (Eight-Ingredient Pill)."

This quotation succinctly points out that dual vacuity of kidney yīn and yáng can cause numerous disease patterns of vacuity-detriment taxation damage.

Debilitation of both yīn and yáng is treated by enriching yīn and boosting the kidney, and by doubly supplementing yīn and yáng. The recommended formula is *zàn huà xuè yú dān* (Human Hair to Assist Transformation Elixir) from the *Jǐng Yuè Quán Shū* ("Jǐng-Yuè's Complete Compendium").

Zàn Huà Xuè Yú Dān 赞化血余丹
Human Hair to Assist Transformation Elixir

xuè yú (血余 Crinis, hair)
shú dì huáng (熟地黄 Rehmanniae Radix Praeparata, cooked rehmannia)
gǒu qǐ zǐ (枸杞子 Lycii Fructus, lycium)
dāng guī (当归 Angelicae Sinensis Radix, Chinese angelica)
lù jiǎo jiāo (鹿角胶 Cervi Cornus Gelatinum, deerhorn glue)
tù sī zǐ (菟丝子 Cuscutae Semen, cuscuta)
dù zhòng (杜仲 Eucommiae Cortex, eucommia)
bā jǐ tiān (巴戟天 Morindae Officinalis Radix, morinda)
xiǎo huí xiāng (小茴香 Foeniculi Fructus, fennel)
fú líng (茯苓 Poria, poria)
ròu cōng róng (肉苁蓉 Cistanches Herba, cistanche)
hé táo rén (胡桃仁 Juglandis Semen, walnut)
hé shǒu wū (何首乌 Polygoni Multiflori Radix, flowery knotweed)
rén shēn (人参 Ginseng Radix, ginseng)

阴阳两衰

阴阳互根互用，偏盛则为害，阳盛则伤阴，阴盛则伤阳，如久病或年老体衰，肾阴虚而及阳，或肾阳虚而及阴，阴阳相互损伤，形成阴阳两衰的病机改变。如《景岳全书•传忠录•天年论》曰：“气为阳，阳主神也; 血为阴，阴主形也。血气若衰，则形神俱败，此营卫之毫厘当惜也”。肾阳虚，阳失温煦，则畏寒怕冷，四肢欠温; 阳气虚不能养心神，神气不足，则头昏眼花，精神不振; 肾阴虚，阴虚内热，则手足心热，咽干舌燥，两颧潮红，骨蒸劳热; 肾其华在发，发又为血之余，肾阴阳两衰，气血不生，发失所养，则须发早白; 阴阳两虚，气血衰败，形体失去气血充养，则形体羸瘦。阴阳两虚，则舌体淡胖或干瘦，脉沉细弱。如《诸病源候论•虚劳客热候》指出：“虚劳之人，血气微弱，阴阳俱虚，劳则生热，热因劳生。”指出了阴阳俱虚，引起虚劳发热的病机特点。《医学入门•内伤•诸虚》曰：“七伤者，惟原劳极之由，久视伤血，久卧伤气，久坐伤肉，久立伤骨，久行伤肝，房劳思虑伤心肾则阴血虚，劳役饥饱伤胃腑则阳气虚，此伤症之于要也。...阴阳俱虚，八物汤、固真饮子或丸、人参养荣汤，或十全大补汤加苁蓉、附子、半夏、麦门冬，或八味丸。"明确提出肾的阴阳两虚，可形成多种虚劳损伤的病证。治法宜滋阴益肾，阴阳双补。方药选用《景岳全书》赞化血余丹（血余、熟地、枸杞子、当归、鹿角胶、菟丝子、杜仲、巴戟天、小茴香、白茯苓、肉苁蓉、胡桃肉、何首乌、人参）。

Literature Review of Debilitation of both Yīn and Yáng

📖 *Wēn Bìng Tiáo Biàn* ("Systematized Identification of Warm Diseases"), "The Lower Burner"

> "Intermittent diarrhea that continues for years without recovery indicates a vacuity of both yīn and yáng in the lower burner. This disables securing and containment and causes qì to bind in the lesser abdomen, resembling concretions and conglomerations. *Shēn fù tāng* (Ginseng and Aconite Decoction) governs it."

The same text further states:

> "Enduring diarrhea with damage to both yīn and yáng, with sagging of the lesser abdomen and anus, and with aching pain in the leg, hip, spine, and thigh is caused by damage to the viscera and bowels that has affected the extraordinary vessels. *Shēn róng tāng* (Ginseng and Velvet Antler Decoction) governs it."

These quotations clearly indicate that enduring illness that has penetrated the lower burner can lead to kidney disease and dual debilitation of yīn and yáng.

📖 *Shí Yòng Zhōng Yī Nèi Kē Xué* ("Practical Chinese Medicine Internal Medicine"), "Dispersion-Thirst: Dual Depletion of Yīn and Yáng"

> "Yīn and yáng are rooted in each other. Despite the fact that dryness-heat damaging yīn is the basic pathology of this disease, if the course of the disease is prolonged, detriment to yīn can affect yáng. Alternatively, improper treatment and overuse of cold bitter medicinals can also damage yáng. In the end, this causes the pattern of dual depletion of yīn and yáng. This means that the root pattern manifests with signs of yīn depletion like heat in the heart of the palms and soles, dry mouth and throat, haggard or drawn facial complexion, and dry helices of the ear However, the patient also suffers from signs of yáng vacuity like lack of warmth in the limbs, fear of cold, and in severe cases yáng wilt."

This quotation clearly indicates the pathomechanism of debilitation of both yīn and yáng.

文献评述

《温病条辩•下焦篇》曰："休息痢，经年不愈，下焦阴阳皆虚，不能收摄，少腹气结，有似癥瘕，参附汤主之。"又曰："痢久阴阳两伤，少腹肛坠，腿胯脊髀酸痛，由脏腑伤及奇经，参茸汤主之"明确提出病久深入下焦，可致肾病阴阳两衰的病机病化。

《实用中医内科学•消渴•阴阳两亏》曰："人之阴阳互根，燥热伤阴虽然为本病的基本病理，但病程日久，阴损及阳，或因治疗失当，过用苦寒伤阳，终致形成阴阳两亏之证。即本证既有手足心热，咽干口燥，面容憔悴，耳轮干枯等阴亏之证，又有四肢欠温，畏寒怕冷，甚则阳萎等阳虚之证。"明确提出阴阳两衰的病机。

Summary of Debilitation of Both Yīn and Yáng

1. Yáng Failing to Warm

   Fear of cold, lack of warmth in the limbs.

2. Heart Spirit Deprived of Nourishment

   Clouded head and flowery vision, devitalized essence-spirit.

3. Yīn Vacuity Internal Heat

   Heat in the hearts of the palms and soles, dry throat and tongue, tidal reddening of the cheeks, steaming bone taxation heat.

4. Hair Deprived of Nourishment

   Premature graying.

5. Formal Body Deprived of Nourishment

   Emaciation.

6. Dual Vacuity of Yīn and Yáng

   Fat pale or dry emaciated tongue, fine weak sunken pulse.

阴阳两衰

阳失温煦—畏寒怕冷，四肢欠温

心神失养—头昏眼花，精神不振

阴虚内热—手足心热，咽干舌燥，两颧潮红，骨蒸劳热

发失所养—须发早白

形体失养—形体瘦羸

阴阳两虚—舌体淡胖或干瘦，脉沉细弱

5.2 Detriment in All Five Viscera

The kidney is the root of earlier heaven. The kidney's original yīn and original yáng are the root of yīn and yáng in the five viscera, and manage yīn and yáng in the entire body. A dual vacuity of the kidney's yīn and yáng over a long time invariably means that qì and blood and yīn and yáng in the heart, lung, liver, and spleen lack the root that engenders them. This manifests in the pathomechanism of detriment in all five viscera.

When kidney vacuity affects the heart, heart qì and blood are not engendered, and the heart spirit is deprived of nourishment. This causes withering of the spirit-mind.

When kidney vacuity affects the lung, which governs qì and is in charge of breathing, lung qì is deprived of nourishment, and its functions of diffusion and depurative downbearing break down. The result is shortness of breath, cough, and hasty panting.

When kidney vacuity affects the liver, which governs the sinews, the liver's blood and qì become insufficient and the sinews and channels are deprived of nourishment. The result is sudden debilitation of strength in the sinews, and heaviness of the lower back and legs.

Kidney vacuity can affect the spleen, which governs the limbs and flesh and the movement and transformation of the subtle essence of food and drink. When the spleen suffers from vacuity detriment, the limbs are deprived of nourishment, food and drink are not transformed, and the subtle essences are not transported. The result is fatigued and emaciated limbs, thinness and weakness, and decreased food intake.

When kidney yīn is vacuous, this engenders internal heat. The result is heat effusion and night sweating.

When kidney yáng is vacuous, it is not secure. The result is seminal emission and white turbidity.

The kidney governs the bones, and the teeth are the surplus of the bone. Kidney vacuity thus results in loose teeth.

The chapter, "Various Symptoms of Vacuity Taxation" in the *Zhū Bìng Yuán Hòu Lùn* ("Origin and Indicators of Disease") points out: "In patients with vacuity taxation, blood and qì are exhausted, yīn and yáng are not guarded, and the bowels and viscera are all debilitated. Therefore, cold arises internally." This quotation describes the pathomechanism by which an exhaustion of yīn and yáng and depletion of the five viscera can lead to internally arising vacuity taxation.

The chapter, "Origin and Development of Vacuity Detriment Consumption" in the *Zá Bìng Yuán Liú Xī Zhú* ("Incisive Light on the Source of Miscellaneous Disease") further states:

> "Vacuity detriment consumption is a disease of the true origin. Vacuity refers to qì and blood being vacuous. Detriment means detriment in the bowels and viscera. When detriment is caused by enduring vacuity, it affects all five viscera... When injury to the qì of the five viscera is prolonged, it will form *láo* consumption. If it is severe, it is called *zhài* consumption. *Láo* consumption refers to taxation, hindrance, and fatigue. *Zhài* consumption refers to emaciation, vanquishing, and destitution.
>
> "The diseases of vacuity detriment and consumption share the same cause and manifest through the five viscera… The source of these two diseases is always taxation of the heart from an excessive liking for sex. This leads to exhaustion of true yáng, exuberance and intensification of evil fire, depletion of true yīn, and scorching of vacuity fire. Because of this, fire steams upward, causing coughing of blood and tidal heat, and stirs in the lower body, causing essence turbidity and diarrhea. All these symptoms swarm like hornets."

This quotation describes in detail the various pathomechanical changes resulting from dual vacuity of kidney yīn and yáng and detriment in all five viscera.

Detriment in all five viscera is treated by simultaneously supplementing yīn and yáng, and by rectifying all five viscera alike. The recommended formula is *zī yīn dà bǔ wán* (Yīn-Enriching Major Supplementation Pill) from the *Jǐng Yuè Quán Shū* ("Jǐng-Yuè's Complete Compendium").

Zī Yīn Dà Bǔ Wán 滋阴大补丸
Yīn-Enriching Major Supplementation Pill

shú dì huáng (熟地黄 Rehmanniae Radix Praeparata, cooked rehmannia)
shān yào (山药 Dioscoreae Rhizoma, dioscorea)
niú xī (牛膝 Achyranthis Bidentatae Radix, achyranthes)
shān zhū yú (山茱萸 Corni Fructus, cornus)
dù zhòng (杜仲 Eucommiae Cortex, eucommia)
bā jǐ tiān (巴戟天 Morindae Officinalis Radix, morinda)
fú líng (茯苓 Poria, poria)

wǔ wèi zǐ (五味子 Schisandrae Fructus, schisandra)
xiǎo huí xiāng (小茴香 Foeniculi Fructus, fennel)
ròu cōng róng (肉苁蓉 Cistanches Herba, cistanche)
yuǎn zhì (远志 Polygalae Radix, polygala)
shí chāng pú (石菖蒲 Acori Tatarinowii Rhizoma, acorus)
gǒu qǐ zǐ (枸杞子 Lycii Fructus, lycium)

五脏俱损

肾为先天之本，肾之元阴元阳，为五脏阴阳之根，统司一身之阴阳。如肾之阴阳两虚，久必可导致心肺肝脾各脏气血阴阳无根以生，出现五脏俱损的病机变化。肾虚及心，心之气血不生，心神失养，故神志萎颓; 肾虚及肺，肺主气，司呼吸，肺气失养，宣发肃降功能失常，则呼吸气短，咳嗽喘促; 肾虚及肝，肝主筋，肝之气血不足，筋经失养，则筋力顿衰，腰脚沉重; 肾虚及脾，脾主四肢肌肉，运化饮食精微，脾之虚损，四肢不养，饮食不化，精微不输，则肢体倦怠羸乏，瘦弱食减; 肾阴虚而生内热，则发热盗汗; 肾阳虚不固，则遗精白浊; 肾主骨，齿为骨之余，则肾虚而牙齿浮动。如《诸病源候论•虚劳病诸候》指出："虚劳之人，血气衰竭，阴阳不守，脏腑俱衰，故内生寒冷也。" 论述阴阳衰竭，五脏亏损可致虚劳内生的病机。《杂病源流犀烛•虚损痨瘵源流》又曰："虚损痨瘵，真元病也。虚者，气血之虚。损者，脏腑之损。虚久致损，五脏皆有。...五脏之气，有一损伤，积久成痨，甚而为瘵。痨者，劳也，劳闲疲惫也。瘵者，败也，羸败凋敝也。虚损痨瘵，其病相因，其实由于五脏如此。...二病之原，皆由劳心好色，以至真阳衰惫，邪火盛炽，真阴亏损，虚火炎烁，由是火蒸于上，则为咳血，为潮热，火动于下，则为精浊，为泄泻，诸症蜂起矣。"对肾之阴阳两虚，五脏俱损导致的各种病机变化进行了详细的阐述。治法宜阴阳并补，五脏同理。方药选用《景岳全书》滋阴大补丸（熟地黄、怀山药、牛膝、山茱萸、杜仲、巴戟天、茯苓、五味子、小茴香、肉苁蓉、远志、石菖蒲、枸杞子）.

Literature Review of Detriment in All Five Viscera

🕮 *Zhū Bìng Yuán Hòu Lùn* ("Origin and Indicators of Disease"), "The Various Symptoms of Vacuity Taxation"

> "Taxation damage in the bowels and viscera results in dual vacuity of qì and blood, insufficiency of qì in the five viscera, and inability to luxuriate the eyes, which causes dim vision."

This quotation points out that insufficiency in the five viscera prevents qì and blood from luxuriating the eyes, which leads to dim vision.

🕮 *Sān Yīn Jí Yī Bìng Zhèng Fāng Lùn* ("A Unified Treatise on Diseases, Patterns, and Remedies According to the Three Causes"), "Patterns and Treatment of Vacuity Detriment"

> "*Yǎng róng tāng* (Construction-Nourishing Decoction) treats accumulated taxation vacuity detriment presenting with heaviness and stagnation in the four limbs, aching pain in the bones and flesh, shortage of qì despite frequent inhalations, panting and cough during activity, hypertonicity during urination, stiffness and pain in the back and lower back, heart vacuity and fright palpitations, dry throat and lips, inability to taste food, debilitation of yīn and yáng, sorrow, anxiety, self-pity, and distress, and increased lying down and reduced getting up. In enduring cases, it lasts for years, in acute cases, for a hundred days. It gradually leads to thinness and whittling of the flesh, and to exhaustion of qì in the five viscera. Recuperation is difficult achieve."

This quotation points out the pathomechanism and manifestations of dual debilitation of yīn and yáng and detriment in all five viscera.

文献评述

《诸病源候论•虚劳诸病候》曰："脏腑劳伤，血气俱虚，五脏气不足，不能荣于目，故令目暗也"。指出了五脏不足，气血不能充于眼目导致目暗的病机变化。

《三因极一病证方论•虚损证治》曰："养荣汤：治积劳虚损，四肢沉滞，骨肉酸疼，吸吸少气，行动喘咳，小便拘急，腰背强痛，心虚惊悸，咽干唇燥，饮食无味，阴阳衰弱，悲忧惨戚，多卧少起，久者积年，急者百日，渐至瘦削，五脏气竭，难可振复。"提出阴阳两衰，五脏俱损的病机及表现。

Summary of Detriment in All Five Viscera

1. Heart Vacuity and Spirit Deprived of Nourishment
   Withering of the spirit mind.
2. Lung Vacuity and Qì Deprived of Nourishment
   Shortness of breath, cough and hasty panting.
3. Liver Vacuity and Sinews Deprived of Nourishment
   Sudden debilitation of strength in the sinews, heaviness of the lower back and legs.
4. Spleen Vacuity and Flesh Deprived of Nourishment
   Fatigued and emaciated limbs, thinness, weakness, and decreased food intake.
5. Kidney Yīn Vacuity and Internal Heat
   Heat effusion and night sweating.
6. Kidney Yáng Vacuity and Insecurity
   Seminal emission and white turbidity.
7. Kidney Vacuity and Bones Deprived of Nourishment
   Loose teeth.

五脏俱损

心虚神失所养—神志萎颓

肺虚气失所养—呼吸气短，咳嗽喘促

肝虚筋失所养—筋力顿衰，腰脚沉重

脾虚肉失所养—肢体倦怠羸乏，瘦弱食减

肾阴虚内热—发热盗汗

肾阳虚不固—遗精白浊

肾虚骨失所养—牙齿浮动

Chapter Six

Kidney Vacuity Verging on Desertion

The kidney stores original yīn and original yáng. Yīn and yáng qì serve each other in growing, declining, and transforming, and in maintaining balance. Just as Yú Zhèn explained Yù Jiā-Yán's point of view, in the chapter, "Dizziness" from the *Gǔ Jīn Yī Àn Àn* ("Commentary on Case Histories Ancient and Modern")

> "In the course of human life, yīn and yáng embrace each other and thereby avoid desertion. Thus, when yáng is about to desert upward, yīn draws it down and thereby stops it from deserting; when yīn is about to desert downward, yáng draws it up and thereby stops it from deserting. It is only after great drunkenness or severe sexual taxation when the five viscera are turned upside down and the hundred vessels stir and shake, that the two qì exuberate and desert each other."

This passage explains that in a normal physiological state, yīn and yáng maintain and regulate their balance, but that after illness or extreme indulgence the pathomechanism of yīn and yáng separating from each other can arise.

If the condition of kidney vacuity continues to develop and the pathomechanism of dual vacuity of kidney yīn and yáng worsens further, yīn and yáng qì are unable to hold to each other and transform into irreconcilable opposites. This can manifest in the pathomechanism of kidney vacuity verging on desertion. This pathomechanism consists either of yīn desertion or yáng desertion and is a critical condition that results when yīn and yáng separate.

肾虚欲脱

肾藏元阴元阳，阴阳二气相互为用，消长转化，保持平衡。如俞震在《古今医案按眩晕》中转述喻嘉言之观点说：“人生之阴阳，相抱而不脱，故阳欲上脱，阴下吸之则不脱。阴欲下脱，阳上吸则之不脱。惟大醉后大犯房劳，五脏翻覆，百脉动摇，二气盛之脱离。"说明了阴阳互相维系、协调平衡的正常生理状态，患病之后，即可形成阴阳脱离的病机变化。如肾虚病情继续发展，肾阴阳两虚之病机进一步恶化，阴阳之气不能相互维系，成为不可调和的对立两方，则可能出现肾虚欲脱的病机变化。肾虚欲脱，不是阴脱即是阳脱，为阴阳离决时的危急病变。

6.1 Yīn Vacuity Verging on Desertion

Yīn is the material basis of the body. Kidney yīn constitutes original yīn and as such governs the engenderment of yīn liquid and blood of the five viscera and six bowels. Because of this, if heat evil has scorched true yīn for a long time, or if great sweating, vomiting, or diarrhea have caused blood collapse and loss of essence, to the point where kidney yīn is greatly reduced and exhausted in the extreme, it is no longer lodged in its proper place. This manifests in the pathomechanism of yīn vacuity verging on desertion.

If kidney yīn is on the verge of desertion, vacuity yáng harasses the upper body, kidney qì fails to absorb, and lung qì ascends counterflow. This manifests in panting and thirst verging on desertion.

When yīn is vacuous to the point of verging on desertion, vacuity yáng harasses the upper body, and the heart spirit is disquieted. The result is vacuity vexation, agitation, harassment, fearful throbbing, and sleeplessness.

When yīn is vacuous to the point of verging on desertion, the sinews are deprived of nourishment, and vacuity wind wants to stir. The result is tugging of the extremities.

When yīn is vacuous and deserts to the outside, hyperactive yáng follows it outward into the hands and feet. The result is warm hands and feet and sweating on the verge of expiry.

Kidney yīn vacuity verging on desertion manifests in a crimson tongue with scant tongue fur, and vacuous weak pulse.

The chapter, "Various Symptoms of Vacuity Taxation Disease; Vacuity Taxation Qì Ascent" in the *Zhū Bìng Yuán Hòu Lùn* ("Origin and Indicators of Disease") states: "The condition of vacuity taxation is either related to damage to both yīn and yáng, or to unilateral detriment to blood or qì. In this case, it is an insufficiency of yīn and superabundance of yáng that causes qì ascent." This quotation discusses how great depletion of kidney yīn and vacuity yáng harassing the upper body lead to hasty panting and qì ascent.

The "Treatise on the Cause and Treatment of Blood Ejection and Spontaneous External Bleeding" in the *Yī Xué Zhōng Zhōng Cān Xī Lù* ("Records of Chinese Medicine with Reference to Western Medicine") further points out:

> "Excessive blood loss causes depletion of the blood aspect. This results in heat effusion due to inability to subdue yáng, and in panting due to inability to absorb qì. In severe cases, surging qì can occur, which, because of the vacuity, interferes in the upper body, causing hiccup, dizziness, and cough. Because heart blood cannot luxuriate internally, we see fearful throbbing, fright palpitations, sleeplessness, and a rapid floating pulse that is forceless under strong pressure…
>
> "Yīn and yáng in the human body originally hold each other together, which is the same as qì and blood in the body holding each other together. Blood ejection and spontaneous external bleeding are due to the fact that yīn blood is depleted and is held together without strength. If originally there is concern about solitary yáng floating astray and *dú shēn tāng* (Pure Ginseng Decoction) is prescribed to assist the floating, this results not only in a tendency of qì to flee upward, but in blood following it upward, causing blood ejection and spontaneous external bleeding. In this clumsy formula where the intent is to treat blood ejection and spontaneous external bleeding, whenever you use *rén shēn* (Ginseng Radix), you must make heavy use of *zhě shí* (Haematitum) to support it through its strength of thrusting downward."

This quotation is an incisive analysis of the pathomechanism and treatment of yīn vacuity verging on desertion.

Yīn vacuity verging on desertion is treated by enriching and rescuing yīn. The recommended formula is *dà dìng fēng zhū* (Major Wind-Stabilizing Pill) from the *Wēn Bìng Tiáo Biàn* ("Systematized Identification of Warm Diseases").

Dà Dìng Fēng Zhū 大定风珠 Major Wind-Stabilizing Pill
bái sháo (白芍 Paeoniae Radix Alba, white peony)
ē jiāo (阿胶 Asini Corii Colla, ass hide glue)
guī bǎn (龟版 Testudinis Plastrum, tortoise plastron)
shēng dì huáng (生地黄 Rehmanniae Radix, rehmannia)
huǒ má rén (火麻仁 Cannabis Semen, cannabis seed)

wǔ wèi zǐ (五味子 Schisandrae Fructus, schisandra)
mǔ lì (牡蛎 Ostreae Concha, oyster shell)
mài dōng (麦冬 Ophiopogonis Radix, ophiopogon)
jī zǐ huáng (鸡子黄 Galli Vitellus, egg yolk)
biē jiǎ (鳖甲 Trionycis Carapax, turtle shell)
zhì gān cǎo (炙甘草 Glycyrrhizae Radix cum Liquido Fricta, mix-fried licorice)

阴虚欲脱

阴为物质基础，肾阴为元阴，主生五脏六腑之阴津血液。因此，如遇热邪久灼真阴，或大汗吐下，亡血失精，肾阴大损，虚竭致极，不恋其位，表现为阴虚欲脱的病机变化。肾阴欲脱，虚阳上扰，肾气不纳，肺气上逆，则表现为喘渴欲脱; 阴虚欲脱，虚阳上扰，心神不宁，则虚烦躁扰，怔忡不寐; 阴虚欲脱，筋脉失养，虚风欲动，则手足瘛疭; 阴虚外脱，亢阳随之外达于手足，则手足虽温而汗出欲绝。肾之阴虚欲脱，则舌绛苔少，脉气虚弱。如《诸病源候论•虚劳诸病候•虚劳上气候》曰："虚劳之病，或阴阳俱伤，或血气偏损，今是阴不足，阳有余，故上气也。"论述了肾阴大亏，虚阳上扰，引起喘促上气的病机变化。又如《医学衷中参西录•论吐血衄血之原因及治法》指出："失血过多，阴分亏损，不能潜阳而作热，不能纳气而作喘，甚或冲气因虚上干，为呃逆、眩晕、咳嗽，心血因不能内荣，为怔忡、惊悸、不寐，脉象浮数，重按无力者。...夫人身之阴阳原相维系，即人身之气血相维系也。吐衄血者，因阴血亏损维系无力，原有孤阳浮越之虞，而复用独参汤以助其浮越，不但其气易上奔，血亦将随之上奔而复吐衄矣。是拙拟治吐衄方中，凡用参者，必重用赭石以辅之，使其力下达也。"对阴虚欲脱的病机改变进行了深刻的分析。治法宜滋阴救阴。方药选用《温病条辨》大定风珠(生白芍、阿胶、生龟板、干地黄、麻仁、五味子、生牡蛎、麦冬、鸡子黄、生鳖甲、炙甘草)。

Literature Review of Yīn Vacuity Verging on Desertion

📖 *Jǐng Yuè Quán Shū* ("Jǐng-Yuè's Complete Compendium"), "Schema of Miscellaneous Patterns: Vacuity Detriment"

"Lì Zhāi once treated Hán Zhōu-Tóng for excessive sexual desire, heat vexation and thirst, incessant drinking of water, dribbling urination,

> fecal block, spittle gushing with phlegm, red face and eyes, sores all over the tongue, cracked lips and generalized heat effusion, at times a prickling sensation without fixed location on the body, a sensation like heat in the heart of the palms and soles, and a surging and forceless pulse in the three positions on the left. This was a case of kidney yīn vacuity, with yáng lacking support and therefore effusing outward. Great heat was aggravated and there was no cold, which meant an absence of water. Such a condition must be treated with drastic supplementation of yīn."

This quotation discusses a condition where kidney yīn depletion has reached an extreme, so that yīn is vacuous and yáng qì without support, leading to vacuous yáng verging on desertion.

🕮 *Lín Zhèng Zhǐ Nán Yī Àn* ("A Clinical Guide with Case Histories"), "Wheezing"

> "When evil is dissipated, panting will also stop and not recur... If panting is caused by a root depletion leading to kidney vacuity, qì counterflow, and upward surging of turbid yīn, this condition must not be allowed to persist for more than one or two days, or the dynamic will become critical."

When yīn is vacuous to the point of verging on desertion, turbid yīn surges upward and causes chaotic counterflow of the qì dynamic and panting.

🕮 *Yī Xué Zhōng Zhōng Cān Xī Lù* ("Records of Chinese Medicine with Reference to Western Medicine"), "Discussing the Treatment of Fire Failing to Return to its Origin"

> "In cases of true yīn vacuity detriment in the lower burner and original yáng lacking something to tie it down and thereby floating astray, the pulse is predominantly stringlike and rapid, and possibly forceless under strong pressure. Its sign is intermittent scorching heat, possibly with bitter taste in the mouth and dry tongue, or repeated panting and cough. It is recommended to use 1 *liǎng* each of *shēng shān yào* (Dioscoreae Rhizoma Crudum) and *shú dì huáng* (Rehmanniae Radix Praeparata)... This is what is called focusing on strengthening water to dam the luster of yáng."

This quotation indicates the pathomechanism by which kidney yīn depletion and hyperactive yáng harassing internally leads to panting, thirst, and scorching heat.

文献评述

《景岳全书•杂证谟•虚损》曰："立斋治韩州同色欲过度，烦热作渴，饮水不绝，小便淋沥，大便闭结，唾痰如涌，面目俱赤，满舌生刺，唇裂身热，或身如芒刺而无定处，两足心如烙，左三部脉洪而无力，此肾阴虚，阳无所附而发于外。盖大热而甚，寒之不寒，是无水也，当峻补其阴。" 这是肾阴亏虚至极，阴虚而阳气无所附，虚阳欲脱所致。

《临证指南医案•哮》曰："邪散则喘亦止，后不复发; …若因根本有亏，肾虚气逆，浊阴上冲而喘者，此不过一二日之间，势必危笃。"阴虚而欲脱，则浊阴上冲而致气机逆乱而喘。

《医学衷中参西录•论火不归原治法》曰："有下焦真阴虚损，元阳无所系恋而浮越者，其脉象多弦数，或重按无力，其证时作灼热，或口苦舌干，或喘嗽连连。宜用生山药，熟地黄各一两，…此所谓壮水之主，以制阳光。"指出了肾阴亏损，亢阳内扰引起喘渴灼热的病机改变。

Summary of Yīn Vacuity Verging on Desertion

1. Vacuity Yáng Harassing the Lung
   Panting, thirst, verging on desertion.
2. Vacuity Yáng Harassing the Heart
   Vacuity vexation, agitation, harassment, fearful throbbing, sleeplessness.
3. Sinews Deprived of Nourishment
   Tugging of the extremities.
4. Yīn Vacuity and Outward Desertion
   Warm hands and feet and sweating on the verge of expiry.
5. Yīn Vacuity Verging on Desertion
   Crimson tongue with scant fur, vacuous weak pulse.

阴虚欲脱

虚阳扰肺—喘渴欲脱

虚阳扰心—虚烦躁扰，怔忡不寐

筋脉失养—手足瘛疭

阴虚外脱—手足虽温而汗出欲绝

阴虚欲脱—舌绛苔少，脉气虚弱

6.2 Yáng Vacuity Verging on Desertion

Kidney yáng is the root of the entire body's yáng qì and is preserved in the Life Gate. When debilitation of kidney yáng reaches an extreme, it departs from yīn and ascends. Vacuous yáng floats upward and the lower origin is exhausted, so that qì floats on the verge of dispersing, while original yáng is on the verge of deserting. This manifests in the pathomechanism of yáng vacuity verging on desertion.

When kidney yáng is debilitated and yáng qì is on the verge of desertion, qì is not contained and absorbed, and vacuous yáng floats upward and accumulates within the lung. Lung qì fails to downbear, and the qì dynamic suffers from chaotic counterflow. The result is phlegm congestion in the chest, qì ascent, and hasty panting.

If yáng qì is debilitated to an extreme, it fails to warm the four limbs. The result is reverse-flow of the limbs.

Yáng failing to contain liquid causes incessant sweating.

When kidney yáng is debilitated, the lower back is not warmed and qì is unable to flow freely. The result is heaviness of the back and lower back.

Debilitation of kidney yáng causes yáng vacuity and insecurity, so that the bladder loses its ability to retain. The result is long voidings of clear urine and frequent and profuse urination at night.

When kidney yáng is debilitated, kidney qì surges up or down in counterflow. This manifests in running piglet, surging counterflow, and possibly cold mounting and abdominal pain.

Kidney yáng debilitation and yáng vacuity verging on desertion manifests in a pale tongue with white fur, and a sunken rapid pulse.

The chapter, "Panting" in the *Yī Guàn* ("Thorough Knowledge of Medicine") points out: "When the true origin is consumed, panting proceeds from the upward flight of kidney qì... This means that qì fails to return to its origin." This quotation describes the pathomechanism by which kidney yáng debilitation and water lacking governance intimidate the heart and shoot into the lung, causing counterflow ascent of lung qì and consequently incessant panting.

The chapter, "Origin and Development of All Sweating" in the *Zá Bìng Yuán Liú Xī Zhú* ("Incisive Light on the Source of Miscellaneous Disease") also points out:

> "If there is profuse incessant sweating, true yáng collapses and deserts. This condition is called yáng collapse. A patient with this condition

> invariably suffers from a cold body, often forming impediment cold or hypertonicity of the limbs. Furthermore, yáng vacuity with inability to sweat is also called yáng collapse. It must lead to dizzy head and shivering of the body... Kidney damage results in yáng debilitation, and debilitation of yáng results in vacuity of the defense. Defense that is vacuous moves into the yīn aspect, and when the person closes their eyes in sleep, there is no qì to secure the exterior. As a result, the interstices open and night sweat is discharged. When awake, defense qì that has moved into yīn returns to the exterior, and night sweating stops."

This quotation analyzes in detail the pathomechanical changes of yáng vacuity verging on desertion.

Yáng vacuity verging on desertion is treated by breaking yīn and rescuing yáng. The recommended formula is *hēi xí dān* (Galenite Elixir) from the *Tài Píng Huì Mín Hé Jì Jú Fāng* (Tài-Píng Imperial Grace Pharmacy Formulas).

Hēi Xí Dān 黑锡丹 Galenite Elixir
hēi xí (黑锡 Galenitum, galenite)
liú huáng (硫黄 Sulphur, sulfur)
ròu guì (肉桂 Cinnamomi Cortex, cinnamon bark)
fù zǐ (附子 Aconiti Radix Lateralis Praeparata, aconite)
mù xiāng (木香 Aucklandiae Radix, costusroot)
chén xiāng (沉香 Aquilariae Lignum Resinatum, aquilaria)
xiǎo huí xiāng (小茴香 Foeniculi Fructus, fennel)
pó gù zhī (婆固脂 Psoraleae Fructus, psoralea)
yáng qǐ shí (阳起石 Actinolitum, actinolite)
hú lú bā (胡芦巴 Trigonellae Semen, fenugreek)
ròu dòu kòu (肉豆蔻 Myristicae Semen, nutmeg)
jī zǐ huáng (鸡子黄 Galli Vitellus, egg yolk)

阳虚欲脱

肾阳为全身阳气之根，存于命门。肾阳虚衰至极，离阴而上，虚阳上浮，下元虚惫，气浮欲散，元阳欲脱，出现阳虚欲脱的病机变化。肾阳虚衰，阳气欲脱，气不摄纳，虚阳上浮，壅积胸中，肺气不降，气机逆乱，则胸中痰壅，上气喘促；阳虚至极，不温四肢，则四肢厥逆；阳不摄津，则冷汗不止；肾阳虚衰，腰府不温，气行不畅，则腰背沉重；肾阳虚衰，阳虚不固，膀胱失约，则小便清长，夜尿频多；肾阳虚衰，肾气冲逆于上下，则表现为奔豚冲逆，或寒疝腹痛。肾阳虚衰，阳虚欲脱，则舌淡苔白，脉沉数。如《医贯•喘》指出："真元耗损，喘出于肾气之上奔，...乃气不归元也。"论述了肾阳衰弱，水无所主，凌心射肺，肺气上逆而喘息不止的病机变化。《杂病源流犀烛•诸汗源流》也指出："若乃汗多不止，真阳亡脱，名曰亡阳症。其身体必冷，多成痹寒或四肢拘急。又阳虚亡阳，汗不得出，亦名曰亡阳症，必致头眩身栗。...盖肾伤则阳衰，阳衰则卫虚，所虚之卫行于阴分，当目瞑之时，无气以固其表，则腠理开而盗汗出，醒则行阴之卫气复于表，而盗汗止。"详细分析了阳虚欲脱的病机变化。治法宜破阴救阳。方药选用《和剂局方》黑锡丹（黑锡、硫磺、肉桂、附子、木香、沉香、茴香、破故纸、水飞阳起石、葫芦巴、肉豆蔻、金铃子）。

Literature Review of Yáng Vacuity Verging on Desertion

🕮 *Sù Wèn* ("Plain Questions"), "On Reversal"

> "Debilitation of yáng qì in the lower body leads to cold reversal... Cold that is related to cold reversal must start from the five toes and rise up to the knees."

This quotation indicates how yáng vacuity and inability to warm the four limbs leads to reverse-flow of the limbs.

🕮 *Zá Bìng Yuán Liú Xī Zhú* ("Incisive Light on the Source of Miscellaneous Disease"), "The Origin and Development of Kidney Disease: Kidney Expiry"

> "A floating and surging pulse, oily sweating of the body, incessant panting, inability to retain water or fluids, insensitivity of the formal body, and alternating tranquility and derangement are signs of expiry of the life gate."

This quotation discusses oily sweating of the body, incessant panting, and expiry of the life gate, which is the same as kidney yáng vacuity verging on desertion.

🕮 *Yī Xué Zhōng Zhōng Cān Xī Lù* ("Records of Chinese Medicine with Reference to Western Medicine"), "Discussing the Treatment of Fire Failing to Return to its Origin"

"There are cases of great vacuity of original yáng in the sea of qì, with deep-lying cold accumulated in the lower burner. This distresses original yáng, like fire that is about to be distinguished, and its flames turn scurrying upward. Patients with this condition have a stringlike, slow, fine, and weak pulse, possibly with seeming force in the superficial aspect of both cùn positions. This pattern manifests with vexation, agitation, and disquietude in the heart, intermittent scorching heat in the upper burner, a sensation of severe cold in the lower burner, and possibly frequent diarrhea."

This quotation discusses how yáng vacuity verging on desertion manifests in the pathomechanical changes of dryness-heat and disquietude.

文献评述

《素问•厥论篇》曰："阳气衰于下，则为寒厥。…寒厥之为寒也，必从五指而上于膝。"指出了阳虚不温四肢，导致四肢厥逆的病机变化。

《杂病源流犀烛•肾病源流•肾绝候》曰："脉浮而洪，身汗如油，喘不休，水浆不下，形体不仁，乍静乍乱者，此为命门绝也。"论述了身汗如油，喘不休，命门绝，即肾阳虚欲脱的病机变化。

《医学衷中参西录•论火不归原治法》曰："有气海元阳大虚，其下焦又积有沉寒锢冷，逼迫元阳如火之将灭，而其焰转上窜者。其脉弦迟细弱，或两寸浮分似有力。其证为心中烦躁不安，上焦时作灼热，而其下焦转觉凉甚，或常作泄泻。"论述了阳虚欲脱，出现燥热不安的病机改变。

Summary of Yáng Vacuity Verging on Desertion

1. Kidney Yáng Failing to Absorb
   Phlegm congestion in the chest, qì ascent, and hasty panting.
2. Limbs Deprived of Warmth
   Reverse-flow of the limbs.
3. Yáng Vacuity Failing to Contain
   Incessant cold sweating.
4. Lack of Warmth in the Lower Back
   Heaviness in the back and lower back.

5. Insecurity of Kidney Yáng
    Long voidings of clear urine, frequent and profuse urination at night.
6. Surging Counterflow of Kidney Qì
    Running piglet surging counterflow, possibly cold mounting and abdominal pain.
7. Yáng Vacuity Verging on Desertion
    Pale tongue with white fur, sunken rapid pulse.

阳虚欲脱

肾阳不纳—胸中痰壅，上气喘促
四肢失温—四肢厥逆
阳虚不摄—冷汗不止
腰府不温—腰背沉重
肾阳不固—小便清长，夜尿频多
肾气冲逆—奔豚冲逆，或寒疝腹痛
阳虚欲脱—舌淡苔白，脉沉数

6.3 Desertion of Both Yīn and Yáng

The kidney stores original yīn and original yáng. Waxing and waning, yīn and yáng maintain their balance with each other. As the chapter, "Yīn and Yáng" in the "Record of Transmitting Loyalty" from the *Jǐng Yuè Quán Shū* ("Jǐng-Yuè's Complete Compendium") states: "Yīn is rooted in yáng, and yáng is rooted in yīn." If between yīn and yáng one party suffers vacuity detriment, also over time it will invariably exhaust the other party, and vacuity desertion of one party will also result in desertion of the other. This manifests in the pathomechanism of desertion of both yīn and yáng.

The treatise, "On Superiority" in the *Líng Shū* ("The Magic Pivot") states: "In patients with habitual failure to store essence, true yīn is consumed. As a result, the root of true yáng is shallow and easily exposed." This quotation indicates the pathomechanism by which yīn desertion affects yáng.

When debilitation of kidney yáng reaches an extreme, it is unable to warm the limbs, body, and hundred vessels. The result is cold shudders and shaking.

Progressing further, yáng fails to support yīn, vacuous yáng deserts to the outside, containment and absorption break down, and lung qì ascends counterflow. The result is shortness of breath, and inability to breathe continuously.

Yáng qì vacuity desertion prevents original qì from securing and containing. The result is blood ejection, spontaneous external bleeding, and frequent bloody stool.

Vacuity desertion of kidney yīn deprives yīn liquid of enrichment and causes vacuity heat to harass the inner body. The result is lack of coolness in the hands and feet, discharge of thick sticky salty sweat, wrinkled shriveled skin, and dry lips and tongue.

Dual vacuity of yīn and yáng results in a red tongue with scant fur, and a faint fine rapid pulse.

The chapter, "Non-Wind" in the *Jǐng Yuè Quán Shū* ("Jǐng-Yuè's Complete Compendium"), "Schema of Miscellaneous Patterns" points out:

> "All cases of this disease are mostly caused by habitual carelessness, perhaps related to internal damage from the seven affects or to excesses of drink or sex, which have first damaged true yīn in the five viscera… Previous depletion of yīn causes detriment to yáng afterwards. Because yīn falls downward and yáng is lacking in the upper body, yīn and yáng lose each other, and essence and qì do not interact. This leads to sudden clouding, fretting, falling, and collapse."

This quotation discusses the pathomechanical changes of desertion of both yīn and yáng and yīn and yáng losing each other.

Desertion of both yīn and yáng is treated by securing both yīn and yáng. The recommended formula is *liù wèi huí yáng yǐn* (Six-Ingredient Yáng-Returning Beverage) from the *Jǐng Yuè Quán Shū* ("Jǐng-Yuè's Complete Compendium").

Liù Wèi Huí Yáng Yǐn 六味回阳饮 Six-Ingredient Yáng-Returning Beverage
rén shēn (人参 Ginseng Radix, ginseng)
fù zǐ (附子 Aconiti Radix Lateralis Praeparata, aconite)
gān jiāng (干姜 Zingiberis Rhizoma, dried ginger)
zhì gān cǎo (炙甘草 Glycyrrhizae Radix cum Liquido Fricta, mix-fried licorice)
shú dì huáng (熟地黄 Rehmanniae Radix Praeparata, cooked rehmannia)
dāng guī (当归 Angelicae Sinensis Radix, Chinese angelica)

阴阳两脱

肾藏元阴元阳，阴阳互相消长而保持平衡。如《景岳全书•传忠录•阴阳篇》曰："阴根于阳，阳根于阴。"而阴阳双方一方的虚损久必导致另一方的衰竭，而一方的虚脱，亦会引起另一方的脱散，呈现阴阳两脱的病机变化。如《灵枢•尚论》云："素不藏精之人，真阴既耗，则真阳之根，浅而易露。"指出了阴脱及阳的病机改变。肾阳衰竭至极，不能温煦肢体百脉，则寒栗而振；进而阳不附阴，虚阳外脱，摄纳无权，肺气上逆，则呼吸短气，不能接续；阳气虚脱，元气不能固摄，则吐血、衄血、便血频作；肾阴虚脱，阴津失滋，虚热内扰，则手足不冷，汗出粘稠、味咸，皮肤皱瘪，唇舌干燥。阴阳两虚，则舌红少苔，脉微细而数。《景岳全书•杂证谟•非风》指出："凡此病者，多以素不能慎，或七情内伤，或酒色过度，先伤五脏之真阴，...阴亏于前而阳损于后，阴陷于下而阳乏于上，以致阴阳相失，精气不交，所以忽尔昏愦，卒然仆倒。"论述了阴阳两脱，阴阳相失的病机变化。治法宜阴阳两固。方药选用《景岳全书》六味回阳饮（人参、制附子、炮干姜、炙甘草、熟地黄、当归）。

Literature Review of Desertion of Both Yīn and Yáng

🕮 *Jǐng Yuè Quán Shū* ("Jǐng-Yuè's Complete Compendium"), "Schema of Miscellaneous Patterns: Vacuity Detriment"

> "Great vomiting and major spontaneous external bleeding, with the six pulses being fine and deserting, and reversal cold of the extremities, which is an extremely critical condition: if the bleeding will not stop, quickly use *zhèn yīn jiān* (Settle Yīn Brew), and the bleeding will stop on its own. If blood desertion is extreme, and qì follows it, causing reverse flow, clouding, and fretting, quickly boost qì to secure vitality. *Liù wèi huí yáng yǐn* (Six-Ingredient Yáng-Returning Beverage) or *sì wèi sì yáng yǐn* (Four Flavors, Four Yangs Beverage) govern this condition. If you use cold medicinals, death will result."

This quotation, while discussing therapy, describes how severe blood loss damages yīn, so that yīn qì is on the verge of desertion, qì follows blood to desert, and yáng qì collapses, resulting in the pathomechanism of desertion of both yīn and yáng.

🕮 *Xuè Zhèng Lùn* ("On Blood Patterns"), "Blood Ejection"

> "When evil moves in, the right must become vacuous, blood loss will increase, and yīn is vacuous all around. Yīn is the guard of yáng, and when yīn is vacuous, yáng is without support. If this endures, yáng

> follows and collapses. Therefore, supplementing vacuity is the therapy that achieves results."

This quotation describes the pathomechanism by which dual vacuity of yīn and yang causes yīn desertion and subsequent collapse of yáng.

文献评述

《景岳全书•杂证谟•虚损》曰："若大吐大衄，而六脉细脱，手足厥冷，危在倾刻，而血犹不止者，速宜用镇阴煎，其血自止。若血脱至甚，气亦随之，因至厥逆昏愦者，速当益气以固生机，宜六味回阳饮，或四味四阳饮主之，若再用寒凉即死。"从讨论治法中论述了大失血伤阴，阴气欲绝，气随血脱，阳气消亡，形成阴阳两脱的病机。

《血证论•吐血》曰："邪之所凑，其正必虚，去血既多，阴无有不虚者矣。阴者阳之守，阴虚则阳无所附，久且阳随而亡，故又以补虚为收功之法"。阐述了阴阳两虚，阴脱而阳随后亡的病机变化。

Summary of Desertion of Both Yīn and Yáng

1. Kidney Yáng Failing to Warm
   Cold shudders and shaking.
2. Vacuity Yáng Deserting Outward
   Shortness of breath, inability to breathe continuously.
3. Yáng Desertion and Lack of Containment
   Blood ejection, spontaneous external bleeding, frequent bloody stool.
4. Vacuity Heat Harassing the Inner Body
   Lack of coolness in the hands and feet, discharge of thick sticky salty sweat, wrinkled shriveled skin, dry lips and tongue.
5. Dual Vacuity of Yīn and Yáng
   Red tongue with scant fur, faint fine rapid pulse.

阴阳两脱

肾阳失温—寒栗而振

虚阳外脱—呼吸短气，不能接续

阳脱不摄—吐血，衄血，便血频作

虚热内扰—手足不冷，汗出粘稠、味咸，皮肤皱瘪，唇舌干燥

阴阳两虚—舌红少苔，脉微细而数

Bibliography 参考文献

[1].上海第一医科大学脏象专题研究组. 对祖国医学肾本质的探讨[J].中华内科杂志，1976；1(2)：80.

[2].沈自尹，等.肾阳虚病人的垂体—肾上腺皮质系统的改变[J].上海中医药杂志，1979；(2)：34.

[3].沈自尹. 中医基础理论研究概况[J].中医杂志，1979；(10)：12.

[4].江部康二，等.肾阳虚和肾阴虚患者中 17-羟类固醇和 17-酮类固醇排泄值[J].国外医学中医中药分册，1982；4(4)：201.

[5].沈自尹，等.从肾阳虚和老年人的不同反馈模式讨论阴阳学说[J].中西结合杂志，1986；6(10)：628.

[6].沈自尹.肾的研究进展与总结[J].中国医药学报，1988；(2)：56.

[7].沈自尹，等.老年人与“肾阳虚”患者的甲状腺轴功能对比观察[J].中西医结合杂志，1982；2(1)：9.

[8].沈自尹，等.“肾阳虚”证的下丘脑-垂体-甲状腺轴的初步观察[J].上海中医药杂志，1982；(2)：42.

[9]. 青姚，等. 肾阳虚患者甲状腺激素水平变化及温补肾阳的疗效观察[J].广西中医学院学报，2001；4（4）：63.

[10]. 王琴琴，等. “甲减”患者肾阳虚与生长激素分泌变化的联系及温肾助阳的疗效[J]. 上海中医药杂志，1996；（6）：19.

[11].邝安堃，等.中医辨证论治对原发性甲状腺功能减退症的疗效及作用机理的初步探讨[J].中西医结合杂志，1983；3(6)：343.

[12].查良伦，等.甲状腺功能减退症与肾阳虚关系探讨[J].中西医结合杂志，1993；13(4)：202.

[13].王文健，等.肾阳虚患者和老年人（男性）的下丘脑-垂体-性腺轴功能初步观察[J].中西医结合杂志，1982；2(3)：149.

[14].沈自尹，等.中医基础理论研究进展[J].中医杂志，1982；23(1)：73.

[15].王琦，等.肾虚型阳痿患者性激素变化的临床观察和实验研究[J].江苏中医，1988；(7)：43.

[16].周智恒，等.补肾法促进睾丸生精原理的实验研究[J].上海中医药杂志，1992；(7)：24.

[17].王学美，等.五子衍宗液对雄性大鼠下丘脑单胺类递质、性激素和生育能力的影响[J].中西医结合杂志，1993；13(6)：349.
[18].方素钦，等.中老年人肾虚证与性激素及免疫功能的研究[J].福建中医药，2002；33(2)：1.
[19].王培训，等.免疫与中医肾的研究进展[J].广州中医学院学报，1991；8(l)：55.
[20].范国荣，等.老年人肾虚证的T细胞亚群及对免疫调控的影响[J].中国中西医结合杂志，1992；（8）：478.
[21].李庆阳，等.老年肾虚T细胞亚群关系[J].福建中医学院学报，2001；11(2)：5.
[22]. 陈小峰，等.免疫灵合剂对肾虚病人T淋巴细胞免疫功能的作用[J].福建中医学院学报，1999；9(3)：5.
[23].陈小峰，等.对肾虚与自然杀伤细胞关系的观察[J].中国医药学报，1996；11(2)：39.
[24].王培训，等.补肾健脾方药免疫药理作用比较[J].中药新药与临床药理，1998；9(2)：84.
[25].王米渠，等.惊恐孕鼠对子代鼠自然杀伤细胞活性的影响[J].成都中药大学学报，1997；20(2)：33.
[26].Siegelg I .Tian linliu.The red-cell immune system[J].Lancet，1981；8246：556.
[27].杨嘉珍.肾虚血瘀证与红细胞免疫的关系[J].湖北中医杂志，1996；18(3)：55.
[28].王米渠，等."恐伤肾"对小鼠红细胞免疫及免疫器官的影响[J].成都中医药大学学报，1996；19(2)：34.
[29].郭峰，等.现代红细胞免疫学[M].上海：第二军医大学出版社，2002.
[30].杜标炎.肾阳虚造型及补肾中药对大鼠免疫功能的影响[J].广州中医药大学学报，1996；13(1)：37.
[31].徐文流，等.肾虚与脾虚模型动物IL-l的比较[J].广州中医药大学学报，1997；14(3)：175.
[32].徐世杰，等.切除卵巢所致肾虚对II型胶原诱导的关节炎小鼠IL-2和IL-6含量的影响[J].中国中医基础医学杂志，1998；4(10)：33.
[33].陈小峰，等.肾虚病人的细胞因子研究[J].福建中医学院学报，2000；10(2)：12.
[34].李文静，等.半硫丸对甲状腺机能减退肾阳虚大鼠血清slL-2R水平影响的实验研究[J].辽宁中医学院学报，2002；4(l)：59.
[35].肖学长，等.中医激光血疗对老年肾虚脑梗死病人免疫功能的影响[J].中国中西医结合杂志，2000；20(4)：264.
[36].朱华宇，等."天一寿"胶囊延缓衰老作用的临床研究[J].云南中医学院学报，2001；24(2)：4.
[37].姜晓红，等.健肾宝补肾壮阳作用的研究[J].浙江省医学科学院学报，1997；8(4)：9.

[38].张文彭，等.老年肾虚证血浆过氧化脂质高密度脂蛋白胆固醇及其亚组分水平变化[J].中医杂志，1989；30(2)：43.
[39].周群，等.动脉粥样硬化和胆石症异病同治的实验研究[J].中国中西医结合杂志，1992；12(7)：417.
[40].许沛虎，等.中医药研究中有关自由基研究近况[J].中国中西医结合杂志，1995；15(3)：185.
[41].陈晏珍，等.肾虚与超氧化物歧化酶关系初探[J].中医杂志，1989；30(4)：42.
[42].播志恒.肾虚本质的现代研究进展[J].上海中医药杂志，1995；(5)：44.
[43].陈玉碧，等.肾虚血瘀II型糖尿病患者红细胞SOD活性、血清LPO水平观察[J].北京中医，1995；14(4)：58.
[44].李承军，等.老年虚症自由基代谢机理研究[J].中医杂志，1998；29(12)：56.
[45].李庆阳，等.老年肾虚证LPO、SOD、血脂及细胞免疫水平变化[J].福建中医学院学报，2001；11(3)：7.
[46].董慧，等.肾阳虚证患者红细胞LPO、SOD和ATP酶活性的变化[J].微循环学杂志，2002；12(3)：10.
[47].刘锐.38例阳虚病人血锌变化规律[J].陕西中医，1984；(4)：8.
[48].柴立，等.肾藏精与微量元素[J].微量元素，1986；(l)：32.
[49].管竞环.中医药理论量化与微量元素[M].湖北科技出版社，1998；263.
[50].侯振江，等.内皮素及其在心脑血管疾病中的作用[J].国外医学，临床生物化学与检测学分册，1997；18（2）：56.
[51].李华，等.48例老年虚证患者血清内皮素观察[J].南京中医药大学学报，1999；（2）：208.
[52].李云杰，等.肾阳虚证的甲皱微循环改变的临床探讨[J].中国民间疗法，1995；（6）：47.
[53].赵伟康，等.老年期肾阴阳虚损大鼠的线粒体能量代谢及其调控机制的研究[J].中国中医基础医学杂志，2001；7（3）：31.
[54].周志东，等."寒体"、"热体"大鼠肝线粒体能量代谢的研究[J].上海中医药大学学报，2000；14(2)：34.
[55].吴瑞荣.阴虚冠心病人尿17羟皮质类固醇昼夜节律变化与脑的关系[J].中西医结合杂志，1982；（2）：100.
[56]邝安堃，等.急性心肌梗塞的中医辨证及其与血浆环核普酸、性激素的关系[J].中西医结合杂志，1983；（3）：151.
[57].王琦.肾虚型阳痿患者性激素变化的临床观察和实验研究[J].江苏中医，1988；（7）：43.
[58].吴水生，等.中老年性激素水平与不同肾虚证型关系研究[J].福建中医药，2000；（2）：4.
[59].朱楣光，等.中医肾虚与下丘脑-垂体-睾丸轴关系的探讨[J].天津医药，1990；（1）：37.

[60].俞谨.肾主生殖与生命网络研究中的启示[J].中国中西医结合杂志，2000；（6）：49.
[61].李恩，等.肾性高血压中医分型与血浆前列腺素、肾素、血管紧张素II、核苷酸变化的观察[J].中西医结合杂志，1983；（3）：195.
[62].蓝健姿，等. 肾虚证型慢性肾性小球肾炎与血清总 T3、T4 含量关系的探讨[J].福建中医药，2001；（3）：35.
[63].聂莉芳.80 例肾脏病患者胰高血糖素观察及临床意义[J].中国医药学报，1990；（4）：40.
[64].陈梅芳，等.尿毒症肾虚与内分泌及免疫状态的关系[J].中西医结合杂志，1983；(6)：328.
[65].朱滨弟，等.慢性原发性肾小球疾病中医辨证分型与实验室指标的关系[J].中国医药学报，1990；（6）：43.
[66].张宏伟，等.肾虚研究概述[J].中国医药学报，1991；（6）：43.
[67].达南.阴阳虚实辨证与血、尿 B2-MG 变化的关系[J].现代中医，1992；（4）：155.
[68].李文雄，等.肾虚与红细胞免疫功能关系的实验观察[J].成都中医学院学报，1989；（4）：33.
[69].吴正治，等.慢性肾炎患者外周血细胞化学 ANAE 变化与中医辨证关系的研究[J].中西医结合杂志，1990；（7）：399.
[70].方素钦，等.中老年人肾虚证与性激素及免疫功能的研究[J].福建中医药，2002；(2)：3.
[71].王鸿.肾虚患者甲皱微循环改变的观察与探讨[J].中医杂志，1980；（9）：677.
[72].刘新，等.慢性肾炎辨证论治和血液流变学观察[J].中医杂志，1988；（11）：44
[73].刘素蓉，等.阴虚阳虚证与血液流变学研究[J].中国医药学报，1989；(1)：12.
[74].申春娣，等.肾虚证与红细胞刚性的研究[J].中国中医基础医学杂志，1995；(2)：28.
[75]. 朱秀英，等，六味地黄冲剂对肾阴虚小白鼠血浆 cAMP、E2、T、Zn++、Cu++含量的影响[J]. 中医药学报，1995；（1）：51.
[76]. 刘晶霞，等.六味地黄汤治疗老年肾阴虚证血浆中锌铜含量的观察[J].中医药信息，1995；（3）：50.
[77].陈德珍，等.脾肾阴虚证血清铜、锌含量的变化[J].辽宁中医杂志，1999；7：291.
[78].丁伟璜，等.从慢性肾炎患者看中医阳虚、阴虚的病理生化学基础[J].上海中医药杂志，1983；(4)：46.
[79].尹永洗，等.肾脏病的中医辨证与继发性高脂蛋白血型的关系[J].中西医结合杂志，1985；(9)：546.
[80].阮诗玮，等. 慢性肾炎及中医证型与血中内皮素、一氧化氮关系探讨[J].福建中医学院学报，1999；(4)：7.

[81]陈德珍，等.脾肾阴虚证血清氧自由基损伤初探[J].华人消化杂志，1998；6(8)：660.
[82].方素钦，等.中老年人肾虚证与性激素及免疫功能的研究[J].福建中医药，2002；(2)：3.

[引用书目]

《素问》.北京：人民卫生出版社，1965.
《灵枢经》.北京：人民卫生出版社，1965.
三画
万 全.《片玉新书》.武汉：湖北人民卫生出版社，1981.
马宝璋.《中医妇科学》.上海：上海科学技术出版社，1997.
方 隅.《医林绳墨》.上海：商务印书馆，1957.
尤在泾.《金匮要略心典》.上海：上海卫生出版社，1975.
尤在泾.《金匮翼》.上海：上海卫生出版社，1957.
王叔和.《脉经》.北京：人民卫生出版社，1956.
王孟英.《温热经纬》.北京：人民卫生出版社，1956.
王怀隐.《太平圣惠方》.北京：人民卫生出版社，1958.
王清任.《医林改错》.上海：上海科学技术出版社，1966.
王肯堂.《证治准绳》.上海：上海卫生出版社，1958.
王 焘.《外台秘要》.北京：人民卫生出版社，1955.
王 晛.《全生指迷方》.北京：人民卫生出版社，1986.
王好古.《医垒元戎》.见东垣十书附一种.明嘉靖间绵纸刻本.
王永炎.《临床中医内科学》.北京：北京出版社.1994.
丹波元坚.《杂病广要》.北京：人民卫生出版社，1958.
五画
叶天士.《临证指南医案》.上海：上海人民出版社，1976.
田维君.《阴虚证治》.南昌：江西科学技术出版社，1990.
六画
吕不韦.《吕氏春秋》.上海：上海古籍出版社.1989.
朱震亨.《丹溪心法》.上海：上海科学技术出版社，1959.
朱震亨.《丹溪手镜》.北京：人民卫生出版社，1982.
朱震亨.《格致余论》.沈阳：辽宁科学技术出版社，1997.
朱震亨.《脉因证治》.北京：人民卫生出版社，1956.
华 佗.《中藏经》.北京：人民卫生出版社，1990.
江涵暾.《笔花医镜》.上海：上海科学技术出版社，1958.
刘完素.《宣明论方》.北京：人民卫生出版社，1956.
孙思邈.《千金要方》.北京：人民卫生出版社，1955.
孙文胤.《丹台玉案》. 上海：上海科学技术出版社，1984.
孙志宏.《简明医彀》. 北京：人民卫生出版社，1984.
成无己.《注解伤寒论》.北京：人民卫生出版社，1972.
成都中医学院.《金匮要略选读》.上海：上海科学技术出版社，1980.

七画
汪绮石.《理虚元鉴》.北京：人民卫生出版社，1988.
汪 昂.《医方集解》.沈阳：辽宁科学技术出版社，1997.
沈金鳌.《杂病源流犀烛》.上海：上海科学技术出版社，1962.
沈金鳌.《妇科玉尺》. 沈金鳌医学全书，北京：中国医药出版社.1999.
李 梴.《医学入门》.天津：天津科学技术出版社，1999.
李 杲.《医学发明》.北京：人民卫生出版社，1959.
李东垣.《兰室秘藏》.北京：人民卫生出版社，1957.
李中梓.《医宗必读》.上海：上海科学技术出版社，1959.
李用粹.《证治汇补》.上海：上海科学技术出版社，1956.
杨士瀛.《直指方》.上海：上海科学技术出版社，1989.
严用和.《济生方》.北京：人民卫生出版社，1956.
吴有性.《温疫论》.北京：人民卫生出版社，1990.
吴鞠通.《温病条辨》.北京：人民卫生出版社，1957.
吴鞠通.《增补评注温病条辨》.上海：科技卫生出版社，1958.
吴谦等.《医宗金鉴》.北京：人民卫生出版社，1963.
何梦瑶.《医碥》.上海：上海科学技术出版社，1982.
何廉臣.《重订广温热论》.北京：人民卫生出版社，1960.
张元素.《医学启源》.北京：人民卫生出版社，1978.
张介宾.《景岳全书》.北京：人民卫生出版社，1990.
张介宾.《类经附翼》.北京：人民卫生出版社，1965.
张景岳.《质疑录》.南京：江苏科学技术出版社，1981.
张仲景.《伤寒论》.北京：人民卫生出版社，1991.
张仲景.《金匮要略》.北京：人民卫生出版社，1991.
张仲景.《金匮玉函经二注》.北京：人民卫生出版社，1955.
张路玉.《张氏医通》.上海：上海科学技术出版社，1963.
张锡纯.《医学衷中参西录》.石家庄：河北人民出版社，1974.
张之文.《温病学》.成都：四川人民出版社.1987.
陈修园.《医学从众录》.上海.上海卫生出版社.1957.
陈士铎.《辨证录》.北京：人民卫生出版社，1965.
陈士铎.《辨证奇闻》.上海：上海锦章书局，1914.
陈士铎.《石室秘录》.北京：北京科学技术出版社，1984.
陈自民.《妇人良方大全》.上海：上海卫生出版社，1956.
陈师文.《太平惠民和剂局方》.北京：人民卫生出版社，1985.
陈 言.《三因极一病证方论》.北京：人民卫生出版社，1957.
陈复正.《幼幼集成》.上海：上海科学技术出版社.1962
陈直撰.《寿亲养老新书 》.上海：上海古籍出版社.1990.
余 霖.《疫疹一得》.南京：江苏科学技术出版社，1985.
八画
林佩琴.《类证治裁》.上海：上海科学技术出版社，1959.

罗 美.《内经博议》.见珍本医书集成第 1 册. 上海：上海科学技术卫生出版社，1985.
周学海.《读医随笔》.南京：江苏科学技术出版社，1983.
郑树珪.《七松岩集》. 石家庄：河北人民出版社.1980.
郑钦安.《医法园通》.成都：巴蜀书社，1988.
九画
赵 佶.《圣济总录》.北京：人民卫生出版社，1962.
赵献可.《医贯》.北京：人民卫生出版社，1959.
赵绍琴.《温热纵横》. 北京：人民卫生出版社.1982
皇甫中.《明医指掌》.北京：人民卫生出版社，1982.
费伯雄.《医醇剩义》.南京：江苏科学技术出版社，1982.
俞震纂.《古今医案按》.上海：上海科学技术出版社，1959.
十画
徐灵胎.《医学源流论》. 徐灵胎医学全书，北京：中国医药出版社.1999.
徐春甫.《古今医统大全》.南京：南京中医学院影印，1984.
秦景明.《症因脉治》.上海：上海科学技术出版社，1990.
秦越人.《难经》.北京：人民卫生出版社，1991.
秦伯未.《中医临证备要》.北京：人民卫生出版社.1963.
钱仲阳.《小儿药证直诀》.北京：人民卫生出版社，1955.
唐蓉川.《血证论评释》.北京：人民卫生出版社，1980.
顾松园.《顾松园医镜》. 郑州：河南人民卫生出版社，1961.
浙江省中医研究所文献所.《重订严氏济生方》.北京：人民卫生出版社，1980.
十一画
黄文东等.《实用中医内科学》.上海：上海科学技术出版社.1986.
龚云林.《寿世保元》.上海：上海科学技术出版社，1959.
龚廷贤.《万病回春》.北京：中国中医药出版社，1998.
巢元方.《诸病源候论》.北京：人民卫生出版社，1955.
寇宗奭.《本草衍义》上海：上海商务印书馆.1957.
十二画
喻 昌.《医门法律》.上海：上海科学技术出版社，1959.
傅青主.《傅青主女科》.南京：江苏科学技术出版社，1982.
程文囿.《医述》.合肥：安徽科技出版社，1981.
程国彭.《医学心悟》.北京：人民卫生出版社，1963.
程绍寰.《肾病证治概要》.北京：中国古籍出版社.1987.
彭静山.《华佗神医秘传》.沈阳：辽宁科学技术出版社.1982
韩 矛心 《韩氏医通》.上海：上海科学技术出版社，1959.
鲁伯嗣.《婴童百问》.北京：人民卫生出版社.1961.
曾世荣.《活幼心书》.天津：天津科学技术出版社.1999.
谢映庐.《谢映庐医案》.上海：上海科学技术出版社，1962.
十三画

虞 抟.《医学正传》.北京：人民卫生出版社，1965.
蒲辅周.《蒲辅周医疗经验》.北京：人民卫生出版社，1976.
十四画
臧达德.《履霜集》.见珍本医书集成第 14 册.上海科学技术卫生出版社
1985.
十五画
潘敏求.《中医内科治疗大成》. 石家庄：河北科学技术出版社.1997.
十六画
薛 己.《保婴撮要》.北京：人民卫生出版社.1983.
十七画
戴思恭.《证治要诀》.北京：中国中医药出版社，1998.

Index

B

C

D

E

G

H

I

J

M

N

O

P

S

T

U

V

X

Y

Z